Statistical Evaluation of Diagnostic Performance

Topics in ROC Analysis

Chapman & Hall/CRC Biostatistics Series

Chapman & Hall/CRC Biostatistics Series

Adaptive Design Theory and Implementation Using SAS and R
Mark Chang

Advanced Bayesian Methods for Medical Test Accuracy
Lyle D. Broemeling

Advances in Clinical Trial Biostatistics
Nancy L. Geller

Applied Statistical Design for the Researcher
Daryl S. Paulson

Basic Statistics and Pharmaceutical Statistical Applications, Second Edition
James E. De Muth

Bayesian Adaptive Methods for Clinical Trials
Scott M. Berry, Bradley P. Carlin, J. Jack Lee, and Peter Muller

Bayesian Analysis Made Simple: An Excel GUI for WinBUGS
Phil Woodward

Bayesian Methods for Measures of Agreement
Lyle D. Broemeling

Bayesian Missing Data Problems: EM, Data Augmentation and Noniterative Computation
Ming T. Tan, Guo-Liang Tian, and Kai Wang Ng

Bayesian Modeling in Bioinformatics
Dipak K. Dey, Samiran Ghosh, and Bani K. Mallick

Causal Analysis in Biomedicine and Epidemiology: Based on Minimal Sufficient Causation
Mikel Aickin

Clinical Trial Data Analysis using R
Ding-Geng (Din) Chen and Karl E. Peace

Clinical Trial Methodology
Karl E. Peace and Ding-Geng (Din) Chen

Computational Methods in Biomedical Research
Ravindra Khattree and Dayanand N. Naik

Computational Pharmacokinetics
Anders Källén

Controversial Statistical Issues in Clinical Trials
Shein-Chung Chow

Data and Safety Monitoring Committees in Clinical Trials
Jay Herson

Design and Analysis of Animal Studies in Pharmaceutical Development
Shein-Chung Chow and Jen-pei Liu

Design and Analysis of Bioavailability and Bioequivalence Studies, Third Edition
Shein-Chung Chow and Jen-pei Liu

Design and Analysis of Clinical Trials with Time-to-Event Endpoints
Karl E. Peace

Design and Analysis of Non-Inferiority Trials
Mark D. Rothmann, Brian L. Wiens, and Ivan S. F. Chan

Difference Equations with Public Health Applications
Lemuel A. Moyé and Asha Seth Kapadia

DNA Methylation Microarrays: Experimental Design and Statistical Analysis
Sun-Chong Wang and Arturas Petronis

DNA Microarrays and Related Genomics Techniques: Design, Analysis, and Interpretation of Experiments
David B. Allsion, Grier P. Page, T. Mark Beasley, and Jode W. Edwards

Dose Finding by the Continual Reassessment Method
Ying Kuen Cheung

Elementary Bayesian Biostatistics
Lemuel A. Moyé

Frailty Models in Survival Analysis
Andreas Wienke

Generalized Linear Models: A Bayesian Perspective
Dipak K. Dey, Sujit K. Ghosh, and Bani K. Mallick

Handbook of Regression and Modeling: Applications for the Clinical and Pharmaceutical Industries
Daryl S. Paulson

Measures of Interobserver Agreement and Reliability, Second Edition
Mohamed M. Shoukri

Medical Biostatistics, Second Edition
A. Indrayan

Meta-Analysis in Medicine and Health Policy
Dalene Stangl and Donal A. Berry

Monte Carlo Simulation for the Pharmaceutical Industry: Concepts, Algorithms, and Case Studies
Mark Chang

Multiple Testing Problems in Pharmaceutical Statistics
Alex Dmitrienko, Ajit C. Tamhane, and Frank Bretz

Sample Size Calculations in Clinical Research, Second Edition
Shein-Chung Chow, Jun Shao and Hansheng Wang

Statistical Design and Analysis of Stability Studies
Shein-Chung Chow

Statistical Evaluation of Diagnostic Performance: Topics in ROC Analysis
Kelly H. Zou, Aiyi Liu, Andriy I. Bandos, Lucila Ohno-Machado, and Howard E. Rockette

Statistical Methods for Clinical Trials
Mark X. Norleans

Statistics in Drug Research: Methodologies and Recent Developments
Shein-Chung Chow and Jun Shao

Statistics in the Pharmaceutical Industry, Third Edition
Ralph Buncher and Jia-Yeong Tsay

Translational Medicine: Strategies and Statistical Methods
Dennis Cosmatos and Shein-Chung Chow

Chapman & Hall/CRC Biostatistics Series

Statistical Evaluation of Diagnostic Performance

Topics in ROC Analysis

Kelly H. Zou
Aiyi Liu
Andriy I. Bandos
Lucila Ohno-Machado
Howard E. Rockette

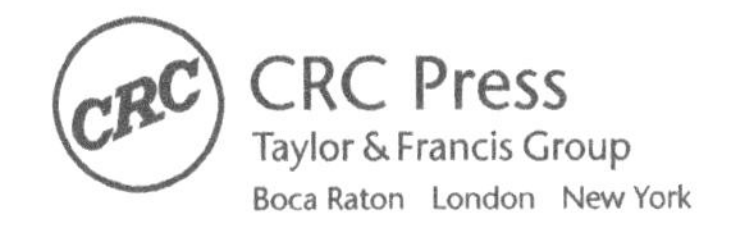

CRC Press is an imprint of the
Taylor & Francis Group, an **informa** business
A CHAPMAN & HALL BOOK

Chapters 4 and 6 have been created by Aiyi Liu, a U. S. Government employee, as part of his official duties. These chapters are U. S. Government work as that term is defined by the U. S. copyright law.

CRC Press
Taylor & Francis Group
6000 Broken Sound Parkway NW, Suite 300
Boca Raton, FL 33487-2742

International Standard Book Number: 978-1-4398-1222-8 (Hardback)

Visit the Taylor & Francis Web site at
http://www.taylorandfrancis.com

and the CRC Press Web site at
http://www.crcpress.com

In memory of Professor Harry Samuel Wieand of the University of Pittsburgh who passed away at the age of 62 due to a recurrence of non-Hodgkin's lymphoma.

Contents

Section III Advanced Approaches and Applications

Authors

Kelly H. Zou, PhD is a director of statistics in the Specialty Care Business Unit at Pfizer, Inc. A native of Shanghai, China, she earned a BA (summa cum laude) in mathematics from Chaminade University of Honolulu, a master's and PhD in statistics from the University of Rochester, and completed a postdoctoral fellowship in biostatistics and radiology from Harvard Medical School and its affiliated Brigham and Women's Hospital. She has been a lecturer on health care policy at Harvard Medical School; an instructor, assistant professor, and associate professor in radiology at Harvard Medical School; the principal statistician in radiology at Brigham and Women's Hospital; and the director of biostatistics at Children's Hospital Boston. In addition to her career in academia, Dr. Zou served as an associate director of rates at Barclays Capital and director of statistics in outcomes research and evidence-based strategies at Pfizer, Inc.

Dr. Zou served as the principal investigator on a number of research grants funded by the National Library of Medicine, National Institute of General Medical Sciences, and the Agency for Healthcare Research and Quality of the U.S. National Institutes of Health. Her work on ROC analysis and statistical classification led her to be the recipient of the Stauffer Award for the best article published in *Academic Radiology*, the first place winner of the American Statistical Association and Biopharmaceutical Statistics Section poster competition at the 2009 Joint Statistical Meetings, and second and third place winner at the 2010 meeting. She was the recipient of the Travel Stipend Award from the Society of Health Services Research in Radiology and received the Reviewer with Special Distinction Award from *Radiology*.

Dr. Zou has published more than 100 peer-reviewed articles listed via *PubMed*. She served as an associate editor of *Statistics in Medicine*, *Radiology*, and *Medical Physics*, and as a referee for more than 10 professional statistical and medical journals. She served as vice chair of the Committee on Applied Statistics American Statistical Association; member of the Corporate Sponsorship Committee, Biopharmaceutical Section, American Statistical Association; chair of Judiciary Committee, Radiology Alliance to Health Services Research, Association of University Radiologists; and member of the Faculty Taskforce, Joint Committee on the Status of Women, Harvard Medical School and Harvard School of Dental Medicine. She was the theme editor on *Mathematical and Statistical Methods for Diagnoses and Therapies*. Her research interests include diagnostic tests, medical imaging, health policy, outcomes research, and clinical trials.

Aiyi Liu, PhD is a senior investigator in the Biostatistics and Bioinformatics Branch, Division of Epidemiology, Statistics and Prevention Research, of the Eunice Kennedy Shriver National Institute of Child Health and Human Development of the National Institutes of Health (NIH). He earned a BA in mathematics and a master's degree in statistics from the University of Science and Technology of China, and subsequently taught for 5 years in the Department of Mathematics at the same university. He earned a PhD in statistics from the University of Rochester, and completed his postdoctoral training at St. Jude Children's Research Hospital in Memphis, Tennessee. Prior to his appointment at NIH, Dr. Liu was an assistant professor of biostatistics in the Department of Biomathematics and Biostatistics, Georgetown University Lombardi Cancer Center, Washington, DC, and taught in the department's master's program and the center's tumor biology program.

Dr. Liu's research interests include general statistical theory and methods, sequential methodology, multivariate data analysis, diagnostic biomarkers, and ROC curve analysis. He has published more than 80 articles in peer-reviewed journals including *Biometrics, Biometrika,* and the *Journal of the American Statistical Association.* He served as a referee for more than 15 journals and organized a number of invited sessions for statistical meetings. Dr. Liu is an associate editor for the *Journal of Statistical Planning and Inference,* and acted as a guest co-editor for *Philosophical Transaction of the Royal Society A.* He is an elected member of the International Statistical Institute, and a member of the American Statistical Association, International Chinese Statistical Association, and Institute of Mathematical Statistics. His tenure as a member of the Committee on Award of an Outstanding Statistical Application of the American Statistical Association started in 2011.

Andriy I. Bandos, PhD is a research assistant professor in the Department of Biostatistics at the University of Pittsburgh. He earned a master's in mathematics from Karazin Kharkiv National University (Ukraine) and a PhD in biostatistics from the University of Pittsburgh. Over the past several years, he has worked extensively on methodology development and analysis of observer performance studies in diagnostic imaging. His work has been published in a number of biostatistical and radiology-related journals.

Dr. Bandos developed and teaches a graduate-level course on ROC analysis at the University of Pittsburgh. He is a reviewer for a number of academic journals and governmental agencies. His current research interests include statistical evaluation of diagnostic performance, ROC analysis, free-response ROC (FROC) methodology, nonparametric methods, and resampling approaches in statistics.

Lucila Ohno-Machado, MD, PhD is a professor of medicine and the founding chief of the Division of Biomedical Informatics at the University of California San Diego, (UCSD). She earned her medical degree from the

University of Sao Paulo, Brazil and her doctorate in medical information sciences from Stanford University. Before joining UCSD, she was the director of the training program of the Harvard–MIT–Tufts–Boston University consortium in Boston, and the director of the Decision Systems Group at Brigham and Women's Hospital, Harvard Medical School.

Dr. Ohno-Machado's research focuses on the development of new evaluation methods for predictive models of disease, with special emphasis on the analysis of model calibration and implications in healthcare. She is an elected member of the American College of Medical Informatics, the American Institute for Medical and Biological Engineering, and the American Society for Clinical Investigation. She is the editor-in-chief of the *Journal of the American Medical Informatics Association* (JAMIA).

Howard E. Rockette, PhD, is a former chair and currently a professor of biostatistics at the University of Pittsburgh Graduate School of Public Health. He is a fellow of the American Statistical Association and a member of the Society for Epidemiological Research and the Society of Clinical Trials. He has written 150 peer-reviewed articles, more than a third of which relate to the development of statistical methodology or its application to the evaluation of diagnostic imaging systems. He served on numerous advisory committees for government and industry, and on the editorial board of *Annals of Epidemiology* and *Academic Radiology*.

Preface

> We now extend the body of literature via the journey of "ROC Trek" into where classifiers have never gone before.
>
> MATT GÖNEN
> *ROC on*

Statistical evaluation of diagnostic performance in general, and receiver operating characteristic (ROC) analysis in particular, are important for assessing the performance of medical tests and statistical classifiers, and also for evaluating predictive models or algorithms. In diagnostic and prognostic tasks, the receiver operating characteristic (ROC) curve plays an essential role by providing a graphic display that illustrates the discrimination performance of a medical diagnostic test. ROC analysis originated during World War II as a method of assessing classification accuracy for differentiating signals from noise in radar detection. Recently, the ROC methodology has been adapted to many disciplines, including several clinical areas that depend heavily on screening and diagnostic tests.

The purpose of this book is to present innovative approaches in ROC analysis that are relevant to a wide variety of clinical applications including medical imaging, cancer research, epidemiology, and bioinformatics. We begin by reviewing the conventional ROC methodology. Monotone transformation models taking data to parametric forms are chosen to improve goodness of fit of modeling approaches. Likelihood-based algorithms for estimating an ROC curve are discussed, along with the associated characteristics of several models for univariate and multivariate data. The covered topics include monotone transformation techniques in parametric ROC analysis, ROC methods for combined and pooled biomarkers, Bayesian hierarchical transformation models, sequential designs and inferences in the ROC setting, predictive modeling, multireader ROC analysis, and free-response ROC (FROC) methodology. The topics highlighted include:

- Methods for statistical validations of diagnostic accuracy using ROC analysis
- Methods for estimation and comparison of diagnostic test characteristics
- Monotone transformation methods, binormality testing, and goodness-of-fit issues
- Bayesian hierarchical models for estimating diagnostic accuracy

- Multireader and multimodality ROC analysis and FROC analysis
- Biomarkers, sequential designs, and bioinformatics

The intended audience of this book includes graduate-level students and researchers in the areas of statistics, biostatistics, epidemiology, public health, biomedical engineering, radiology, medical imaging, biomedical informatics, and other closely-related fields. Additionally, clinical researchers and practicing statisticians in academia, industry, and government may benefit from the presentation of such important and yet frequently overlooked topics.

The CA19-9 and CA125 cancer marker data were provided by Professor H. Samuel Wieand, of the University of Pittsburgh, who passed away on June 10, 2006 from a recurrence of non-Hodgkin's lymphoma. This book is in memory of Professor Wieand for his important contribution to the field of ROC analysis following his classical work examining the nonparametric statistics for comparing diagnostic markers with paired or unpaired data.

The authors wish to express our deepest gratitude to Rob Calver, the senior statistics acquisitions editor at Taylor & Francis Group, who tirelessly provided tremendous assistance in making this project a reality. We are most grateful to two anonymous experts who reviewed earlier chapters. We especially thank the many authors who have contributed extensively to the body of ROC literature including widely used software programs.

The authors were partially funded by Grants R03-HS13234, R01-LM007861, R01-GM074068, R01-EB002106, R01-EB006388, R01-LM009520, and U54-HL108460 from the U.S. National Institutes of Health (NIH). Dr. Aiyi Liu's research was supported by the Intramural Research Program of the Eunice Kennedy Shriver National Institute of Child Health and Human Development (NICHD) of the NIH.

By gaining an in-depth understanding and accurate validation of complex biomarkers and high-dimensional modality data, we hope that appropriate therapies and improved outcomes may ultimately be achieved using methods described in this book.

ROC ROCKS!

K.H.Z., A.L., A.I.B., L.O.-M., and H.E.R.

Section I

Introduction

1

Background and Introduction

1.1 Background Information

Receiver operating characteristic (ROC) methodology was developed during the Second World War to evaluate new signal detection technology. Since the 1950s, it has been used extensively in radar detection and psychophysical research. The classic textbooks are by Green and Swets (1966) and Egan (1975). Since 1982, both interest and applications have increased in the fields of radiology, preventive medicine, and clinical evaluative sciences. Comprehensive textbooks over the past two decades included those authored by Swets and Pickett (1982), Macmillan and Creelman (1991), Zhou et al. (2002), Pepe (2003), Gönen (2007), and Krzanowski and Hand (2009). New methodological developments in biomedical contexts frequently appear in medical and statistical journals. Hence, the ROC methodology has been adapted to several clinical areas heavily dependent on screening and diagnostic tests, in particular, laboratory testing, epidemiology, radiology, and bioinformatics.

ROC analysis is a useful tool for evaluating the performance of diagnostic tests, and more generally, for evaluating the accuracy of a statistical model (e.g., logistic regression and discriminant analysis) that classifies subjects into one of two classes, labeled as the diseased or nondiseased (or healthy) categories. Earlier ROC literature focused mostly on ordinal rating data that take on only discrete values indicating levels of subjective uncertainty of disease. Increasingly, ROC methods are applied to continuous data (Krzanowski and Hand, 2009).

The function of the ROC curve as a simple graphical tool for displaying the accuracy of a medical diagnostic test is one of the best known applications. In practice, diagnostic testing plays a useful role in clinical practice (e.g., finding serum markers of myocardial necrosis and cardiac imaging tests). Besides the aspect of validating diagnostic modalities, predictive modeling to estimate expected outcomes such as mortality or adverse cardiac events based on patient risk characteristics also is common in cardiovascular research, where ROC analysis is useful in such situations.

A variety of software packages are available for conducting ROC analyses to evaluate either the performance of a single diagnostic test or the comparative performances of repeated or multiple tests. Well-cited ROC software has been developed by Professor Charles E. Metz at the Kurt Rossmann Laboratories for Radiologic Image Research of the University of Chicago (please visit the web link at: http://www-radiology.uchicago.edu/krl/KRL_ROC/software_index6.htm).

1.2 Gold Standard, Decision Threshold, Sensitivity, and Specificity

Evaluation of a medical technology may be carried out by application to a sample of nondiseased subjects and a sample of diseased subjects, obtaining measurements for each subject. In many settings, determination of who is healthy and who is diseased is no easy task. In order to estimate classification accuracy via standard ROC methods, the disease status for each patient is assumed to be measured without error. The true disease status often is referred to as the gold standard (GS), labeled D. Such a "truth" or "true disease status" may be determined from clinical follow-up, clinical verification, and autopsy. In some cases, status is adjudicated by a gold standard committee. To determine the gold standard, two potential problems arise: verification bias and measurement error. Verification bias results when the accuracy of a test is likely to be evaluated among those with known disease status. Measurement errors may result when a true gold standard is absent or an imperfect standard is used for comparison.

Screening or diagnostic (Dx) tests are common in clinical practice because they play an important role in the selection of therapy. Suppose the outcome of a medical test results in a continuous measurement T. Let ξ be a positivity threshold (i.e., cutoff value) used to classify patients, such that a subject is classified as healthy (H) if $T \le \xi$ and diseased (D) if $T > \xi$. For any set of test results, the following 2×2 contingency table at some ξ may be formed. The accuracy of such a diagnostic test is commonly assessed using the probability that the test correctly classifies a healthy subject as healthy, namely the true negative fraction $TNF = 1 - FPF$, or specificity, and the probability that the test correctly classifies a diseased subject as diseased, namely the true positive fraction TPF, or sensitivity. Both FPF and TPF depend on the test threshold ξ, that varies, as do FPF and TPF (Tables 1.1. and 1.2).

TABLE 1.1

A 2 × 2 Contingency Table Classifying Test Results at Arbitrary Threshold, ξ

Diagnosis (Dx) or Screening Test	Gold Standard (GS)		
	Healthy (*H*)	**Diseased (*D*)**	**Total**
Negative (–)	*TN*	*FN*	$\#\{T \le \xi\}$
Positive (+)	*FP*	*TP*	$\#\{T > \xi\}$
Total	n^0	n^1	$N = n^0 + n^1$

TN = *true negative. FP* = *false positive. FN* = *false negative. TP* = *true positive.*

TABLE 1.2

Joint Proportions of Choices between Diagnosis and Gold Standard

Diagnosis (Dx) or Screening Test	Gold Standard (GS)		
	0	***1***	**Marginal**
0	p_{00}	p_{01}	$p_{0.}$
1	p_{10}	p_{11}	$p_{1.}$
Marginal	$p_{.0}$	$p_{.1}$	*1*

$p_{.0} = p_{00} + p_{10}$.
$p_{.1} = p_{01} + p_{11}$.
$p_{00}\, p_{.0}$ = *TNF* = true negative fraction.
$p_{10}\, p_{.0}$ = *FPF* = false positive fraction.
$p_{01}\, p_{.1}$ = *FNF* = false negative fraction.
$p_{11}\, p_{.1}$ = *TPF* = true positive fraction.

1.3 Kappa Statistics

The kappa statistic is a measure of agreement between two ordinal-categorical variables such as the diagnosis and the gold standard. Fleiss (1980) presented the formula for computing the kappa statistic by computing the overall proportion of observed agreement:

$$\hat{\kappa} = \frac{2(p_{00}p_{11} - p_{01}p_{10})}{p_{.0}p_{1.} + p_{0.}p_{.1}}. \tag{1-1}$$

The overall kappa is between [–1, 1]. If $\hat{k} = +1$, there is complete agreement (i.e., the diagnosis is as accurate as the gold standard). Landis and Koch (1977)

TABLE 1.3

Interpretations of Agreement Based on Ranges of Kappa Statistic Values

Kappa Statistic	Interpretation
< 0.00	Poor agreement
0.00 to 0.20	Slight agreement
0.21 to 0.40	Fair agreement
0.41 to 0.60	Moderate agreement
0.61 to 0.80	Substantial agreement
0.81 to 1.00	Almost perfect agreement

devised interpretations based on ranges of the kappa statistic values listed in Table 1.3.

Although the kappa statistic is widely used for assessing the agreement among several tests, particularly by human observers, one must be careful when interpreting the agreement between a diagnostic test and the underlying gold standard. The main caution lies in the dependence of kappa on sample prevalence. For example, a very accurate diagnostic test with both sensitivity and specificity of 0.95 can assume any value of kappa in the range of 0.0 to 0.9, spanning most categories of the "strength of agreement" Landis and Koch (1977) propose in Table 1.3. For the same reason, the kappa statistic can be misleading in comparison to diagnostic tests evaluated on the samples with different prevalences. For example, when the aforementioned test ($FPF = 0.05$ and $TPF = 0.95$) is assessed in a sample with prevalence $p(D = 1) = 0.004$, it will have a smaller kappa statistic than an inferior test ($FPF = 0.05$ and $TPF = 0.15$) assessed in a sample with prevalence of $p(D = 1) = 0.20$. Other nonparametric measures of association may be found in the literature to have specific correspondence and relationship with the ROC-specific indices (Kendall and Gibbons, 1990).

1.4 Receiver Operating Characteristic Curve

The ROC curve displayed in Figure 1.1 is a useful way to demonstrate the performance of a medical diagnostic test for detecting whether a subject has a disease. By considering all possible values of the threshold, ξ, the ROC curve can be constructed as a plot of sensitivity (TPF) versus 1-specificity (FPF) pairs. This figure shows the ROC curve from a perfect diagnostic test, a curve from a diagnostic test that is no better than chance, and an idealized curve.

The ROC curve is closely related to the Lorenz curve and the Gini index (Gastwirth, 1972; Figure 1.2), c-statistic (Ash and Swartz, 1999), Sommers' D

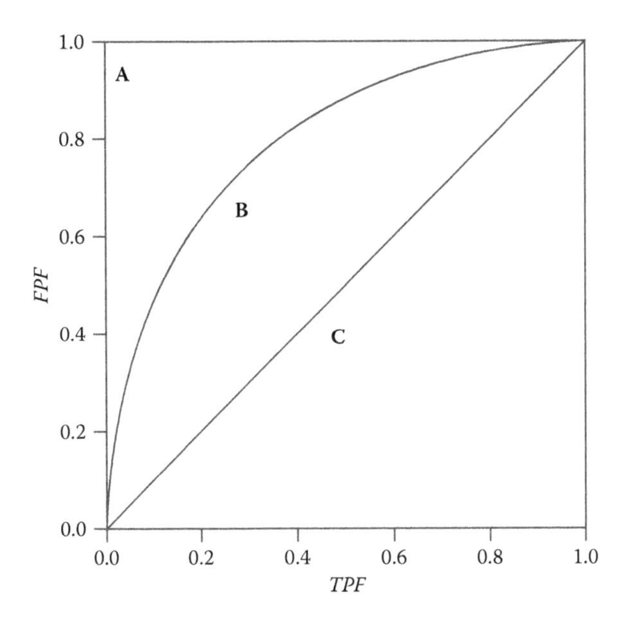

FIGURE 1.1
Three decision outcomes (A, B, C) to differentiate "good" and "bad" signals, reflected in different idealized ROC curve signals. The upper axis and left axis represent the truth and diagonal line C represents chance. Medical decisions generally fall on a typical curve like B between A and C.

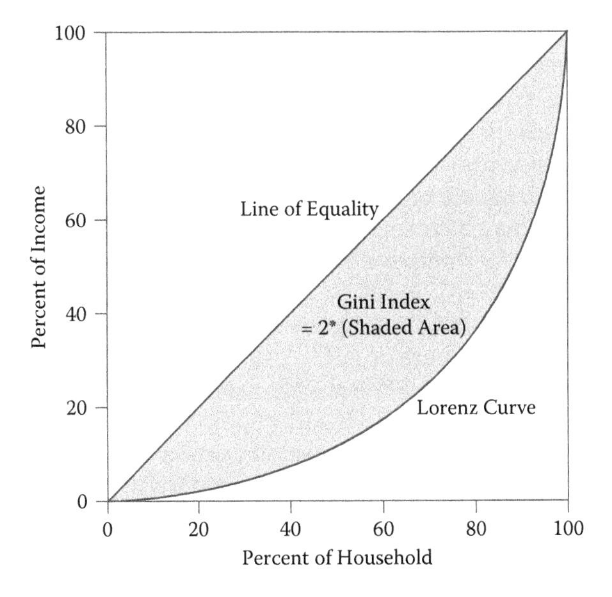

FIGURE 1.2
Lorenz curve and Gini index.

index (Siegel and Castellan, 1988), and the cumulative accuracy profile (CAP) curve (Sobehart and Keenan, 2001). For example, the Gini index is defined as twice the shaded area. Likewise, explanations of the identity of line of equality between sensitivity and specificity in the figure and the chance line in the legend are needed.

There is a parallelism with statistical hypothesis testing concepts (Zou et al., 2009). For example, consider a simple hypothesis about a subject Y: H_0: $Y \in H$ versus H_1: $Y \in H$. A statistical test rejects H_0 if $T > \xi$, where T is a pre-specified critical value, yielding significance level (Type 1 error) of $\alpha = FPF$ and power (1–Type 2 error) of $1 - \beta = TPF$. Varying all possible values of ξ would essentially yield different (α, β) pairs. Plotting power versus significance levels for all possible critical values in essence constitutes the ROC curve. It is worth noting that a correspondence between *FPF*, *TPF* and α, $1 - \beta$ depends on whether a null or alternative hypothesis is put into correspondence with the "diseased" category of the gold standard. If the null hypothesis were termed as "diseased" (correspondingly "non-reject" would correspond to a "positive" test result), α would correspond to *FNF* (or $1 - TPF$) and β would correspond to *FPF*. However, due to different levels of control of two types of mistakes in traditional statistical testing, especially when testing for a composite hypothesis, the hypothesis of interest to detect (i.e., naturally corresponding to the concept of "disease") is taken as null, thus leading to the first type of correspondence between *FPF* versus *TPF* and α versus β, respectively.

Several other terms are relevant. The probability of disease is called the prevalence or prior probability. The ratio of *TPF* and *FPF* is the likelihood ratio positive LR^+ and the ratio of *TNR* and *FNR* is the likelihood ratio negative LV^-. The probability of disease given a positive test result is the predictive value positive PV^+, and the probability of healthy given a negative test result is the predictive value negative PV^-. Using the Bayes theorem for any constant disease prevalence, the predictive values, sometimes called the posterior probabilities, are monotone functions of their corresponding likelihood ratios. They may also serve as indices of the accuracy of a diagnostic test and as a basis for comparison when several diagnostic tests are conducted (Biggerstaff, 2000).

The crudest method for creating an ROC plot based on continuous test results involves plotting pairs of *TPF* versus *FPF* at all possible values for the decision threshold. *TPF* and *FPF* are calculated using the empirical survival distributions for the diseased and healthy subjects. This method is referred to as empirical or nonparametric because no parameters are needed to model the behavior of the plot and the unknown underlying distributions for the two groups are left unstructured (Zweig and Campbell, 1993). This approach has the advantage of being free of structural assumptions. However, the curve is usually unsmooth (technically empirical survival functions lead to a disjoint set of ROC points and any type of curve connecting these points implies some type of continuous estimate of survival function). The efficiency is reduced relative to test results utilizing structured assumptions if they are valid (Gönen, 2007).

A different nonparametric method with a kernel density function was introduced by Zou et al. (1997) and Lloyd (1998) based on a smooth nonparametric ROC curve derived from kernel density or survival estimates of the two test distributions. The degree of smoothness is determined by the choice of kernel and bandwidth. Varying the bandwidth of the kernel trades global smoothness for local fit. The optimal bandwidths were compared by Zhou and Harezlak (2002) and smooth semiparametric curves were constructed by Wan and Zhang (2007).

A real data example was shown in Wieand et al.'s seminal article in 1989. Pancreatic cancer data from the Mayo Clinic were collected using sera from $m = 51$ patients with pancreatitis (considered nondiseased or healthy in subsequent ROC analysis) and $n = 90$ diseased patients with pancreatic cancer (considered diseased). The data were studied with carbohydrate antigen (CA19-9) and cancer antigen (CA125) assays and illustrated by Su and Liu (1993) and Pepe (2003). The subjects between the two antigens were paired across these two tables, respectively, for the healthy and diseased samples. The corresponding fully nonparametric ROC curves for these two antigens are displayed in Figure 1.3. Figure 1.4 demonstrates a mixture of parametric

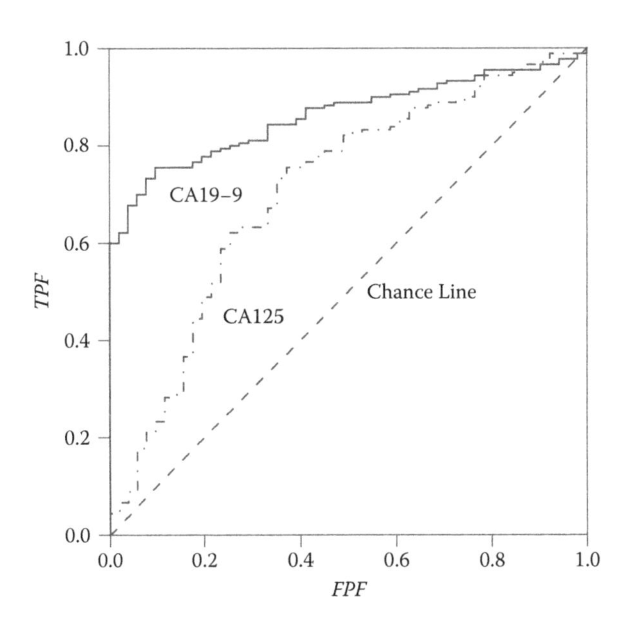

FIGURE 1.3
Nonparametric empirical ROC curves constructed based on CA19-9 and CA125 antigen data.

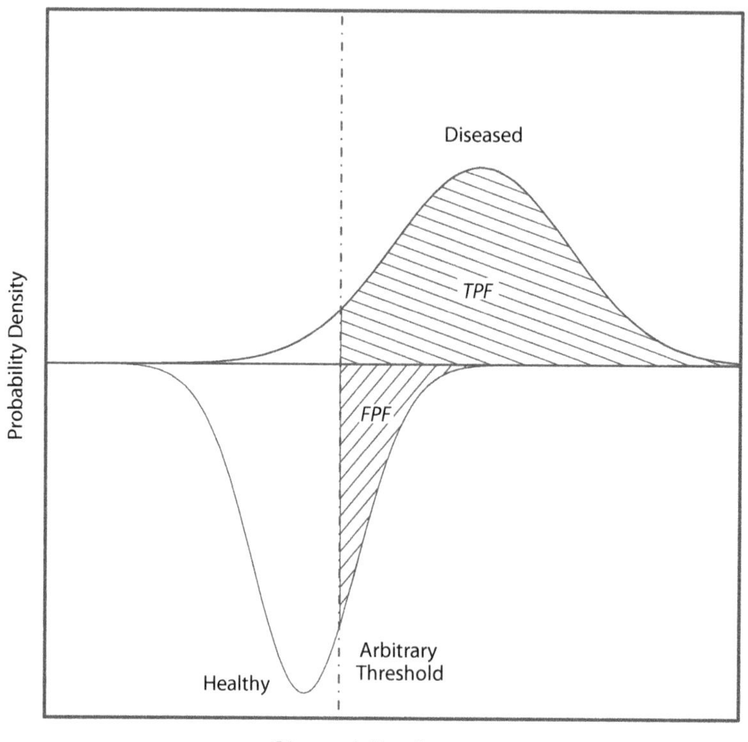

FIGURE 1.4
Two probability density functions on log scale for hypothetical diagnostic marker. After log transformation, distributions are binormal, with N [0,1] and N [1.5, 1.87^2] for healthy and diseased populations, respectively.

distributions on a log scale under the transformed binormal model. The resulting ROC curve at the arbitrarily prespecified threshold is displayed in Figure 1.5.

1.5 Area and Partial Area under ROC Curve

The area under the curve (AUC) is a global summary measure of diagnostic accuracy. It ranges from 0.5 for accuracy of chance to 1 for perfect accuracy. It is possible for an AUC to be less than 0.5, indicating an accuracy worse than random guessing of the diagnosis, at least for some choices of the threshold. The AUC for a truly continuous test result also corresponds to the probability of a pair of independent healthy and diseased measurement values,

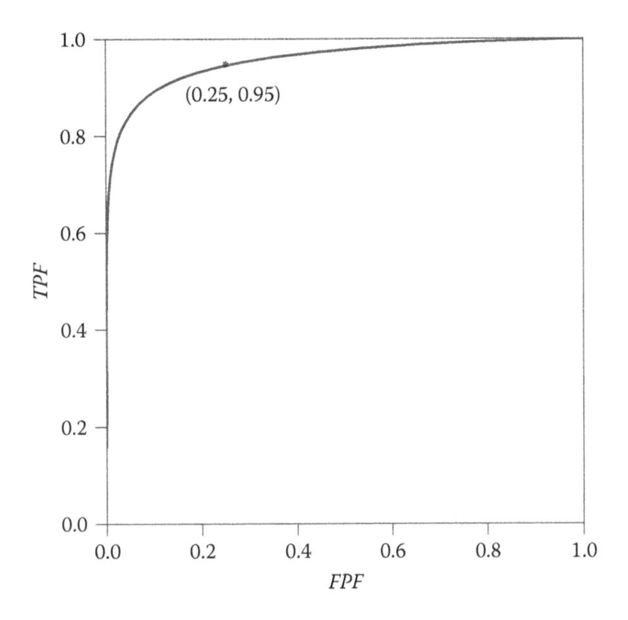

FIGURE 1.5
Corresponding ROC curve using diagnostic marker where underlying ROC curve remains unchanged via any monotone transformation of the measurement scale—known as the invariance property of an ROC curve.

X and Y, respectively, in the correct order, i.e., $P(X < Y) + P(X = Y)/2$ or $P(X < Y)$ without ties stochastically.

The AUC is a simple and convenient overall measure of diagnostic test accuracy. However, it gives equal attention to the full ranges of *TPF* and *FPF*, although only limited ranges may be of practical interest. Also, areas under two ROC curves that cross provide little discriminating information. Partial area under the curve (pAUC) is sometimes used instead (Walter, 2005). It is the area under the ROC curve between two fixed *a priori* values for specificities. It may also be calculated by numerical integration. When estimated parametrically, both the full AUC and pAUC may be computed more easily (McClish, 1989).

1.6 Confidence Intervals, Regions, and Bands

A vertical (or horizontal) confidence interval for *TPF* (or *FPF*) for *a priori* specified *FPF* (or *TPF*) may be constructed first in an unrestricted space such as a probit or logit space in R^2, which may then be transformed back to the ROC space within [0,1] × [0,1]. The reason for the transformation is that normal approximations work better in such an unrestricted space, in contrast to ROC space where values are confined to the [0,1] interval. For example, for sensitivity, the probit transformation is $Probit\ (TPF) = \Phi^{-1}(TPF)$ using the inverse of the cumulative distribution function (CDF) of a standard normal distribution. The logit transform is $logit(TPF) = \log(TPF/1 - TPF)$, where the transformed value is undefined at both ends when p = 0 and 1. Schäfer (1993) constructs vertical nonparametric confidence bounds based directly on the standard errors obtained by Greenhouse and Mantel (1950) rather than using the above transformation. The use of a transformation may improve the accuracy of a large-sample normality approximation.

One difficulty with vertical confidence intervals for a given *FPF* by either method is that we can estimate only the threshold that will yield this *FPF*. When estimating nonparametrically, perhaps of more direct interest is a confidence region for the *FPF* and *TPF* pair on the ROC curve corresponding to a given threshold on the measurement scale. Confidence rectangles, and alternatively, ellipses were proposed based on the nonparametric Greenhouse and Mantel formula in Zou et al. (1997). Hilgers (1991), and Kestler (2001) constructed confidence regions based on distribution-free tolerance intervals, with the extra advantage of conservative small-sample validity. Simultaneous inference is desired when sensitivity is examined over a range of specificities or vice versa. Hall and Ma (1993) constructed simultaneous confidence bands for an ROC curve by mapping out Working–Hotelling bands for a regression line in probit space using a binormal parametric model. Komogolrov–Smirnov type fixed-width nonparametric bands were developed by Campbell (1994) and Jensen et al (2000).

1.7 Point of Intersection and Youden Index

Moses et al. (1993) and Reitsma et al. (2005) adopted a point of intersection of the ROC curve and the line on which the sum of any *FPF* and *TPF* pair is 1 (a diagonal line from [1,0] to [0,1] (see, for example, Figure 1.6). In other words, it is the ROC point at which the sensitivity and specificity become equal. This common sensitivity value also reflects test accuracy: the higher the value, the more accurate the test.

The Youden index is defined as $(Se + Sp - 1) = TPF - FPF$, where Se = sensitivity and Sp = specificity (Biggerstaff, 2000; Fluss et al., 2005). O'Malley et al. (2004) and O'Malley and Zou (2006) computed a measure they called "maximal improvement of sensitivity over chance," defined as the gain the sensitivity beyond the diagonal chance line. Their measure is equivalent to the Youden index computed at a corresponding threshold (Figure 1.7).

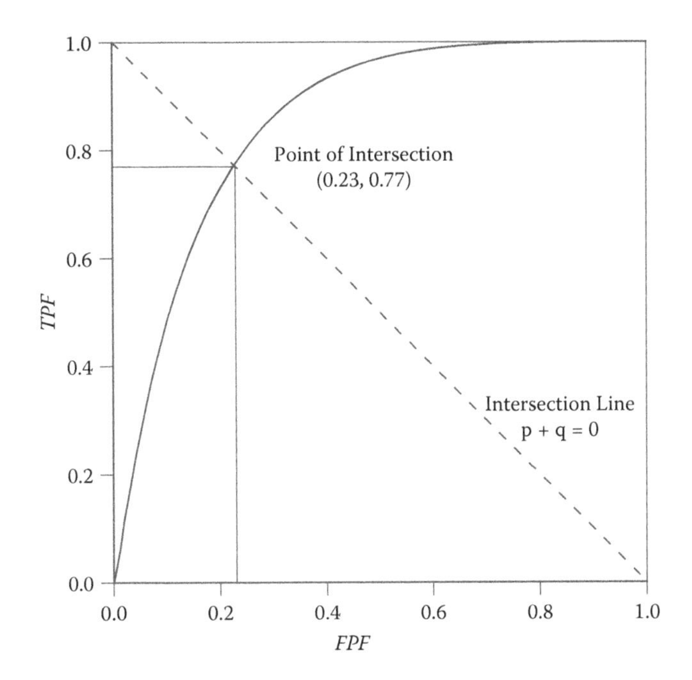

FIGURE 1.6
Point of intersection on ROC curve simulated from N [0,1] and N [1.5, 1.87^2].

1.8 Comparison of Two or More ROC Curves

An important problem concerns the comparison of two or more diagnostic tests. If the tests are performed on the same set of subjects, then results are usually correlated. For example, two different diagnostic tests are administered on the same set of patients, or a single set of test results is interpreted by different clinicians or instruments. A less common situation is to have a different group of subjects for each test, resulting in independent test results. The correlated design is more efficient in that it controls for subject-to-subject variation.

Several authors developed methods for estimating and comparing ROC curves derived from correlated data. For paired tests, Linnet (1987) compared the sensitivities at a common fixed level of specificity. Delong et al. (1988) compared areas using the correlated Mann–Whitney–Wilcoxon U-statistics. Beam and Wieand (1991) compared the performances of correlated tests, one of which is a discrete test and the rest continuous tests, by comparing the sensitivities at a fixed specificity corresponding to a natural threshold of the discrete test. Hanley and McNeil (1983) provided a less computer-intensive approximate procedure to estimate the correlation of two AUCs. Wieand et al. (1989) proposed a family of nonparametric comparisons based on a weighted

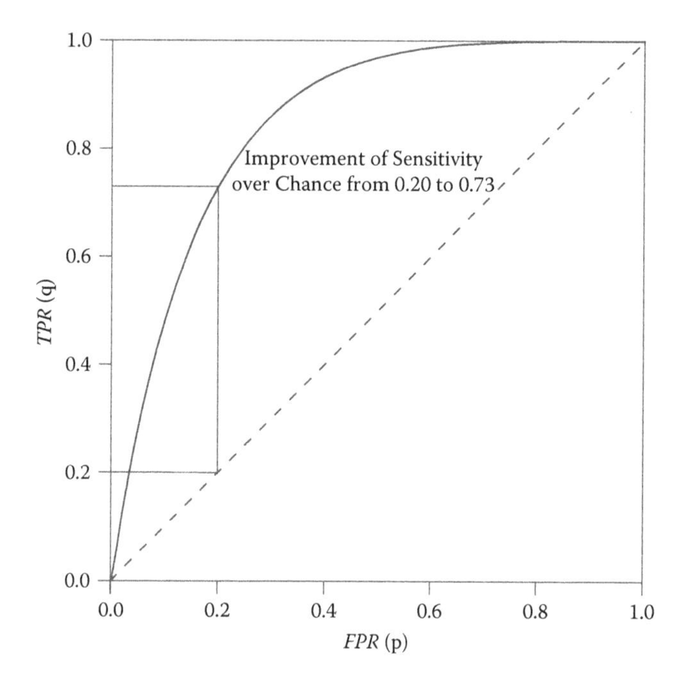

FIGURE 1.7
Maximal improvement of sensitivity over chance at *FPF* 0.20, where specificity = 0.80 simulated from N [0,1] and N [1.5, 1.87^2].

average of sensitivities in which both full AUC and sensitivity at any given specificity become special cases. Venkatraman and Begg (2000) compared two diagnostic tests using permutation. Confidence bands for the difference between two ROC curves (or a portion of them) were presented in Chen and Su (1995). Metz et al. (1997) created a computer algorithm for bivariate extensions to binning methods. Their programs group continuous data into bins, defined primarily by runs of measurements from the two samples, and then use estimation methods for binned data (see: http://www-radiology.uchicago.edu/krl/KRL_ROC/software_index6.htm).

For further readings, see Dorfman et al. (1992), Obuchowski (1995), Obuchowski and Rockette (1995), Pepe (1998; 2000; 2003), Tosteson and Begg (1998), Toledano and Gatsonis (1999), Hillis and Berbaum (2005), Hillis et al. (2005), and Hillis (2007).

1.9 Approaches to ROC Analysis

In this monograph, we summarize various approaches to ROC analysis with a special focus on both univariate and multivariate data in Part II. We discuss the rating scales frequently used in diagnostic studies in Chapter 2. As we have shown the invariance properties of ROC curves, monotone transformation methods are provided in Chapter 3. Under nonparametric methods, rank-based inferences are made; for parametric methods, transformations to various known distributions are discussed. Chapter 4 develops methods for analyzing and combining biomarkers. Methods will be developed for optimally combining different markers and specimens. We introduce Bayesian ROC methods in Chapter 5.

Part III presents some advanced approaches for ROC analysis. Chapter 6 covers sequential methods, including group sequential tests for single and multiple ROC curves using approximation and exact procedures. Chapter 7 elaborates on methods for correlated studies including multireader and multimodality comparisons. Chapter 8 extends the traditional methods to free-response ROC (FROC) analysis for target detection and localization (Bandos et al., 2009). In Chapter 9, methods for machine learning and predictive modeling are discussed.

Finally, Chapter 10 in Part IV provides new applications such as calibration of predictive models, medical imaging, genomics, and time-dependent ROC analysis. Now that ROC analysis is increasingly popular and available, new challenges and unresolved problems in accuracy and reliability analysis may arise.

References

Ash, A. and Schartz, M. 1999. R^2: a useful measure of model performance when predicting a dichotomous outcome. *Statistics in Medicine* 18: 375–384.

Bandos, A.I., Rockette, H.E., Song, T. et al. 2009. Area under the free-response ROC curve (FROC) and a related summary index. *Biometrics* 65: 247–256.

Beam, C.A. and Wieand, H.S. 1991. A statistical method for the comparison of a discrete diagnostic test with several continuous diagnostic tests. *Biometrics* 47: 907–919.

Biggerstaff, B.J. 2000. Comparing diagnostic tests: a simple graphic using likelihood ratios. *Statistics in Medicine* 19: 649–663.

Campbell, G. 1994. Advances in statistical methodology for the evaluation of diagnostic and laboratory tests. *Statistics in Medicine* 13: 499–508.

Chen, H. and Su, J.Q. 1995. Simultaneous confidence bands for comparing diagnostic markers. *Communications in Statistics: Theory and Methods* 24: 375–393.

DeLong, E.R., DeLong, D.M., and Clarke-Pearson, D.L. 1988. Comparing the areas under two or more correlated receiver operating characteristic curves: a nonparametric approach. *Biometrics* 44: 837–845.

Dorfman, D.D., Berbaum, K.S., and Metz, C.E. 1992. Receiver operating characteristic rating analysis: generalization to the population of readers and patients with the jackknife method. *Investigative Radiology* 27: 723–731.

Egan, J.P. 1975. *Signal Detection Theory and ROC Analysis*. New York: Academic Press.

Fleiss, J.L. 1986. *The Design and Analysis of Clinical Experiments*. New York: Wiley.
Fluss, R., Faraggi, D., and Reiser, B. 2005. Estimation of the Youden index and its associated cutoff point. *Biometrical Journal* 47: 458–472.
Gastwirth, J.L. 1972. The estimation of the Lorenz curve and Gini index. *Review of Economics and Statistics* 54: 306–316.
Gönen, M. 2007. *Analyzing Receiver Operating Characteristic Curves with SAS®*. Cary, NC: SAS Institute Inc.
Green, D.M. and Swets, J.A. 1974. *Signal Detection Theory and Psychophysics*. Huntington, NY: Robert E. Krieger Publishing.
Greenhouse, S.W. and Mantel, N. 1950. Evaluation of Diagnostic Tests. *Biometrics* 6: 399–412.
Hanley, J.A. and McNeil, B.J. 1983. A method of comparing the areas under receiver operating characteristic curves derived from the same cases. *Radiology* 148: 839–843.
Hilgers, R.A. 1991. Distribution-free confidence bounds for ROC curves. *Methods of Information in Medicine* 30: 96–101.
Hillis, S.L. and Berbaum, K.S. 2005. Monte Carlo validation of the Dorfman–Berbaum–Metz method using normalized pseudovalues and less data-based model simplification. *Academic Radiolology* 12: 1534–1541.
Hillis, S.L., Obuchowski, N.A., Schartz, K.M. et al. 2005. A comparison of the Dorfman–Berbaum–Metz and Obuchowski–Rockette methods for receiver operating characteristic (ROC) data. *Statistics in Medicine* 24: 1579–1607.
Hillis, S.L. 2007. A comparison of denominator degrees of freedom methods for multiple observer ROC analysis. *Statistics in Medicine* 26: 596–619.
Jensen, K., Müller, H.H., and Schäfer, H. 2000. Regional confidence bands for ROC curves. *Statistics in Medicine* 19: 493–509.
Kendall, M. and Gibbons, J.D. 1990. *Rank Correlation Methods*, 5th ed. New York: Oxford University Press.
Kestler, H.A. 2001. ROC with confidence: a Perl program for receiver operator characteristic curves. *Computer Methods and Programs in Biomedicine* 64: 133–136.
Krzanowski, W.J. and Hand, DJ. 2009. *ROC Curves for Continuous Data*. Boca Raton: Taylor & Francis.
Landis, J.R. and Koch, G.G. 1977. The measurement of observer agreement for categorical data. *Biometrics*. 33: 159–174.
Linnet, K. 1987. Comparison of quantitative diagnostic tests: type I error, power, and sample size. *Statistics in Medicine* 6: 147–158.
Lloyd, C.J. 1988. The use of smoothed ROC curves to summarize and compare diagnostic systems. *JASA* 93: 1356–1364.
Ma, G. and Hall, W.J. 1993. Confidence bands for receiver operating characteristic curves. *Medical Decision Making* 13: 191–197.
Macmillan, N.A. and Creelman, C.D. 1991. *Detection Theory: A User's Guide*. Cambridge: Cambridge University Press.
McClish, D.K. 1989. Analyzing a portion of the ROC curve. *Medical Decision Making* 9: 190–195.
Metz, C.E., Herman, B.A., and Shen, J.H. 1998. Maximum likelihood estimation of receiver operating characteristic (ROC) curves from continuously-distributed data. *Medical Decision Making* 17: 1033–1053.

Moses, L.E., Shapiro, D., and Littenberg, B. 1993. Combining independent studies of a diagnostic test into a summary ROC curve: data-analytic approaches and some additional considerations. *Statistics in Medicine* 12: 1293–1316.

Obuchowski, N.A. 1995. Multireader receiver operating characteristic studies: a comparison of study designs. *Academic Radiology* 2: 709–716.

Obuchowsi, N.A. and Rockette, H.E. 1995. Hypothesis testing of diagnostic accuracy for multiple readers and multiple tests: an ANOVA approach with dependent observations. *Communications in Statistics Simulations* 24: 285–308.

O'Malley, A.J., Zou, K.H., Fielding, J.R. et al. 2001. Bayesian regression methodology for estimating a receiver operating characteristic curve with two radiologic applications: prostate biopsy and spiral CT of ureteral stones. *Academic Radiology* 8: 713–725.

O'Malley, A.J. and Zou, K.H. 2006. Bayesian multivariate hierarchical transformation models for ROC analysis. *Statistics in Medicine* 25: 459–479.

Pepe, M.S. 1998. Three approaches to regression analysis of receiver operating characteristic curves for continuous test results. *Biometrics* 54: 124–135.

Pepe, M.S. 2000. An interpretation for the ROC curve and inference using GLM procedures. *Biometrics* 56: 352–359.

Pepe, M.S. 2003. *The Statistical Evaluation of Medical Tests for Classification and Prediction*. Oxford: Oxford University Press.

Reitsma, J.B., Glas, A.S., Rutjes, A.W. et al. 2005. Bivariate analysis of sensitivity and specificity produces informative summary measures in diagnostic reviews. *Journal of Clinical Epidemiology*. 58: 982–990.

Schäfer, H. 1994. Efficient confidence bounds for ROC curves. *Statistics in Medicine* 13: 1551–1561.

Siegel, S. and Castellan, N.J. 1988. *Nonparametric Statistics for the Behavioral Sciences*, 2nd ed. New York: McGraw-Hill.

Sobehart, J.R. and Keenan, S.C. 2001. Measuring default accurately, credit risk special report. *Risk* 14: 31–33.

Su, J.Q. and Liu, J.S. 1993. Linear combinations of multiple diagnostic markers. *JASA* 88: 1350–1355.

Swets, J.A. and Pickett, R.M. 1982. *Evaluation of Diagnostic Systems: Methods from Signal Detection Theory*. New York: Academic Press.

Toledano, A.Y. and Gatsonis, C. 1999. Generalized estimating equations for ordinal categorical data: arbitrary patterns of missing responses and missingness in a key covariate. *Biometrics* 55: 488–496.

Tosteson, A.N. and Begg, C.B. 1988. A general regression methodology for ROC curve estimation. *Medical Decision Making* 8: 204–215.

Venkatraman, E.S. 2000. A permutation test to compare receiver operating characteristic curves. *Biometrics* 56: 1134–1138.

Walter, S.D. 2005. The partial area under the summary ROC curve. *Statistics in Medicine* 24: 2025–2040.

Wan, S. and Zhang, B. 2007. Smooth semiparametric receiver operating characteristic curves for continuous diagnostic tests. *Statistics in Medicine* 26: 2565–2586.

Wieand, S., Gail, M.H., James, B.R. et al. A family of nonparametric statistics for comparing diagnostic markers with paired or unpaired data. *Biometrika* 76: 585–592.

Zhou, X.H. and Harezlak, J. 2002. Comparison of bandwidth selection methods for kernel smoothing of ROC curves. *Statistics in Medicine* 21: 2045–2055.
Zhou, X.H., Obuchowski, N.A., and McClish, D.K. 2002. *Statistical Methods in Diagnostic Medicine*. New York: Wiley.
Zou, K.H., DeTora, L.M., Haker, S.J. et al. 2009. Revisiting the p-value: a comparison of statistical evidence in clinical and legal medical decision making. *Law, Probability and Risk* 8: 159–170.
Zou, K.H., Hall, W.J., and Shapiro, D.E. 1997. Smooth non-parametric receiver operating characteristic (ROC) curves for continuous diagnostic tests. *Statistics in Medicine* 16: 2143–2156.

Section II

Methods for Univariate and Multivariate Data

2

Diagnostic Rating Scales

2.1 Introduction

Traditional ROC analysis focuses on assessment of the ability of a diagnostic system to reproduce the results of a "binary gold standard." In the simplest scenario, a binary gold standard indicates the presence or absence of a specific condition (e.g., abnormality) in a specific subject. In other scenarios, it may indicate the locations of multiple abnormalities within an subject, hence associating any specific location with a binary indication of the presence or absence of a certain abnormality (see Chapter 8). In this chapter, we discuss a simple case in which the gold standard indicates a binary truth (normal or abnormal) for each subject (see Chapter 1). Note that the principles and concepts discussed here extend to more general scenarios.

Many diagnostic systems can provide the result of assessment of an subject in a form of a rating (e.g., confidence rating in regard to the presence of an abnormality) that may have more than two values. The rating provided by the system can be continuous (or interval), pseudocontinuous (integers from 0 to 100), ordered-categorical (ordinal), and unordered-categorical (nominal).

The ratings provided by diagnostic systems are frequently used for making decisions regarding further management of the subjects tested (e.g., referral for an additional diagnostic work-up as a result of screening). For these types of diagnostic system utilizations, regardless of the type of scale natural for a given system, its ratings are often categorized to be consistent with the gold standard—dichotomized into positive or negative in accordance with a binary standard. This categorization creates a natural framework for making decisions related to follow-up actions appropriate for handling subjects with a specific true status.

In more complex scenarios, diagnostic tasks may accommodate more than two types of decisions or sets of actions and the diagnostic ratings can be categorized into an appropriate number of categories for implementation in practice. One well known example in diagnostic imaging is the BIRADS scale of 1 through 5 for diagnostic mammography (0 is reserved for incomplete assessment and 6 for a known prior cancer) with guidelines on recommended further actions. If finer ratings than required are available, the categorization process follows the same general principle as for the dichotomization process described below.

The first step in dichotomization may include ordering of the rating scale so that results with higher orders are more indicative of abnormality. When the rating scale used by a diagnostic system has a natural order (ordinal or interval scale), no additional ordering may be necessary, although optimal ordering does not always coincide with the natural one (Egan, 1975). The diagnostic ratings with natural order are most common in practice and include different types of scales (continuous or pseudocontinuous probability scales, categorical Likert scales). In rare cases when the results of diagnostic tests are nominal, additional characteristics of the nominal categories must be derived for the purpose of ordering the categories. The optimal ordering of test results is based on the likelihood ratio (Egan, 1975), defined as the ratio of the probabilities of observing a given test result in abnormal and normal populations of subjects. The optimality of likelihood-ratio ordering of the ratings of a diagnostic test follows the Neyman–Pearson lemma (Neyman and Pearson, 1933).

After the rating scale of a diagnostic system is ordered, dichotomization can be achieved by grouping values exceeding a given value threshold into the positive category and values below or equal to the same threshold into the negative category. Selection of the threshold is a separate (and often complicated) problem that should be guided by the nature of the diagnostic task and the question of interest. In diagnostic medicine, a threshold is frequently guided by the severity and prevalence of a disease, costs of incorrect diagnosis, and other aspects of decision making in the medical arena (Zhou et al., 2002).

Once the specific dichotomization is defined, the accuracy of a diagnostic test can be assessed based on the proportions of positive test results among abnormal (sensitivity) or normal (1-specificity) subjects. The accuracy of the diagnostic system for all thresholds simultaneously may be conveyed with an ROC curve (see Chapter 1).

Thus, regardless of the type of result of a diagnostic system, the approaches for assessing its accuracy are well established and widely known. However, prior to performing such analyses, investigators must sometimes make the important decision of which rating scale to use for data collection. Some related issues are summarized in Zhou et al. (2002). Here we focus on the relative merits of different scales from the perspective of assessing the performance of a diagnostic test. We place a special emphasis on the distinction between the diagnostic procedures that include human observers as integral parts of the system and interpreter-free diagnostic systems.

2.1.1 Frequent Need for Finer Scale

When faced with the problem of selecting a rating scale, the natural question is why not select a scale of the same type as the targeted gold standard—a binary scale in the case of a binary gold standard. Indeed such a scale would seem to not require additional preprocessing related to ordering and selecting thresholds. The problem, however, lies in the general absence of a uniformly accepted set of thresholds. The performance characteristics of a binary test obtained by dichotomizing results of a given diagnostic system can vary substantially, depending on the specific threshold. Different studies may consider different thresholds as optimal for a perceived diagnostic condition.

As a result of the absence of a uniform threshold, implementations of the same diagnostic system with different thresholds may appear as implementations of intrinsically different diagnostic systems. Consideration of raw (noncategorized) test results helps avoid this problem (e.g., by considering the ROC curves summarizing performance of the diagnostic systems for all thresholds simultaneously).

This may lead to thinking that the use of the finest scale possible is the best decision for evaluating performance of a diagnostic test. While this may be true for many scenarios, exceptions exist. One notable exception arises in studies of diagnostic systems that include human observers as integral parts of the system. In addition, some analytical approaches may superimpose categorizations for technical reasons.

2.2 Interpreter-Free Diagnostic Systems

The use of the finest possible scale is often justified in performance assessments of interpreter-free (completely automated) diagnostic systems that produce results using a single algorithm that is not affected by the diagnostic environment. In these instances, the use of the artificial categorization of the scale may lead to downward bias, especially when a nonparametric analysis is undertaken (Zhou et al., 2002). In addition, along with possible problems with a binary scale, superimposition of a categorical scale may lead to mistaking different implementations of the same diagnostic system as intrinsically different systems (Pepe, 2003). The superimposed categorization of test results may also lead to increased variability due to loss of information (Wagner et al., 2001).

Categorization of diagnostic test results may sometimes be implemented for technical purposes. For example, categorization of continuous data may be used for fitting an ROC curve of a given parametric form using a latent variable approach (Metz et al., 1998; Pepe, 2003). One of the advantages of such an approach is the reduction of dependence on the distribution of the observed data achieved by exploiting the principle of invariance of an ROC curve with respect to any order-preserving transformation (see Chapter 1). If the assumed parametric shape of the ROC curve is correct, the latent variable approach permits a reduction in bias and an increase in precision. However, both bias and precision depend on the appropriateness of the assumed model and categorization (Walsh, 1997). The approaches for categorization-free and distribution-free fitting of smooth ROC curves for continuous data continue to be developed (Zou and Hall, 2000), thereby reducing the need for use of categorization for solely technical reasons.

Thus, when assessing performance of an established interpreter-free diagnostic system, the best approach frequently is using the finest scale available. However, this conclusion does not automatically generalize to observer performance studies.

2.3 Human Interpreter as Integral Part of Diagnostic System

The categorical scale is essential in studies of diagnostic systems that involve human observers as integral parts of a diagnostic process. Many diagnostic systems, particularly in medicine, require interpretation of the test results by a human observer (e.g., radiologists interpreting mammograms, cardiologists interpreting cardiograms). One of the primary problems in performance assessment of such diagnostic systems is that the diagnostic ratings may depend on a large number of factors that may affect human behavior. Furthermore, depending on the diagnostic task, training, overall experience, and other characteristics of human observers may constitute different intrinsic abilities to rate subjects. An observer's intrinsic scale cannot be observed directly. Investigators must assume that the ratings provided by observers on the suggested scale accurately reflect their intrinsic ratings. These issues result in nontrivial challenges for selecting appropriate scale for the collection of diagnostic ratings in observer-performance studies.

Psychological studies indicate that human ability to consistently order subjects is limited to only a few categories for many tasks (Miller, 1956). Traditional observer-performance studies were recommended to be performed on a five-category scale (Swets and Pickett, 1982). Conversely, in some scenarios, humans can handle a large number of categories without damaging diagnostic performance and may even improve it (Rockette et al., 1992; Wagner et al., 2001). One of the complexities of observer-performance studies is the possibility of requesting human observers to express diagnostic results using a type of scale that is different from the scale natural for the given diagnostic task.

The superimposition of a coarser-than-natural rating scale in observer-performance studies may prove disadvantageous and lead to consequences similar to those in studies of interpreter-free systems discussed previously. However, one of the potential advantages of using a coarser scale in observer-performance studies is the potential for improved repeatability of the results. Furthermore, the use of a categorical scale may increase the immediate practical (clinical) relevance of the results of performance assessment when the same categorical scale is routinely used in practice and relates to specific recommended actions for similar diagnostic tasks. However, the appropriateness of using categorical scales solely due to the potential practical relevance should be carefully evaluated, since a categorization adopted by readers may depend on a number of factors including familiarity with task, the scale used, and maintenance of a realistic diagnostic environment.

Along with the drawback of superimposition of a coarser categorical scale in observer-performance studies, the converse problem may result from superimposition of an artificially finer scale. In some diagnostic tasks, human observers naturally tend to classify subjects in only a few categories (e.g., detection of pneumothorax or a rib fracture on x-ray images, Gur et al., 2007), yet during a performance assessment study, observers may be asked to report their ratings on a substantially more refined scale (0 to 100). If indeed the intrinsic opinion of a human observer for a given task is limited to only a few categories, the reported ratings may be contaminated with random noise. This could result in bias and loss of precision, which are typically present in ROC analysis in the presence of measurement errors (Coffin and Sukhatme, 1997; Feraggi, 2000).

Superimposition of a finer-than-natural scale may also be problematic at the stage of analysis of the data collected under a naturally coarser scale. For example, a problem could arise if the intrinsic rating ability of a human observer was limited to five categories and a five-category scale was used for data collection and the performed analysis estimated a smooth ROC curve corresponding to a continuous latent variable. In this case, the estimated ROC curve would tend to be biased upward. Assuming the parametric assumptions used for construction of a smooth ROC curve are correct, the absolute magnitude of the bias is exactly the same as that of the bias resulting from categorization of an intrinsically continuous diagnostic rating.

2.4 Remarks and Further Reading

In general, for assessment of performance of diagnostic systems, the "best" scale for collected test results coincides with the intrinsic ability of the system to rate subjects. Failure to select such a scale could lead to both bias and loss of precision. The inappropriate categorization of a scale may lead to underestimation of diagnostic ability and increase the variability of the estimates. The inappropriate superimposition of a finer scale may also lead to both bias (frequently upward in this case) and an increase of variability. Variability may further increase in observer-performance studies due to a decrease in repeatability of the results.

For interpreter-free diagnostic systems, using the finest possible scale is often the most appropriate choice. For diagnostic systems that require interpretation of results by a trained observer, the appropriateness and/or usefulness of the scale adopted in a performance assessment study depend highly on the specific diagnostic task in question. In some cases, the finest possible scale may be appropriate; in others, the categorical or binary scale may be a better choice. In addition, a fine rating scale can be used for data collection for some diagnostic tasks, but the binary responses (corresponding to latent reader-specific dichotomization of the scale) may provide important information on how the test could be used in practice.

Books by Swets and Pickett (1982) and Zhou et al. (2000) provide further discussion of practical aspects of selecting a rating scale for assessment of performance of a diagnostic system for a binary gold standard. The extensions of ROC analysis for scenarios with more than dichotomous truths are discussed in several papers focused on specific types of gold standards such as nominal (Mossman, 1999), ordered categorical (Nakas and Yiannoutsos, 2004) and continuous (Obuchowski, 2006).

References

American College of Radiology. 2003. Breast Imaging Reporting and Data System Atlas (BI-RADS® Atlas). *Mammography,* 4th ed. Reston, VA: American College of Radiology. www.acr.org (accessed 12/17/2010).

Coffin, M. and Sukhatme, S. 1997. Receiver operating characteristic studies and measurement errors. *Biometrics* 53: 823–837.

Egan, J.P. 1975. *Signal Detection Theory and ROC Analysis.* New York: Academic Press.

Faraggi, D. 2000. The effect of random measurement error on receiver operating characteristic (ROC) curves. *Statistics in Medicine* 19: 61–70.

Gur, D., Rockette, H.E., and Bandos, A.I. 2007. "Binary" and non-binary detection tasks: are current performance measures optimal? *Academic Radiology* 14: 871–876.

Metz, C.E., Herman, B.A., and Shen, J. 1998. Maximum likelihood estimation of receiver operating characteristic (ROC) curves from continuously distributed data. *Statistics in Medicine* 17: 1033–1053.

Miller, G.A. 1956. The magical number seven, plus or minus two: some limits on our capacity for processing information. *Psychological Review* 63: 81–98.

Mossman, D. 1999. Three-way ROCs. *Medical Decision Making* 19: 78–89.

Nakas, C.T. and Yiannoutsos, C.T. 2004. Ordered multiple-class ROC analysis with continuous measurements. *Statistics in Medicine* 23: 3437–3449.

Neyman J. and Pearson, E. 1933. On the problem of the most efficient tests of statistical hypotheses. *Philosophical Transactions of the Royal Society of London Series A* 231: 289–337.

Obuchowski, N.A. 2006. An ROC-type measure of diagnostic accuracy when the gold standard is continuous scale. *Statistics in Medicine* 25: 481–493.

Pepe, M.S. 2003. *The Statistical Evaluation of Medical Tests for Classification and Prediction*. Oxford: Oxford University Press.

Rockette, H.E., Gur, D., and Metz, C.E. 1992. The use of continuous and discrete confidence judgment in ROC studies of diagnostic imaging techniques. *Investigative radiology* 27: 169–172.

Swets, J.A. and Pickett, R.M. 1982. *Evaluation of Diagnostic Systems: Methods from Signal Detection Theory*. New York: Academic Press.

Wagner, R.F., Beiden, S.V., and Metz, C.E. 2001. Continuous versus categorical data for ROC analysis: some quantitative considerations. *Academic Radiology* 8: 328–334.

Walsh, S.J. 1997. Limitations to the robustness of binormal ROC curves: effects of model misspecification and location of decision threshold on bias, precision, size and power. *Statistics in Medicine* 16: 669–679.

Zhou, X.H., Obuchowski, N.A., and McClish D.K. 2002. *Statistical Methods in Diagnostic Medicine*. New York: Wiley.

Zou, K.H. and Hall, W.J. 2000. Two transformation models for estimating an ROC curve derived from continuous data. *Journal of Applied Statistics* 27: 621–631.

3

Monotone Transformation Models

3.1 Introduction

The previous chapters have summarized the notations and assumptions for ROC analysis. In this chapter, the special feature that an ROC curve is invariant to any monotone transformation is utilized. That is, a single diagnostic test is evaluated on random samples of subjects of two underlying populations governed by the gold standard.

The relevant assumptions are presented in Section 3.2. Empirical methods for fully estimating an ROC curve nonparametrically based on the ranks of the two-sample measurements in a combined ranking are described in Section 3.3, followed by a nonparametric kernel-smoothed version in Section 3.4. In Section 3.5, it is assumed that transformed test results via a normality transformation of the two samples follow a particular parametric model, namely the binormal model. Section 3.6 presents the corresponding characteristic, i.e., confidence intervals for several measures of interests. Beyond univariate diagnostic tests, bivariate data on the same set of subjects are analyzed in Section 3.7. Their concordance following a monotone transformation is evaluated. Besides accuracy and concordance, Section 3.8 presents methods for evaluating the agreement between two or more tests using an intraclass correlation coefficient (ICC).

3.2 General Assumptions

As introduced in Chapter 1, from the H and D populations, there are independent and identically distributed (i.i.d.) random samples of sizes n^0 and n^1, respectively. Let ξ be an arbitrary threshold or, given *a priori FPF* value, here denoted as *fpf*, and the underlying ROC curve is defined as:

$$\left(S_X(\xi), S_Y(\xi)\right), \forall\xi \in R, \text{ or } \left(fpf, S_Y \circ S_X^{-1}(fpf)\right), \tag{3-1}$$

labeled as 1-specificity and sensitivity, respectively. A special feature of an ROC curve is that it is invariant to any monotonically increasing transformation of the threshold scale, i.e., if $X' = h(X)$ and $Y' = h(Y)$ with threshold $\xi' = h(\xi)$ for some monotone increasing transformation h. Then the invariance property means that:

$$FPF = S_X\left(h^{-1}(\xi')\right) \text{ and } TPF(fpf) = S_Y \circ h^{-1} \circ h \circ S_X^{-1}(fpf) = S_Y \circ S_X^{-1}(fpf). \quad (3\text{-}2)$$

Both estimation and hypothesis testing procedures with regard to the characteristics of these two populations may be conducted. For univariate problems with special reference to ROC curves, estimation is generally of more interest. Nonetheless, much of the classical two-sample literature focuses on hypothesis testing to detect the presence of differences between these two populations, rather than estimate the actual difference.

Several methods have been developed for inference of the location difference between two populations. The model employed is the two-sample location-shift model that assumes that the underlying distributions have a common shape. For example, nonparametric rank-based estimation and testing procedures are found in classical text books by Lehmann (1975, 1986) and Hettmansperger (1991), in which small and large sample methods were derived and efficiency studies were discussed. Robustness aspects of the procedures may be found in Rieder (1982) and Lambert (1982).

For distribution-free tests methods as the permutation test, see Maritz (1981) and Pesarin (2001). Parametric procedures are found in Krzanowski (1988). For the case of unequal variances, the Behrens–Fisher t-test problem may be considered. When both locations and scales are allowed to differ between the two populations, a location–scale model may be used. Kochar (1977) presented a class of distribution-free tests under this model. Goria (1982) derived asymptotic relative efficiencies of some rank tests. Parametric procedures such as ANOVA techniques were described in Nair (1982).

3.3 Empirical Methods

Plotting *TPF* versus *FPF* pairs at all possible values of a decision threshold may be achieved using empirical distributions that are essentially unsmoothed histograms based on the H and D samples. This is the simplest nonparametric method without parameters to model the data, and the underlying distributions for both populations are fully unstructured. The advantages of this approach are its robustness and freedom from structural assumptions. The main disadvantage is that the resulting ROC curve is jagged.

Example: 2-h plasma glucose (mmol/L) in diabetes — Lasko et al. (2004) generated hypothetical 2-h plasma glucose measurements taken from

TABLE 3.1

Empirical *FPFs* and *TPFs* at Various Thresholds Using 2-Hour Plasma Glucose Data

2-Hour Plasma Glucose (mmol/L)		Joint Rank		Arbitrary Threshold ξ (mmol/L)	Estimated 1-Specificity $FPF(\xi)$	Estimated Sensitivity $TPF(\xi)$
Healthy	Diseased	Healthy	Diseased			
				<4.86	1.0	1.0
4.86	*	1	1	4.86	0.9	1.0
5.69	*	2	2	5.69	0.8	1.0
6.01	*	3	3	6.01	0.7	1.0
6.06	*	4	4	6.06	0.6	1.0
6.27	*	5	5	6.27	0.5	1.0
6.37	*	6	6	6.37	0.4	1.0
6.55	*	7	*	6.55	0.3	1.0
7.29	7.29	8.5	8.5	7.29	0.2	0.9
7.82	*	10	*	7.82	0.1	0.9
*	9.22	*	11	9.22	0.1	0.8
*	9.79	*	12	9.79	0.1	0.7
*	11.28	*	13	11.28	0.1	0.6
*	11.83	*	14	11.83	0.1	0.5
12.06	*	15	*	12.06	0.0	0.5
*	18.48	*	16	18.48	0.0	0.4
*	18.50	*	17	18.50	0.0	0.3
*	20.49	*	18	20.49	0.0	0.2
*	22.66	*	19	22.66	0.0	0.1
*	26.01	*	20	≥26.01	0.0	0.0

* = *No diagnostic data. FPF = 1-specificity =* $(\#X>\xi)/n^0$. *TPF = sensitivity =* $(\#Y>\xi)/n^1$.

10 healthy controls and 10 diseased patients with diabetes. Sample H consists of n^0= 10 measurements {4.86, 5.69, 6.01, 6.06, 6.27, 6.37, 6.55, 7.29, 7.82, 12.06}. Sample D also consists of n^1= 10 measurements {7.29, 9.22, 9.79, 11.28, 11.83, 18.48, 18.50, 20.49, 22.66, 26.01}. The empirical survival functions are computed in Table 3.1 given any natural threshold values in the combined H and D samples and their joint ranks. The ROC curve is displayed in Figure 3.1.

3.4 Nonparametric Kernel Smoothing

Zou et al. (1997) proposed using a kernel-based estimate of the *PDFs* for the H and D samples. The *PDFs* are approximated by:

$$\hat{f}_X(\xi) = \frac{1}{n^0 w_X} \sum_{i=1}^{n^0} k\left(\frac{\xi - X_i}{w_X}\right) \text{ and } \hat{f}_Y(\xi) = \frac{1}{n^1 w_Y} \sum_{j=1}^{n^1} k\left(\frac{\xi - X_j}{w_Y}\right), \tag{3-3}$$

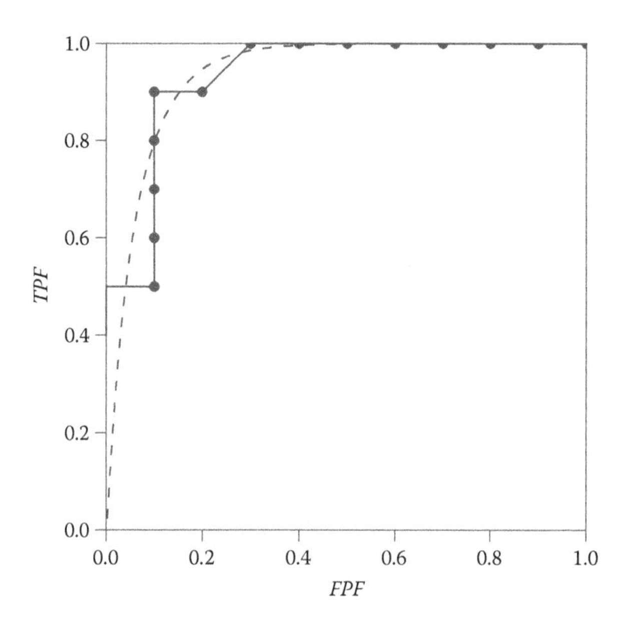

FIGURE 3.1
Empirical and binormal ROC curves based on glucose data. ROC curve parameters are estimated on a log scale with a = 3.12 and b = 1.79 after a test of log normality yielding p = 0.07 and 0.45 using the Shapiro-Wilk test.

where w_X and w_Y are the bandwidths computed from the H and D samples, respectively; $k(\times)$ is the common kernel that is a nonnegative function integrating to unity with a corresponding distribution function $K(\times)$. Instead of smoothing the empirical density functions (i.e., essentially raw histograms), the distribution functions may be smoothed using $K(\times)$ directly to yield approximated sensitivity against 1-specificity along the smoothed ROC curve.

Various optimal bandwidths for the choices of kernel and degree of smoothness were investigated by Hsieh and Turnbull (1996), Zou et al. (1997), Lloyd (1998), Zhou and Harezlak (2002), and Krzanowski and Hand (2009). A default function "density" in the software R may be used to obtain smoothed *PDF*s at 100 equally spaced and prespecified threshold values throughout the entire domain of the combined H and D data. The survival functions may be approximated via Reimann sums using numerical integrations.

Example: dermoscope scoring for detecting malignant melanoma — Venkatraman and Begg (1996) analyzed the features of skin lesions based on asymmetry, border irregularity, coloration, and size to derive a scoring system. They inspected a total of 72 lesions (51 benign versus 21 malignant) without and with a dermoscope to evaluate the added value of the instrument. The smoothed histograms are shown in Figure 3.2. At any arbitrary thresholdξ, the estimated *FPF* and *TPF* are given by:

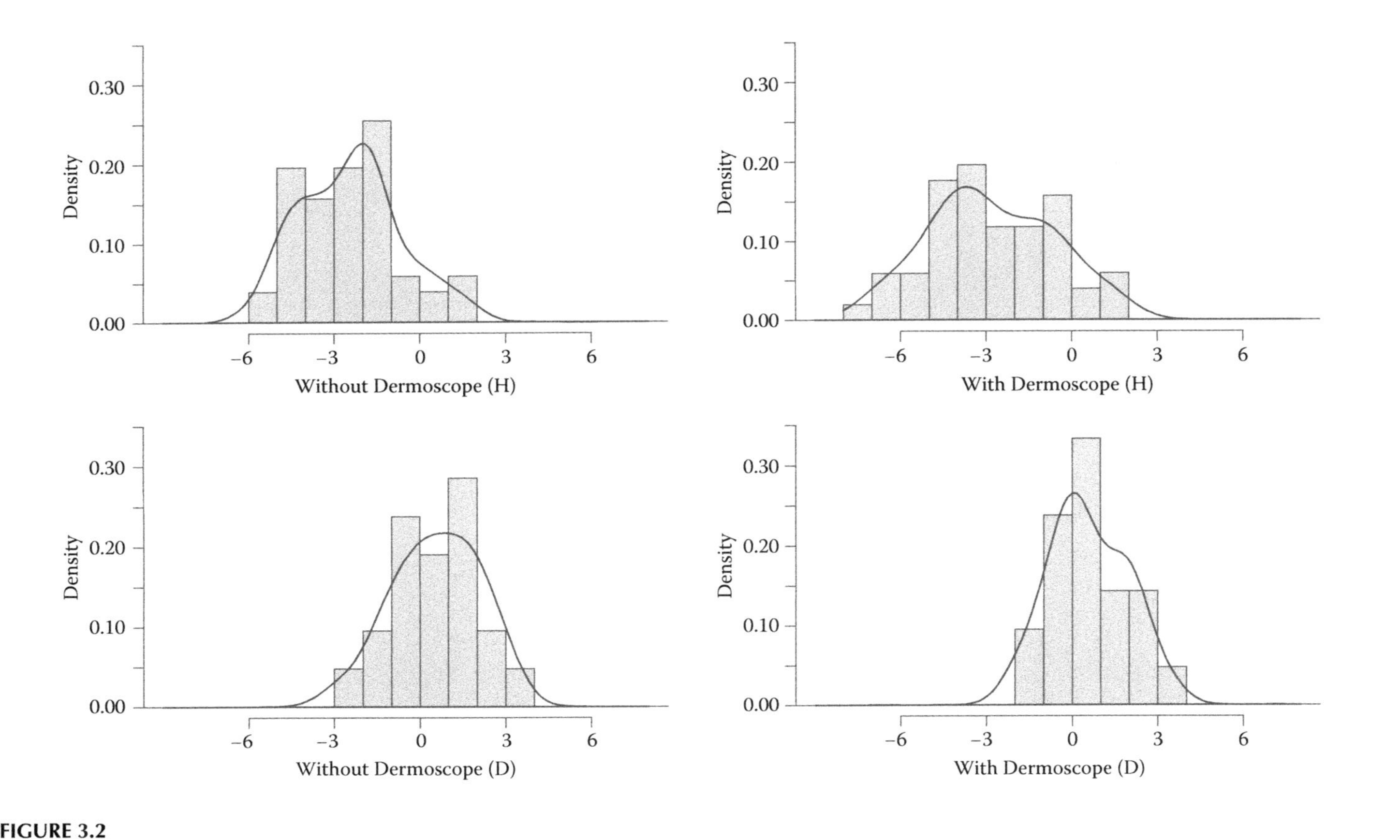

FIGURE 3.2
Histograms along with kernel-smoothed versions of scores for healthy subjects without malignant melanoma (upper left) and diseased subjects with malignant melanoma (lower left) without dermoscope, and similarly for healthy subjects (upper right) and diseased subjects (lower right) with dermoscope.

$$\widehat{FPF}(\xi) = \hat{S}_X(\xi) = \frac{1}{n^0}\sum_{i=1}^{n^0} S_k\left(\frac{\xi - X_i}{w_X}\right) \text{ and } \widehat{TPF}(\xi) = \hat{S}_Y(\xi) = \frac{1}{n^1}\sum_{j=1}^{n^1} S_k\left(\frac{\xi - Y_j}{w_Y}\right). \tag{3.4}$$

We demonstrated the simple methods described here based on kernel smoothing of the underlying distributions. In contrast, Du and Tang (2009) proposed curve smoothing based directly on the empirical ROC points rather than distributions. Alternatively, smoothing of *CDF*s rather than *PDF*s may be conducted (Lloyd, 1998). Zhou and Harezlak (2002) used simulations to demonstrate that direct smoothing of the *CDF*s performed well.

3.5 Parametric Models and Monotone Transformations to Binormal Distributions

The most frequently-used binormal model assumes that the measurements have two independent normal distributions with different means and standard deviations (SDs). The binormal model is a specific case of a bivariate model but assumes independent distribution of components. Suppose each of F_x and F_y belongs to a location–scale family, i.e., $F_X(\bullet) = F_{0X}\{(\bullet - \mu_X)/\sigma_X\}$ and $F_Y(\bullet) = F_{0Y}\{(\bullet - \mu_Y)/\sigma_Y\}$, where F_{0X} and F_{0Y} are known *CDFs* with corresponding survival functions S_{0X} and S_{0Y}, respectively. The underlying ROC curve becomes:

$$(FPF,\ TPF) = \left(S_{0,X}(\xi), S_{0,Y}\left(\frac{\xi - a}{\frac{1}{b}}\right)\right). \tag{3-5}$$

Metz et al. (1988) defines the ROC parameters as follows:

$$a = \frac{\mu_Y - \mu_X}{\sigma_Y} \text{ and } b = \frac{\sigma_X}{\sigma_Y}. \tag{3-6}$$

These two ROC parameters fully determine the shape of the ROC curve because of any invariance to monotone transformation. An Excel PLOTROC.xls macro may be downloaded to plot ROC curves given any ROC parameters (http://xray.bsd.uchicago.edu/krl/roc_soft.htm).

An assumption of a specific form for both F_{0X} and F_{0Y} results in a parametric model that presents the further advantage of facilitating the incorporation of covariates into ROC curve fitting (Pepe, 1998, 2000 and 2003). The most popular is the binormal model where $F_{0X} = F_{0Y} = \Phi$, which is the *CDF* of a standard normal distribution (Metz, 1998).

Goodness-of-fit (GoF) tests for univariate or bivariate normality may be conducted under the transformation-to-normality model. Pearson (1900) devised the oldest testing procedure for GoF. A review of various GoF tests may be found in D'Agostino and Stephens (1986). For univariate normality, a simple quantile–quantile (Q-Q) plot, a useful graphical method (Wilk and Gnanadesikan, 1968), can be used. Also see Madansky (1988) for a review of available formal tests for univariate normality, including those by Shapiro-Wilk (1965), Filliben (1975), and D'Agostino (1971; 1972). Lin and Mudholkar (1980) developed the z-test for univariate normality based on a characterization that the mean and variance of a sample are independent if and only if the population is normal. The Nortest R package provides five omnibus tests for a composite hypothesis of normality (http://cran.r-project.org/web/packages/nortest).

In the dermoscope scoring example, the sores are normally distributed. The Shapiro-Wilk normality confirmed, with nonsignificant p-values at 0.4719 (H, without dermoscope), 0.9084 (D, without dermoscope), 0.5433 (H, with dermoscope), and 0.9784 (D, with dermoscope), respectively. Hence, the ROC parameters may be estimated appropriately using sample means and standard deviations. The corresponding sample mean (SD) values are –2.426 (1.760), 0.557 (1.523), –2.814 (2.180), 0.575 (1.357). The corresponding ROC parameters are $\left(\widehat{a_1}, \widehat{b_1}\right) = (1.694, 0.865)$ versus $\left(\widehat{a_2}, \widehat{b_2}\right) = (1.357, 1.555)$, without versus with a dermoscope, respectively. See Figure 3.3.

Transformation models may be considered to improve GoF. This model assumes a parametric monotone transformation of the measurement scale that simultaneously makes both H and D distributions marginally normal. They further assume that a transformation takes the data into a specified parametric family, regardless of the true model for the data on the original measurement scales. See Bickel (1986) and Bickel et al. (1993). Barndorff-Nielsen et al. (1989) used the transformation model term differently to describe any parametric model invariant under some group of transformations—what Lehmann (1986) calls an invariant model. If the transformation is specified by a parametric form, the transformation model is said to be parametric. Parametric transformation models that take data into normal models were introduced by Box and Cox (1964).

Denote T as the result of a diagnostic test. A monotone transformation h is applied to the result, leading to the transformed version T'. Following this transformation h for both the healthy and diseased samples, let $X' = h(X)$ be an actually negative diagnostic unit equivalent to $(T'|D = 0)$ after h. Similarly, let $Y' = h(Y)$ be an actually positive diagnostic unit equivalent to $(T'|D = 1)$ following the same transformation. To parameterize the transformation, a family of power transformations assumes that the support of the X and Y data is the positive real line R^+. For the support of R other than

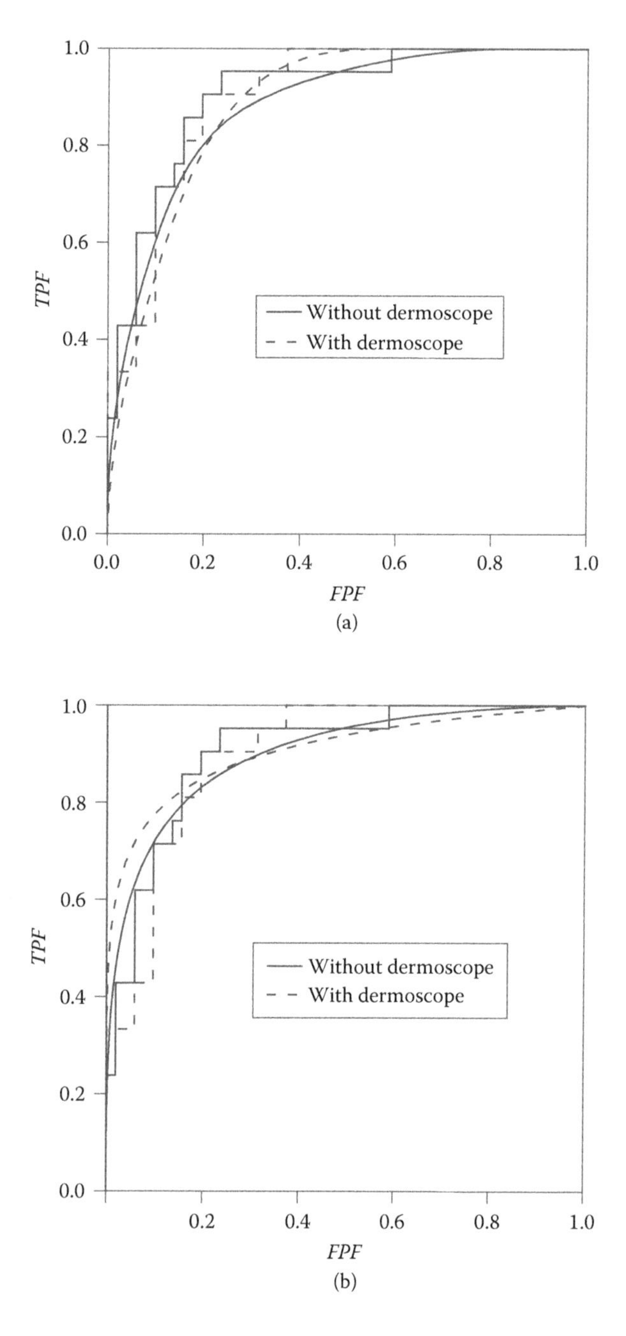

FIGURE 3.3
Kernel-smoothed (a) and binormal (b) ROC curves for detecting malignant melanoma without (solid line) and with (dashed line) use of dermoscope. Diagnostic performances appeared similar to corresponding two ROC curves crossing.

R^+, we may exponentiate the measurements or add a positive shift δ. For probabilistic classification data in [0,1], the measurements may be transformed using a probit $(x) = \Phi^{-1}(x)$ or logit $(x) = \log[x/(1-x)]$, with the natural log transformation or directly fitting the data using a beta distribution (Zou et al., 2004; 2010).

Positively valued diagnostic data may be transformed to normality in two steps. A Box–Cox (1964) transformation with a power coefficient λ is applied first to the measurements in both samples.

$$X_i'(\lambda) = h_\lambda(X_i) = \begin{cases} \dfrac{X_i^\lambda - 1}{\lambda}, & if\ \lambda \neq 0, \\ \log(X_i^\lambda), & otherwise, \end{cases} \quad \forall_i = 1, \ldots, n^0. \tag{3-7}$$

Similarly, $Y_i'(\lambda) = h_\lambda(Y_j)$, $\forall_j = 1, \ldots, n^0$. The transformed random variables X' and Y, follow independent normal distributions $\Phi(\mu_X, \sigma_X^2)$ and $\Phi(\mu_Y, \sigma_Y^2)$, respectively. A second step further standardizes X' linearly to $N(0,1)$ and Y' to $N(a/b, 1/b^2)$. To jointly estimate the three parameters (λ, a, b), the log likelihood function associated with X' is given by Hernandez and Johnson (1980). Zou and Hall (2001) proposed maximizing the profile log likelihood shown below, which is to be maximized with respect to λ.

$$l(\lambda \mid x, y) = -n^0 \log[s(x')] - n^1 \log[s(y')] + (\lambda - 1)\left[\sum_{i=1}^{n^0} \log(x_i') + \sum_{j=1}^{n^1} \log(y_j')\right] + \text{constant}, \tag{3-8}$$

where the *constant* term is free of λ. The nonlinear minimization routine *nlm* in R may be run to derive the estimated power coefficient $\hat{\lambda}$. Gönen (2007) described implementation of the Box–Cox transformation techniques using standard routines in SAS.

Theoretical studies on several aspects of the Box–Cox transformation were conducted. Hinkley (1975) and Hernandez and Johnson (1980) investigated the asymptotic properties of the parameter estimates for the one-sample problem. Bickel and Doksum (1981) examined the behavior of the asymptotic variances of parameter estimates for both regression and analysis of variance (ANOVA) situations. Conditionals were investigated by Hinkley and Runger (1984), Doksum (1987), and Carroll and Ruppert (1988).

After estimating this optimal transformation to normality, apply $\hat{\lambda}$ to both x and y samples to yield the corresponding x' and y'. The estimated ROC parameters $(\hat{a}, \hat{b})$ are computed using sample means and SDs.

$$\hat{a} = \frac{\hat{\mu}_{Y'} - \hat{\mu}_{X'}}{\hat{\sigma}_{Y'}} = \frac{\overline{y'} - \overline{x'}}{s(y')},$$

$$\hat{b} = \frac{\hat{\sigma}_{X'}}{\hat{\sigma}_{Y'}} = \frac{s(x')}{s(y')}. \tag{3-9}$$

The 4×4 variance and covariance matrix Σ of the sample mean and standard deviation are given by:

$$\sum\left(\hat{\mu}_{X'}, \widehat{\sigma}^2_{X'}, \hat{\mu}_{Y'}, \widehat{\sigma}^2_{Y'}\right) = Diag\left(\frac{\sigma^2_X}{n^0}, \frac{\sigma^2_X}{2n^0}, \frac{\sigma^2_Y}{n^1}, \frac{\sigma^2_Y}{2n^1}\right). \tag{3-10}$$

Using the delta method (Rao, 1973), the 2×2 large-sample variance and covariance matrix of the estimated ROC parameters is $\Sigma(\hat{a},\hat{b}) = u\Sigma\ (\hat{\mu}_{X'}, \hat{\sigma}^2_{X'}, \hat{\mu}_{Y'}, \hat{\sigma}^2_{Y'})$ u^T, with T representing the transpose of a matrix and u containing the following elements:

$$u = \begin{pmatrix} -\frac{1}{\sigma_{Y'}} & 0 & \frac{1}{\sigma_{Y'}} & \frac{\mu_{X'} - \mu_{Y'}}{\sigma^2_{Y'}} \\ 0 & \frac{1}{\sigma_{Y'}} & 0 & -\frac{\sigma_{X'}}{\sigma^2_{Y'}} \end{pmatrix}. \tag{3-11}$$

The estimated variances and the covariance of $(\hat{a}, \hat{b})$ are:

$$v(\hat{a}) = \frac{n^0(\hat{a}^2 + 2) + 2n^1\hat{b}^2}{2n^0n^1},$$

$$v(\hat{b}) = \frac{n^0 + n^1}{2n^0n^1}\hat{b}^2, \tag{3-12}$$

$$\text{cov}(\hat{a},\hat{b}) = \frac{\hat{a}\hat{b}}{2n^1}.$$

Example: ureteral stone image features — O'Malley et al. (2001) analyzed 100 unenhanced spiral computed tomographic (CT) scans to evaluate flank pain in patients with obstructing ureteral stones documented by means of chart review. The size of a ureteral stone may be treated as the outcome variable. The treatment option, here a binary gold standard, includes spontaneous passage ($n^0 = 71$) as sample H versus surgical intervention ($n^1 = 29$) as sample D (Table 3.2 and Table 3.3) respectively. Prior analyses suggested that in-plane stone size (in millimeters), followed by stone location (for simplicity, in or not in the UVJ), are the most predictive features for intervention.

TABLE 3.2

Healthy Sample with Stones via Spontaneous Passage ($n^0 = 71$)

Size (mm)	1	2	3	4	5	6	7	8	9	10
Count	2	13	17	14	11	5	1	3	4	1

TABLE 3.3

Diseased Sample with Stones Requiring Surgical Interventions ($n^1 = 29$)

Size (mm)	3	4	5	6	7	8	9	10	11	16
Count	2	3	4	6	2	4	2	3	2	1

TABLE 3.4

p-Values from Shapiro-Wilk Test in Ureteral Stone Example

	p-Value from Test of Normality		
Gold Standard	**No Transformation**	**Log**	**Box–Cox ($\hat{\lambda} = 0.110$)**
Healthy	1.886e-05	0.010	0.014
Diseased	0.045	0.677	0.700

The estimated power coefficient is $\hat{\lambda}= 0.110$, which is close to 0. Thus both the optimal Box–Cox and log (when $\hat{\lambda} = 0$) are considered. By applying the Shapiro–Wilk normality test, the resulting p-values are given in Table 3.4. Therefore, the parametric transformation makes the distribution of D closer to normal, but not for the distribution of H. The log and Box–Cox transformations yielded similar results (Figure 3.4). By applying a log transformation, the estimated ROC parameters are $(\hat{a}, \hat{b}) = (1.141, 0.800)$. The estimated standard error (SE) and correlation are $SE(\hat{a}) = 0.213$, $SE(\hat{b}) = 0.125$, and $corr(\hat{a}, \hat{b}) = 0.125$.

Example: prostate-specific antigen in staging local versus advanced prostate cancer — O'Malley and Zou (2006) illustrated multivariate regression methods on data from a multicenter collaborative Radiologic Diagnostic Oncology Group trial. Magnetic resonance imaging was performed in 213 men with prostate cancer, prior to which their prostate-specific antigen (PSA) levels and Gleason scores were obtained in 180 cases. Radical prostatectomy was performed in all cases to provide a binary gold standard, and all patients were classified into two groups. One group included 66 men who had local disease (Stage A or B); the other consisted of 114 men with advanced disease with periprostatic invasion of tumor and spread of disease to the seminal vesicles and lymph nodes (Stage C_1, C_2, or D).

The PSA level was treated as the outcome variable. By applying the Shapiro-Wilk normality test, the p-values are given in Table 3.5. The estimated power coefficient is $\hat{\lambda} = 0.335$. The Box–Cox transformation considerably improves

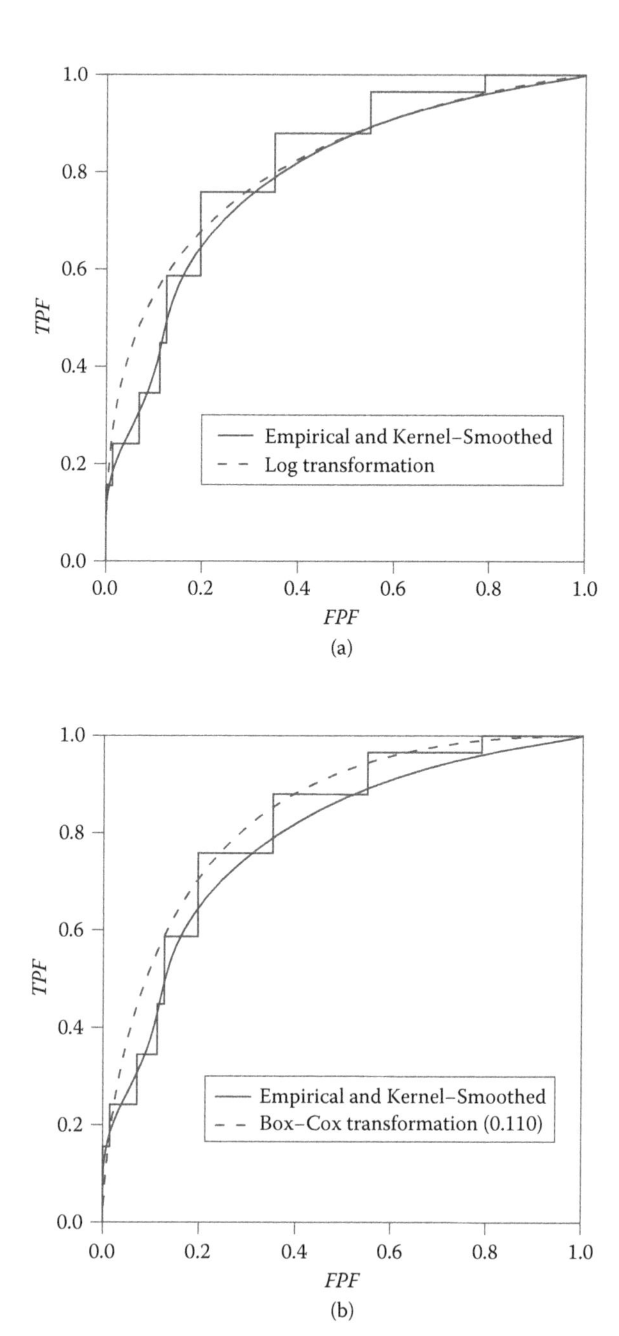

FIGURE 3.4
Empirical and kernel-smoothed with log binormal (a) and Box–Cox transformed (b) ROC curves for discriminating between ureteral stones of spontaneous passage and those requiring surgical intervention based on sizes of the stones.

TABLE 3.5
p-Values from Shapiro-Wilk Test in PSA Example

	p-Value from Test of Normality		
Gold Standard	**No Transformation**	**Log**	**Box–Cox ($\hat{\lambda}$ = 0.335)**
Healthy	0.002	3.469e-7	0.081
Diseased	1.382e-9	0.153	0.201

over the log transformation. Using the optimal Box–Cox transformation, the estimated ROC parameters are $(\hat{a}, \hat{b})$ = (1.203, 1.304). The estimated SE and correlation are $SE(\hat{a}) = 0.203$, $SE(\hat{b}) = 0.143$, and $corr(\hat{a}, \hat{b}) = 0.411$. However, local normality may not guarantee the global fit of the entire ROC curve. See Figure 3.5.

Back to the cancer antigen assay example in Chapter 1, two different marginal Box–Cox transformations are applied to CA 19-9 and CA 125. The estimated power coefficients are, respectively, $\widehat{\lambda_1} = -0.021$ for CA19-9 (suggesting a log transformation) and $\widehat{\lambda_2} = -0.429$ for CA125 (suggesting a departure from log transformation). The different transformations may also indicate that the two assays are different. Applying the Shapiro-Wilk test, the p-values are given in Table 3.6; see also Figure 3.6. However, the normality assumption is not satisfactory for the healthy samples of both assays. Therefore, a nonparametric method may be appropriate.

With regard to the transformation-to-normal models, Doksum (1987) provided an introduction and description in a general regression setting such as homoscedasticity. He used Höeffding's (1951) theorem to obtain the likelihood of the ranks and proposed a Monte Carlo calculation using the term likelihood sampler to evaluate and maximize this likelihood. Doksum's approach was a regression model with a broader array of applications beyond two-sample problems, but the model requires a common error variance. Hsieh and Turnbull (1996) proposed a minimum distance estimator for continuous measurements via the empirical process approach.

Alternative parametric models such as the bigamma were considered by Dorfman et al. (1997) and bi-beta by Zou et al. (2004). Hsieh (1995), Hsieh and Turnbull (1996), Cai and Pepe (2002), Cai (2004), Cai and Moskowitz (2004), and Li and Zhou (2009) developed semiparametric methods.

3.6 Confidence Intervals

3.6.1 Sensitivity or Specificity at Specific Threshold

A 100(1 – α)% confidence interval (CI) for $FPF(\xi)$ and $TPF(\xi)$ may be constructed using binomial proportions independently for healthy and

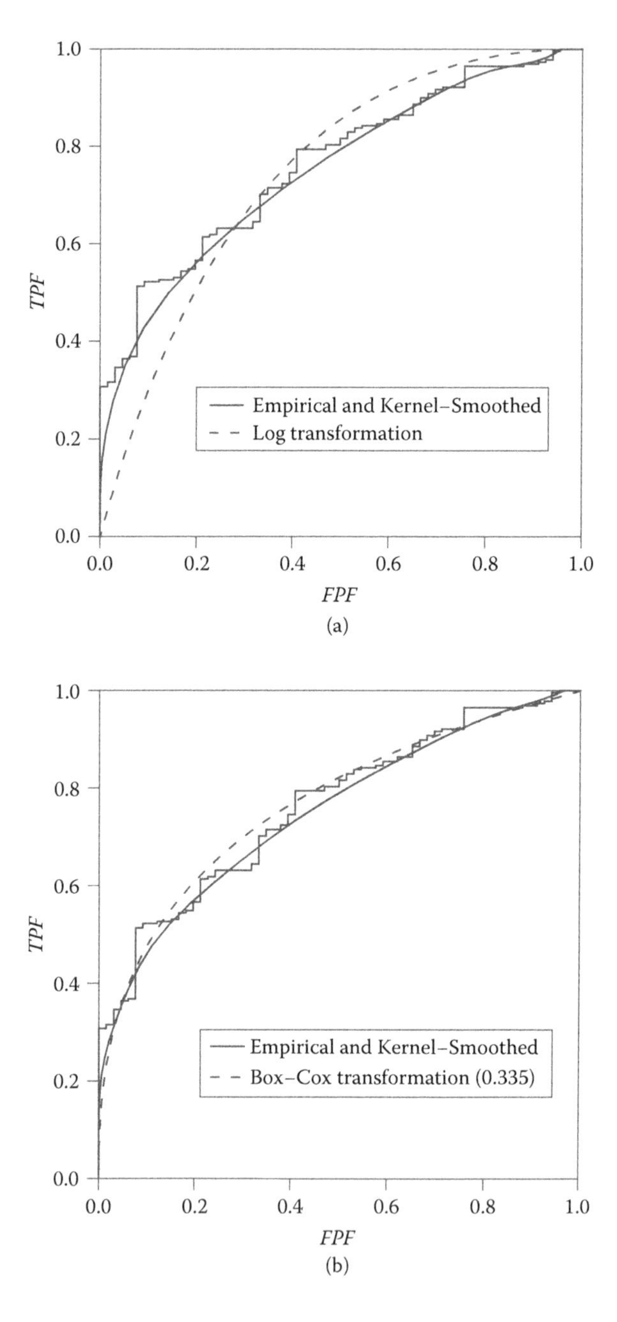

FIGURE 3.5
Empirical and kernel-smoothed with log binormal (a) and with Box–Cox transformed (b) ROC curves for staging local versus advanced prostate cancer.

TABLE 3.6

p-Values from Shapiro-Wilk Test in Pancreatic Cancer Example

Assay	Gold Standard	p-Value from Test of Normality		
		No Transformation	Log	Box–Cox[a]
CA 19-9	Healthy	1.602e-9	0.021	0.027
	Diseased	8.766e-16	0.066	0.054
CA 125	Healthy	9.577e-12	4.153e-5	0.044
	Diseased	2.200e-16	1.078e-4	0.794

[a] Box–Cox $\widehat{\lambda_1} = -0.021$ for CA19-9 and $\widehat{\lambda_2} = -0.429$ for CA125.

diseased samples at an *a priori* threshold ξ. Traditional CIs are simple to compute for the analysis of a proportion. To calculate a sample proportion or percentage, the count of success (number of *TP*s or number of *TN*s) and the corresponding sample size are recorded. There are two ways to assess proportion. One is a Wald (1943) CI. Essentially, the sample estimates are assumed to be consistent, asymptotically normal, and asymptotically independent. To construct a large-sample CI, the central limit theorem ensures that the sum of a sufficiently large number of i.i.d. random variables, each with finite mean and variance, is approximately normally distributed. The law of large numbers states that given a random variable with a finite expected value, if its values are repeatedly sampled as the number of these observations increases, their mean will tend to approach the expected value (Tijms, 2007).

Using the Wald method, *W*, the maximum likelihood estimate of a general proportion parameter π is compared with a prespecified value π_0. The assumption is that the difference between the two will be approximately normal. For a binomial proportion in a univariate case, *n* independent Bernoulli trials are observed with a constant success rate, say, the *TPF*. The Wald statistic is $\widehat{TPF} = TP/n^1$. Methods illustrated herein are applicable to interval estimation for the *FPF*. A Wald CI may be computed based on the asymptotic normality under the central limit theorem and the law of large numbers, such that $(\widehat{TPF} - TPF_0)/SE\ (\widehat{TPF}) \sim AN(0,1)$. The lower and upper bounds of a $(1 - \delta)\%$ CI are computed as follows:

$$\widehat{TPF} \pm \Phi^{-1}(1-\delta/2) \times \sqrt{\widehat{V}}, \tag{3-13}$$

where $\widehat{V} = \widehat{TPF}(1-\widehat{TPF})/n^1$.

However, in the case of rare events or a high number of successes (high sensitivity or specificity), the normal distribution may not be useful for approximating the distribution of the sample proportion. To correct for such bounds, a naïve method, here labeled as the corrected Wald (CW), may be employed to simply truncate the 95% CI at such a limit of either 0 for a rare

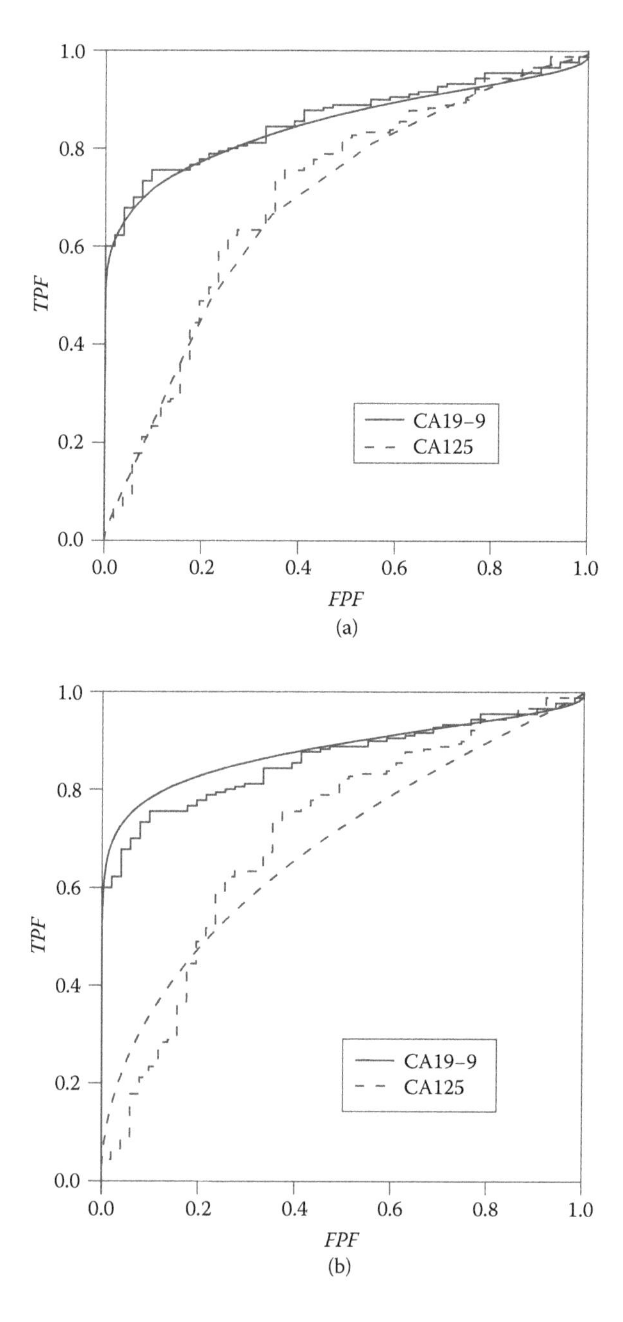

FIGURE 3.6
Empirical and kernel-smoothes ROC curves (a) and optimally transformed curves with log transformation for CA19-9 and Box–Cox transformation with a power coefficient −0.429 for CA125 (b) for detecting pancreatic cancer.

event rate or 1 for a high success rate. Nevertheless, this approach leads to a lower coverage than the nominal 95%, even when sampling is repeated a sufficiently large number of times. A plausible solution is to employ a monotone transformation (e.g., a logit or a probit) to map the sample proportion within [0,1] to an unrestricted domain between $(-\infty,\infty)$. After the CI is constructed on the latter scale to improve large-sample approximations, one may invert back to the original domain. Finally, the confidence bounds in the logit space are inversely transformed back to [0,1].

$$\begin{aligned}
\log it(\widehat{TPF}) &= \log\left[\widehat{TPF}/(1-\widehat{TPF})\right], \\
\widehat{V}(\hat{\pi}) &= \frac{1}{n\widehat{TPF}(1-\widehat{TPF})}, \\
l &= \log it(\widehat{TPF}) - \Phi^{-1}(1-\delta/2)\times\sqrt{\widehat{V}}, \\
u &= \log it(\widehat{TPF}) + \Phi^{-1}(1-\delta/2)\times\sqrt{\widehat{V}}, \\
\widehat{TPF}_l &= \log it^{-1}(l) = \frac{1}{1+\exp(-l)}, \\
\widehat{TPF}_u &= \log it^{-1}(u) = \frac{1}{1+\exp(-u)}.
\end{aligned} \tag{3-14}$$

Example: diseased sample including hypothetical true positives ($n^1 = 100$) — For simplicity, we assume 100 diseased subjects of whom 99 are true positives, yielding $\widehat{TPF} = 0.99$. By constructing a Wald CI, the lower bound is 0.97, while the upper bound is slightly over the domain of the proportion, now at 1.01. The upper bound of the Wald CI exceeds the domain of the proportion data. The modified CIs are computed by an ad hoc correction. A manually corrected Wald truncates this upper bound to 100%. More plausibly, the logit-transformed CI assumes an asymmetric CI, such that the upper bound is 99.9%. Additionally, the Wilson score CI (1927) is an alternative to the traditional large-sample CI for a sample size:

$$\left\{\widehat{TPF} + \frac{[\Phi^{-1}(1-\delta/2)]^2}{2n^1} \pm \Phi^{-1}(1-\delta/2) \times \sqrt{\frac{\widehat{TPF}(1-\widehat{TPF})}{n^1} + \frac{[\Phi^{-1}(1-\delta/2)]^2}{4(n^1)^2}}\right\} \Bigg/ \left(1 + \frac{[\Phi^{-1}(1-\delta/2)]^2}{(n^1)^2}\right). \tag{3-15}$$

The Wilson score CI yields an upper bound of 99.8%. See Table 3.7. The lower bounds of the 95% CIs using these methods show that the logit transform

TABLE 3.7

Hypothetical True Negatives with 95% Wald CI Exceeding Upper Domain of Proportion Data

Diseased Sample Size	True Negatives	Sensitivity	Method	95% CI
100	99	99%	Wald	(97.0%, 101.0%)
			Corrected Wald	(97.0%, 100%)
			Logit transform	(93.2%, 99.9%)
			Wilson score	(94.6%, 99.8%)

Note: CIs employ corrected Wald, logit transform, and Wilson score methods.

and Wilson score CIs exhibit lower bounds at 93.2 and 94.6%, respectively—below the lower bound value of the Wald CI at 97.0%.

Enduring problems in radiological diagnostic studies are the costs of imaging and the time-consuming tasks of reading and analysis. Consequently, small sample sizes are often used. The associated CIs are wide and the normal approximation does not perform well, partly due to the need for continuity correction. A hypothetical scenario involves three independent samples, each of size $n^1 = 5$ in the diseased sample; 3, 2, and 4 are diagnosed as diseased and the corresponding *TPFs* are 0.6, 0.4, and 0.8. The Wald CIs exceed the domain boundaries within [0,1] for two of the three samples. The upper bounds are 1.03, 0.83, and 1.15; the lower bounds are 0.17, −0.03, and 0.45, respectively.

The Wald CI may not be ideal for fewer than 30 samples. Thus, an adjustment to the traditional Wald CI may be applied. Agresti and Coull (1998) proposed using an ad hoc adjusted Wald CI by simply adding two counts to the successes, $TP' = TP + 2$, and similarly two counts to the failures, $FN' = FN + 2$. The adjusted Wald CI may be constructed using the correct counts.

$$\widehat{TPF} \pm \Phi^{-1}(1-\delta/2) \times \sqrt{\widehat{V}},$$
$$\widehat{TPF} = \frac{TP+2}{n^1+4}. \tag{3-16}$$

Example: diseased sample including hypothetical true positives ($n^1 = 10$) — Assume 10 diseased subjects of whom 7 are true positives, yielding a sample event rate at 0.30. The 95% Wald CI is [0.016, 0.584]. See Table 3.8.

3.6.2 Confidence Intervals for Sensitivity (Specificity) at Given Specificity (Sensitivity)

Zou et al. (1997) proposed a CI for *TPR* at an *a priori fpf* in the logit space for any *TPR* away from 0 or 1 before transforming the confidence bounds back to the ROC space. Normal approximations work better in an unrestricted space,

TABLE 3.8

Hypothetical True Positives for Finite Small Sample (10 Diseased Subjects)

Diseased Sample Size	True Positives	Sensitivity	Method	95% CI
10	7	30%	Wald	(42.6%, 98.4%)
10(+2)	7(+2)		Adjusted Wald	(50.5%, 99.5%)
10	7		Wilson score	(39.7%, 89.2%)

Note: 95% Wald, adjusted Wald, and Wilson score CIs.

in contrast to ROC space where the values are restricted in [0,1]. Similarly, the CI for *FPR* at an *a priori tpf* may be constructed. Assume that for any specified *FPF*, there is a corresponding transformed value *TPF′* in the logit space. Let:

$$FPF' = \text{logit}(FPF) = \log\left(\frac{FPF}{1-FPF}\right) \text{ and } TPF' = \text{logit}(TPF) = \log\left(\frac{TPF}{1-TPF}\right). \tag{3-17}$$

Assume that *TPF* is a function of a given value of *fpf* in the logit space and the estimated $\widehat{TPF}'$ at any given $fpf \in (0,1)$ has the following estimated variance:

$$\hat{V}(\widehat{TPF}'(fpf)) = \frac{\frac{1}{n^0} fpf(1-fpf)\left\{\frac{\hat{f}_Y[F_X^{-1}(fpf)]}{\hat{f}_X[F_X^{-1}(fpf)]}\right\}^2 + \frac{1}{n^1}\widehat{tpf}(1-\widehat{tpf})}{\left[\widehat{tpf}(1-\widehat{tpf})\right]^2}, \tag{3-18}$$

where $\hat{l} = \widehat{fpf}' - \Phi^{-1}(1-\delta/2)\sqrt{\hat{V}}$, $\hat{u} = \widehat{tpf}' + \Phi^{-1}(1-\delta/2)\sqrt{\hat{V}}$, $\widehat{tpf_l} = \text{logit}^{-1}(l)$, and $tpf_u = \text{logit}^{-1}(u)$. The lower and upper bounds of *TPF* in the ROC space are illustrated by the cancer antigen assays CA19-9 and CA125 cited in Chapter 1 and earlier in Wieand et al. (1988). At the arbitrary given *fpf* ranging from 0.05 to 0.80, the resulting estimated *TPF(fpf)* and associated 95% CIs are reported in Table 3.9 and Figure 3.7.

3.6.3 Confidence Intervals for Area under Curve (AUC)

If the discrete test results are based on binning of a truly continuous but unobserved test result and the latent result is of interest, the AUC obtained by linear interpolation of the empirical points will underestimate that

TABLE 3.9

95% Vertical CIs for TPFs at given FPF values for log CA19-9 and Box–Cox Transformation with a Power Coefficient −0.429 for CA125 for Detecting Pancreatic Cancer.

	CA19-9			CA125		
Pre-Specified *FPF*	Estimated *TPF*	Lower Bound	Upper Bound	Estimated *TPF*	Lower Bound	Upper Bound
0.05	0.742	0.642	0.821	0.193	0.124	0.288
0.10	0.783	0.685	0.857	0.302	0.215	0.405
0.20	0.828	0.728	0.897	0.460	0.356	0.568
0.40	0.878	0.764	0.941	0.678	0.560	0.777
0.60	0.912	0.796	0.965	0.828	0.714	0.903
0.80	0.942	0.850	0.979	0.934	0.843	0.974

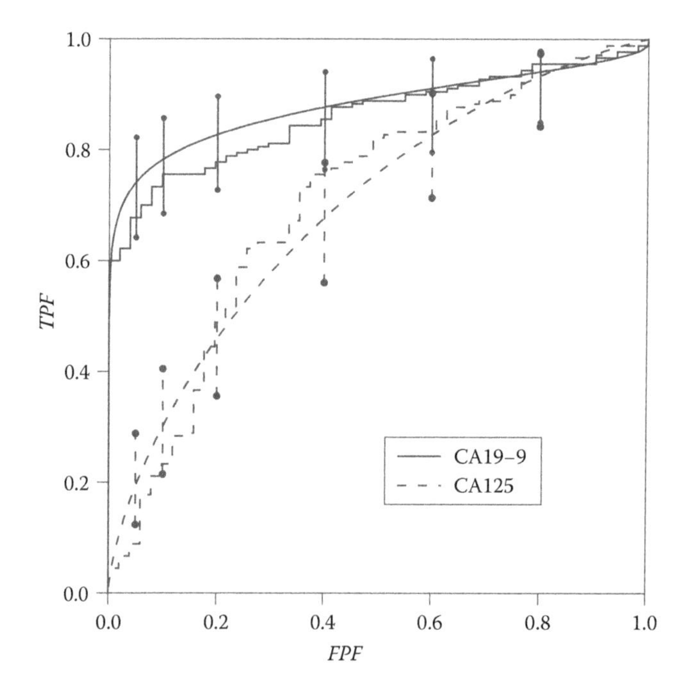

FIGURE 3.7
Empirical and binormal ROC curves along with vertical 95% confidence intervals of *TPFs* at given *FPFs* for log CA19-9 and Box–Cox transformation with power coefficient −0.429 for CA125 for detecting pancreatic cancer.

corresponding to the latent continuous test results. Researchers often presume that an underlying ROC curve is a function of a continuous latent decision variable. Underestimation of the true AUC may result from the trapezoidal rule as an approximation. However, fitting discrete data to a concave curve may result in an overestimation of the true AUC. An alternative to direct integration is to use values of the curve at midpoints of intervals multiplied by interval widths; this will slightly overestimate the true AUC for largely concave curves.

When estimated nonparametrically, the AUC is proportional to the Mann–Whitney U statistic (Mann and Whitney, 1947; Bamber, 1975). Without any ties, Bamber showed that $AUC = P(X < Y)$, which may be calculated using SAS Software's PROC NPAR1WAY (Gönen, 2007). More generally:

$$AUC = P(X < Y) + \frac{1}{2}P(X = Y) = E[I(X,Y)],$$
$$\text{where } I(X,Y) = \begin{cases} 1, & \text{if } X < Y \\ \frac{1}{2}, & \text{if } X = Y \\ 0, & \text{if } X > Y \end{cases} . \tag{3-19}$$

Assume that $X_1, \ldots, X_{n0}$ and $Y_1, \ldots, Y_{n1}$ are samples from a common distribution function $F_X(x)$ and $F_Y(y\text{-}\Delta)$, respectively. To test the hypotheses H_0: $\Delta = 0$ versus H_1: $\Delta > 0$, Wilcoxon (1945) developed the following two-sample Wilcoxon rank-sum test that ranks the combined x and y sample data and computes the sum of the ranks for the y-sample. Let $R_1,\ldots,R_{n^1}$ be the ranks of $Y_1,\ldots,Y_{n^1}$, using the combined $[X,Y]$ data. Since these are the counts of members in the combined two-sample data less than or equal to Y_j, then R_j may be expressed as $R_j = \#(X_i < Y_j) + \#(Y_k < Y_j)$, $\forall i = 1,\ldots n^0$; $\forall (k,j) = 1,\ldots n^1$, yielding the sum of these ranks as the Wilcoxon rank-sum test statistic W:

$$W = \sum_{1}^{n^1} R_j = U + \frac{n^1(n^1+1)}{2}, \tag{3-20}$$

where $U = \#(X_i < Y_j)$, $\forall\, i = 1,\ldots n^1$ *and* $\forall (k,j) = 1,\ldots n^1$.

The U is the U-test statistic of Mann and Whitney (1945). The corresponding two-sample test for the location-shift model is generally called the Mann–Whitney Wilcoxon test. Bamber (1975) showed the relationship between the empirical AUC and W, where:

$$\widehat{AUC} = \frac{W}{n^0 n^1}. \tag{3-21}$$

Nonparametrically, the AUC may be directly approximated via numerical integration, e.g., using the trapezoidal rule. For example, the *integrate* function in R may be used for such a purpose. When dealing with continuous data where both sample sizes are large, such estimates should have little bias but are inefficient. To compute the AUC variance, Hanley and McNeil (1982) showed that

$$V(\widehat{\mathrm{AUC}}) = \frac{\mathrm{AUC}(1-\mathrm{AUC})+(n^0-1)(Q_1-AUC^2)+(n^1-1)(Q_2-AUC^2)}{n^0 n^1}, \quad (3\text{-}22)$$

where $Q_1 = (AUC/2 - AUC)$ and $Q_2 = (2AUC2/1 + AUC)$. Recall that without any ties, the area is an explicit function of ROC parameters under a binormal model, where:

$$AUC = p(X < Y) = \Phi\left(\frac{a}{\sqrt{1+b^2}}\right). \quad (3\text{-}23)$$

The delta method (Rao, 1979) may be used by computing the Jacobian, which is a row vector of length 2 with respect to the ROC parameters $[a,b]$:

$$\begin{aligned} J(a,b) &= \left(\frac{\partial(AUC)}{\partial a}, \frac{\partial(AUC)}{\partial b}\right), \\ \frac{\partial(AUC)}{\partial a} &= (1+b^2)^{-1/2}\phi\left(a/(1+b^2)^{-1/2}\right), \\ \frac{\partial(AUC)}{\partial b} &= -ab(1+b^2)^{-3/2}\phi\left(a/(1+b^2)^{-1/2}\right), \end{aligned} \quad (3\text{-}24)$$

where ϕ is the *PDF* of $N[0,1]$ distribution. The variance of the estimated binormal AUC becomes

$$\begin{aligned} &V(\widehat{\mathrm{AUC}}) \\ &= \mathrm{J(a,b)} \sum \mathrm{(a,b)}\ \mathrm{J(a,b)^T} \\ &= \phi\left(\frac{a}{\sqrt{1+b^2}}\right)^2 \left[\frac{v(a)}{1+b^2}V(a) - \frac{2ab}{(1+b^2)^2}Cov(a,b) + \frac{a^2b^2}{(1+b^2)^3}V(b)\right]. \end{aligned} \quad (3\text{-}25)$$

The variance of the nonparametric partial area was given in Zou and Hall (1997) and the binormal partial area in McClish (1989). The six real-data examples yielded the AUCs in Table 3.10.

TABLE 3.10

Estimated Nonparametric and Binormal AUCs after Optimal Box–Cox Transformation for Six Diagnostic Test Examples

	Nonparametric Estimated		Binormal Estimate with Box–Cox Transformation		
Diagnostic Test	$\widehat{AUC}$	$SE(\widehat{AUC})$	Box–Cox $\hat{\lambda}$	$\widehat{AUC}$	$SE(\widehat{AUC})$
Glucose for diabetes	0.935	0.245	−0.672	0.949	0.101
CA19-9 for pancreatic cancer	0.961	0.173	≈0	0.881	0.084
CA125 for pancreatic cancer	0.706	0.209	−0.429	0.695	0.058
Scoring for malignant melanoma (without dermoscope)	0.906	0.214	N/A	0.900	0.060
Scoring for malignant melanoma (with dermoscope)	0.900	0.218	N/A	0.907	0.048
Ureteral stone size for intervention	0.811	0.229	≈0	0.813	0.059
PSA for prostate cancer	0.763	0.187	0.335	0.768	0.058

3.7 Concordance Measures in Presence of Monotone Transformations

Transformation methods are useful when measuring an underlying correlation or agreement between a set of bivariate variables X_1 and X_2 among healthy controls, and similarly between Y_1 and Y_2 among diseased patients. Without loss of generality, the methods introduced below are for bivariate *X*s and may be extended to bivariate *Y*s. One may measure the linear or monotone relationships between two samples. The linear relationship is measured by the sample correlation coefficient, possibly after a parametric transformation of the data. The sample correlation coefficient is invariant to any linear transformations of the marginal data.

Three classical rank correlation coefficients are the difference sign (also known as Kendall's tau), rank (Spearman's rho), and normal scores (Fisher–Yates) correlations. Rank correlation coefficients are invariant to any monotone transformations of marginal data. A parametric structure such as a bivariate normal may be assumed, possibly after specified or unspecified transformations of the bivariate measurements. All correlation coefficients can be used to make inference on the population correlation coefficient parameter ρ_X in this bivariate structure.

Here we focus on rank-based correlation coefficients and leave the transformations unspecified. Extensive reviews of these methods may be found in Höeffding (1947), Kruskal (1958), and Kendall and Gibbons (1990). The sample correlation coefficient was introduced by Galton (1877 and 1888) and developed by Pearson (1896):

$$r_X = \sum_{i=1}^{n^0} [(x_{1i} - \overline{x_1})(x_{2i} - \overline{x_2})] \bigg/ \left[\sum_{i=1}^{n^0} (x_{1i} - \overline{x_1})^2 \sum_{i=1}^{n^0} (x_{2i} - \overline{x_2}) \right]^{1/2}, \quad (3\text{-}26)$$

where $\overline{x_1}$ and $\overline{x_2}$ are the sample means of x_{1i} and x_{2i}, $\forall I = 1, \ldots, n^0$. The sample correlation coefficient is an asymptotically unbiased and consistent estimate of the population correlation coefficient given by:

$$\rho_X = \frac{cov(X,Y)}{[V(X)V(Y)]^{1/2}}. \quad (3\text{-}27)$$

Under the assumption that X_1 and X_2 have a bivariate normal distribution with correlation coefficient ρ_X, the sample version r_X is the parametric MLE of ρ_X. Fisher (1915) derived the distribution of r_X, and asymptotically, r_X is normal and centered at ρ_X, with the following variance:

$$V(r_X) = (1 - \rho_X)^2 / n^0. \quad (3\text{-}28)$$

The difference sign correlation concept was introduced by Esscher (1924) and later by Kendall (1938), and is commonly known as Kendall's tau. Obuchowski (2005) demonstrated the relationship between generalized Kendall's tau and the AUC when the gold standard is a continuous, ordinal, and nominal scale. Definitions of the population version τ (see Kruskal, 1951) and the sample statistic t_X are as follows:

$$\tau_X = 2\varpi_{X,I} - 1,$$

$$t_X = \frac{1}{\binom{n^0}{2}} \sum\sum_{i<i'} \text{sgn}[(x_{1i'} - x_{1i})(x_{2i'} - x_{2i})]. \quad (3\text{-}29)$$

The sign function $(x_1) = 1$, 0, and –1 for $(x_1 > 0)$, $(x_1 = 0)$, and $(x_1 < 0)$, respectively, and $\varpi_{X,I}$ is the probability of concordance of Type I, i.e., the probability that two pairs of observations, say, (X_{11}, X_{21}) and (X_{12}, X_{22}) are concordant:

$$\varpi_{X,I} = P[(X_{11} - X_{21})(X_{21} - Y_{22}) > 0]. \quad (3\text{-}30)$$

Alternatively, t_X may be computed from the concomitant ranks (x_1) and (x_2) by:

$$1 - \frac{4}{n^0(n^0-1)} \sum\sum_{i<i'} I\left[rank_i(x_1) - rank_{i'}(x_2) > 0\right], \tag{3-31}$$

where $I(\times)$ is the indicator function. It can be shown (Kendall and Gibbons, 1990) that the relationship between τ_X and the transformation correlation coefficient ρ_X in the bivariate normal model, is:

$$\tau_X = \frac{2}{\pi}\sin^{-1}(\rho_X),$$
$$\rho_X = \sin\left(\frac{\pi}{2}\tau_X\right). \tag{3-32}$$

The estimate t_X is unbiased for τ_X with large-sample variance:

$$V(t_X) = \frac{1}{\binom{n^0}{2}}\left\{2(n^0-2)\left\{\frac{1}{9} - \left[\frac{2}{\pi}\sin^{-1}\left(\frac{\rho_X}{2}\right)\right]\right\} + (1-\tau_X^2)\right\},$$
$$= \frac{4}{n^0}\left\{\frac{1}{9} - \left[\frac{2}{\pi}\sin^{-1}\left(\frac{\rho_X}{2}\right)\right]\right\}, \tag{3-33}$$

and asymptotically normal (Höeffding, 1947). Esscher (1924) proposed estimating ρ_X by:

$$\widehat{\rho_{X,DS}} = \sin\left(\frac{\pi}{2}t\right), \tag{3-34}$$

and by assuming bivariate normality. Via the delta method (Rao, 1979), the variance of $\widehat{\rho_{X,DS}}$ is:

$$V(\hat{\rho}_{X,DS}) = \frac{\pi^2}{9n^0}(1-\rho^2)\left\{1 - \left[\frac{6}{\pi}\sin^{-1}\left(\frac{\rho_X}{2}\right)\right]^2\right\}. \tag{3-35}$$

The rank correlation concept was originally introduced by Spearman (1904) and the corresponding coefficient is often called Spearman's correlation coefficient. The population version (see Kruskal, 1951) is:

$$\rho_{X,S} = 6\varpi_{X,II} - 3, \tag{3-36}$$

where $\varpi_{X,II}$ is the probability of concordance of Type II, i.e., the probability that, among three pairs of observations, say, (X_{11},X_{21}), (X_{12},X_{22}), and (X_{13},X_{23}), at least one is concordant with the remaining two:

$$\varpi_{X,II} = P[(X_{11} - X_{12})(X_{21} - X_{23}) > 0]. \tag{3-37}$$

The sample version $r_{X,S}$ is computed using the product–moment correlation coefficient of the paired marginal rank data of the samples. Alternatively, $r_{X,S}$ may be expressed in terms of the concomitant ranks, (x_1) and (x_2), and is given by:

$$r_{X,S} = 1 - \frac{12}{n^0(n^{02} - 1)} \sum\sum_{i<i'} (i' - i) I[rank_i(x_1) - rank_{i'}(x_2) > 0]. \tag{3-38}$$

In the case of bivariate normal, the correlation coefficient is:

$$\rho_{X,S} = \frac{6}{\pi}\sin^{-1}\left(\frac{\rho_X}{2}\right) \quad with \ \rho_X = 2\sin\left(\frac{\pi}{6}\rho_{X,S}\right). \tag{3-39}$$

The estimate $r_{X,S}$ is biased, but is not asymptotic with the bias equal to $3(\tau_X - \rho_{X,S})/(n^0 + 1)$ where τ_X is Kendall's tau defined earlier. It is asymptotically normal, with a large-sample variance given by the Taylor series expansion (Kendall and Gibbons, 1990):

$$V(r_{X,S}) \approx \frac{1}{n^0}(1 - 1.5635\rho_X^2 + 0.3047\rho_X^4 + 0.1553\rho_X^6 + 0.0616\rho_X^8 + 0.0242\rho_X^{10} + \ldots). \tag{3-40}$$

Other expansions have been proposed in the literature (Fieller et al., 1957; Fieller and Pearson, 1961). Hence, an estimate for the bivariate normal transformation correlation coefficient based on the rank correlation coefficient is:

$$\widehat{\rho_{X,R}} = 2\sin\left(\frac{\pi}{6} r_{X,S}\right). \tag{3-41}$$

The delta method (Wald, 1979) leads to

$$V(\widehat{\rho_{X,R}}) \approx \frac{\pi^2}{9}\left(1 - \frac{\rho_X^2}{4}\right) V(r_{X,S}), \tag{3-42}$$

where the variance $v(r_{X,S})$ is approximated in Equation (3-40).

The normal scores correlation concept was developed by Fisher and Yates (1948)—known as the Fisher–Yates correlation. The normal score for the i-th observation for X_1 is defined as $NS_i = E[X_{1(i)}]$, where $X_{1(1)} < \ldots < X_{1(n^0)}$ are the order statistics generated from $N[0,1]$ (Hájek and Sĭdájk, 1967). The normal scores correlation coefficient $\widehat{\rho_{X,NS}}$ may be obtained by replacing the paired data, or equivalently the paired ranks, by scores defined marginally, then calculating the product–moment correlation coefficient. One needs not subtract the means since they are automatically zero, but the covariance must be rescaled by an appropriate variance since the variance of the normal scores is not exactly unity. In practice, however, it is easier to use van der Waerden's (1952) definition, that is, the score for the observation with rank i is:

$$NS_{X_1,i} = \Phi^{-1}\left[\frac{rank_i(X_1)}{n^0+1}\right]; NS_{X_2,i} = \Phi^{-1}\left[\frac{rank_i(X_2)}{n^0+1}\right]. \tag{3-43}$$

Under bivariate normality, pairs of normal scores in samples of size n^0 are asymptotically equivalent to standard bivariate normal samples (Madansky, 1988). Hence, the normal scores correlation coefficient is a consistent estimate of ρ_X:

$$\widehat{\rho_{X,NS}} = \sum_{i=1}^{n^0}\left(NS_{X_1,i} - \overline{NS_{X_1}}\right)\left(NS_{X_2,i} - \overline{NS_{X_2}}\right) \Bigg/ \left\{\sum_{i=1}^{n^0}\left(NS_{X_1,i} - \overline{NS_{X_1}}\right)^2 \sum_{i=1}^{n^0}\left(NS_{X_1,i} - \overline{NS_{X_2}}\right)\right\}^{1/2}, \tag{3-44}$$

by assuming bivariate normality. It is asymptotically normally distributed around ρ_X with the same asymptotic variance as the sample product–moment correlation coefficient r_X, i.e.,

$$v(\widehat{\rho_{X,NS}}) = \frac{\left(1-\rho_X^2\right)^2}{n^0}. \tag{3-45}$$

The above correlation methods for the x samples from healthy controls may be readily applicable to the bivariate y samples from diseased patients. The four correlation coefficients as estimates of ρ_X and ρ_y, are illustrated on

CA19-9 versus CA125 data for pancreatic cancer and scoring for malignant melanoma without and with a dermoscope (Table 3.11 and Table 3.12, respectively).

Fisher (1915) developed Fisher's z transformation as follows:

$$z(r_X) = \frac{1}{2}\log\left[\frac{1+r_X}{1-r_X}\right] = \tanh^{-1}(r_X). \quad (3\text{-}46)$$

TABLE 3.11

Difference Sign, Rank, Transformation, and Normal Scores Correlation Coefficient Methods for Estimating Correlation Coefficients between Log CA19-9 and Box–Cox Transformation with Power Coefficient –0.429 for CA125 in Detecting Pancreatic Cancer

Samples	Method	$\hat{\rho}$	$SE(\hat{\rho})$
Healthy (n^0= 51)	Difference sign	–0.151	0.143
	Rank	–0.159	0.155
	Transformation	–0.133	0.137
	Normal scores	–0.128	0.138
Diseased (n^1= 90)	Difference sign	0.110	0.109
	Rank	0.107	0.104
	Transformation	0.116	0.104
	Normal scores	0.132	0.104

TABLE 3.12

Difference Sign, Rank, Transformation, and Normal Scores Correlation Coefficient Methods for Estimating Correlation Coefficients among Scores without Dermoscope versus with Dermoscope in Detecting Malignant Melanoma

Samples	Method	$\hat{\rho}$	$SE(\hat{\rho})$
Healthy (n^0 = 51)	Difference sign	0.817	0.050
	Rank	0.748	0.041
	Transformation	0.794	0.052
	Normal scores	0.792	0.052
Diseased (n^0 = 21)	Difference sign	0.571	0.156
	Rank	0.528	0.121
	Transformation	0.547	0.153
	Normal scores	0.572	0.147

Note: No transformation applied to data when bivariate normality assumption was satisfactory.

Its asymptotic distribution was derived by Hawkins (1989). The z transformation provides an efficient basis for inference about ρ_X after the transformation to construct a 95% CI since:

$$V\left(z(\widehat{\rho_X})\right) = \frac{1}{\left(1-\rho_X^2\right)^2} V(\rho_X). \tag{3-47}$$

3.8 Intraclass Correlation Coefficient

After the data undergo an optimal monotone normality transformation, various multifactor designs may be assumed in reliability studies. For example, in intrarater or interrater reliability studies, a single rater or diagnostic modality may generate repeated assessments on the same group of subjects. Alternatively, in interrater reliability studies, many raters or different modalities (CT, MRI, or ultrasound) may yield a single assessment on such subjects.

Suppose that each of a random sample of n^r raters independently rates a random sample of n^0 subjects, and that X_{ik} is the rating by the k-th rater on the i-th subject in a two-way random-effects model via ANOVA:

$$X_{ik} = \mu_X + s_{Xi} + r_k + e_{Xik}(i = 1,\ldots,n^0; k = 1,\ldots,n^r), \tag{3-48}$$

where μ_X is the grand mean of the error-free measurements X_{ik} in the healthy population. Here, s_{Xi} represents the i-th subject, assumed to be normally distributed with mean 0 and variance $\sigma_{X,S}^2$; r_k represents the i-th rater, assumed to be normally distributed with mean 0 and variance σ_r^2; e_{Xik} represents the random error, assumed to be normally distributed with mean 0 and variance $\sigma_{X,e}^2$. All the random variables $\{s_{Xi}, r_k, e_{Xik}\}$ are assumed to be mutually independent.

The intraclass correlation coefficient (ICC) is a measure of interrater reliability by the proportion of the variability in the observed scores that can be accounted for by the subject-to-subject variability in the true (unobserved) scores. The ANOVA corresponding to the two-way random effects model is summarized in Table 3.13.

$$ICC = \frac{\sigma_{X,S}^2}{\sigma_{X,S}^2 + \sigma_r^2 + \sigma_{X,e}^2}. \tag{3-49}$$

Rajaratnam (1960) and Bartko (1966) proposed the following estimate of the ICC:

$$\widehat{ICC} = \frac{s_{X,S}^2}{s_{X,S}^2 + s_r^2 + s_{X,e}^2},$$
$$= \frac{n^0(SMS - EMS)}{n^0 SMS + n^r RMS + (n^0 n^r - n^0 - n^r)EMS}. \quad (3\text{-}50)$$

The ICCs based on the pancreatic cancer and dermoscope examples are reported in Table 3.14 and Table 3.15.

TABLE 3.13

Two-Way ANOVA Table for Random Effects Model

Source of Variation	Degrees of Freedom	Mean Squares (MS)	E(MS)
Between subjects	$n^0 - 1$	$SMS = \frac{n^r \sum_{i=1}^{n^0} (X_{i.} - \overline{Y}_{..})^2}{n^0 - 1}$	$\sigma_{X,e}^2 + n^r \sigma_{X,S}^2$
Between raters	$n^r - 1$	$RMS = \frac{n^0 \sum_{k=1}^{n^r} (X_{.k} - \overline{Y}_{..})^2}{n^r - 1}$	$\sigma_{X,e}^2 + n^0 \sigma_r^2$
Errors	$(n^0 - 1)(n - 1)$	$EMS = \frac{\sum_{i=1}^{n^0} \sum_{k=1}^{n^r} (X_{ik} - X_{k.} - X_{.k} + X_{..})^2}{(n^0 - 1)(n^r - 1)}$	$\sigma_{X,e}^2$

TABLE 3.14

Two-Way ANOVA Table for CA19-9 and CA125 Testing for Pancreatic Cancer with Resulting Intraclass Correlation Coefficients (ICCs)

Sample	Source of Variation	df	MS	*F* Statistic	*P* Value	ICC
Healthy	Between subjects	50	2.965	0.833	0.740	–0.055
	Between tests	1	114.110	32.043	7.335e-7	
	Error	50	3.561			
Diseased	Between subjects	89	12.494	1.328	0.0912	0.135
	Between tests	1	51.614	5.488	0.0214	
	Error	89	9.405			

TABLE 3.15

Two-Way ANOVA Table for Scoring without and with Dermoscope for Malignant Melanoma with Resulting Intraclass Correlation Coefficients

Sample	Source of Variation	df	MS	F Statistic	P Value	ICC
Healthy	Between subjects	50	6.973	7.937	6.87e-12	0.765
	Between tests	1	3.834	4.364	0.0418	
	Error	50	0.878			
Diseased	Between subjects	20	2.142	2.119	0.0214	0.355
	Between tests	2	1.321	1.308	0.2818	
	Error	40	1.011			

3.9 Remarks and Further Reading

In summary, this chapter has demonstrated the useful features of monotone transformations in analyzing continuous diagnostic data. Rank-based and parametric transformation methods have been studied and illustrated. Optimal threshold estimation using the Youden index by considering normality transformations may be found in Fluss (2005). For estimation methods based on continuous data, see Krzanowski and Hand (2009). Multivariate regression and semiparametric analysis may be found in Alonzo et al. (2002), Pepe (2003), Cai (2004), and Janes et al. (2009).

For reliability analysis, Fleiss and Shrout (1978) proposed a method for approximating the confidence intervals for ICC based on Satterthwaite's (1946) two-moment approximation. Several authors used decomposition of the variance components and derived confidence intervals based on approximating the sum of squares using chi-square distributions (Zou and McDermott, 1999; Cappelleri and Ting, 2003). Ramasundarahettige et al. (2008) constructed a CI for the difference between correlated ICCs.

References

Agresti, A. and Coull, B.A. 1998. Approximate is better than "exact" for interval estimation of binomial proportions. *American Statistician* 52: 119–126.

Alonzo, T.A. and Pepe, M.S. 2002. Distribution-free ROC analysis using binary regression techniques. *Biostatistics* 3: 421–432.

Bamber, D. 1975. The area above the ordinal dominance graph and the area below the receiver operating graph. *Journal of Mathematical Psychology* 12: 387–415.

Barndorff-Nielsen, O.E., Blæsild, P., and Eriksen, P.S. 1989. *Decomposition and Invariance of Measures, and Statistical Transformation Models.*, New York: Springer.

Bartko, J.J. 1966. The intraclass correlation coefficient as a measure of reliability. *Psychological Reports* 19: 3–11.

Bickel, P.J. and Doksum, K.A. 1981. An analysis of transformations revisited. *Journal of the American Statistical Association* 76: 296–311.

Bickel, P.J., Klaassen, C.A.J., Ritov, Y. et al. 1998. *Efficient and Adaptive Estimation for Semiparametric Models*. New York: Springer.

Bickel, P.J. 1986. Efficient testing in a class of transformation models. In *Papers on Semiparametric Models at the ISI Centenary Session*. Amsterdam, Report MS-R8614. Amsterdam: Centrum voor Wiskunde en Informatica, pp. 63–81.

Box, G.E.P. and Cox, D.R. 1964. An analysis of transformations. *Journal of the Royal Statistical Society Series B* 42: 71–78.

Cai, T and Moskowitz, C. 2004. Semiparametric estimation of the binormal ROC curve. *Biostatistics* 5: 573–586.

Cai, T. and Pepe, M.S. 2002. Semi-parametric ROC analysis to evaluate biomarkers for disease. *Journal of the American Statistical Association* 97: 1099–1107.

Cai, T. 2004. Semi-parametric ROC regression analysis with placement values. *Biostatistics* 5: 45–60.

Cappelleri, J.C. and Ting, N. 2003. A modified large-sample approach to approximate interval estimation for a particular intraclass correlation coefficient. *Statistics in Medicine* 22: 1861–1877.

Carroll, B.J. and Ruppert D. 1988. *Transformation and Weighting in Regression*. New York: Chapman & Hall.

D'Agostino, R.B. and Stephens, M.A. 1986. *Goodness-of-Fit Techniques*. New York: Marcel Dekker.

D'Agostino, R.B. 1971. An omnibus test of normality for moderate and large size samples. *Biometrika* 58: 341–348.

D'Agostino, R.B. 1972. Small sample probability points for the D test of normality. *Biometrika* 59: 319–321.

Doksum, K.A. 1987. An extension of partial likelihood methods for proportional hazard models to general transformation models. *The Annals of Statistics* 15: 325–345.

Dorfman, D.D., Berbaum, K.S., Metz, C,E. et al. 1997. Proper receiver operating characteristic analysis: the bigamma model. *Academic Radiology* 4: 138–149.

Du, P. and Tang, L. 2009. Transformation-invariant and nonparametric monotone smooth estimation of ROC curves. *Statistics in Medicine* 28: 349–359.

Esscher, F. 1924. On a method of determining correlation from the ranks of variates. *Skandinavisk Aktuarietidskirift* 7: 201–219.

Fieller, E.C., Hartley, H.O., and Pearson, E.S. 1957. Tests for rank correlation coefficients I. *Biometrika* 44: 470–481.

Fieller, E.C. and Pearson, E.S. 1961. Tests for rank correlation coefficients II. *Biometrika* 48: 29–40.

Filliben, J.J. 1975. The probability plot correlation coefficient test for normality. *Technometrics* 17: 111–118.

Fisher, R.A. and Yates, F. 1948. *Statistical Tables for Biological, Agricultural, and Medical Research*. New York: Hafner.

Fisher, R.A. 1915. Frequency distributions of the values of the correlation coefficient in samples from an indefinitely large population. *Biometrika* 10: 507–521.

Fleiss, J.L. and Shrout, P.E. 1978. Approximate interval estimation for a certain intraclass correlation coefficient. *Psychometrika* 43: 259–262.

Galton, F. 1988. Correlations and their measurement, chiefly from anthropometric data. *Proceedings of the Royal Society of London* 45: 219–247.

Galton, F. 1877. Typical laws of heredity. *Proceedings of the Royal Institution of Great Britain* 8: 282–301.

Gönen, M. 2007. *Analyzing Receiver Operating Characteristic Curves with SAS®*. Cary, NC: SAS Institute.

Goria, M.N. 1982. A survey of two-sample location-scale problem, asymptotic relative efficiencies of some rank tests. *Statistica Neerlandica* 36: 3–13.

Hájek, J. and Sĭdájk, Z. 1967. *Theory of Rank Tests*. New York: Academic Press.

Hanley, J.A. and McNeil, B.J. 1983. A method of comparing the areas under receiver operating characteristic curves derived from the same cases. *Radiology* 148: 839–843.

Hawkins, D.L. 1989. Using U statistics to derive the asymptotic distribution of Fisher's Z statistic. *The American Statistician* 43: 235–237.

Hernandez, F. and Johnson, R.A. 1980. The large-sample behavior of transformations to normality. *Journal of the American Statistical Association* 75: 855–861.

Hettmansperger, T.P. 1991. *Statistical Inference Based on Ranks*. Malabar: Krieger Publishing.

Hinkley, D.V. and Runger, G. 1984. The analysis of transformed data. *Journal of the American Statistical Association* 79: 302–309.

Hinkley, D.V. 1975. On power transformations to symmetry. *Biometrika* 62: 101–111.

Höeffding, W. 1947. On the distribution of the rank correlation coefficient τ when the variates are not independent. *Biometrika* 34: 183–196.

Hsieh, F. and Turnbull, B.W. 1996. Nonparametric and semiparametric estimation of the receiver operating characteristic curve. *The Annals of Statistics* 24: 25–40.

Hsieh, F. 1995. The empirical process approach for semiparametric two-sample models with heterogeneous treatment effect. *Journal of the Royal Statistical Society Series B* 57: 735–748.

Janes, H., Longton, G. and Pepe, M. 2009. Accommodating covariates in ROC analysis. *The Strata Journal* 9: 17–39.

Kendall, M. and Gibbons, J.D. 1990. *Rank Correlation Methods*. New York: Oxford University Press.

Kendall, M.G. 1938. A new measure of rank correlation. *Biometrika* 30: 81–93.

Kochar, S.C. 1979. A class of distribution-free tests for the two sample location-scale problem. *Bulletin of International Statistical Institute* 47: 288–291.

Kruskal, W.H. 1958. Ordinal measures of association. *Journal of the American Statistical Association* 53: 814–861.

Krzanowski, W.J and Hand, D.J. 2009. *ROC Curves for Continuous Data*. Boca Raton: Taylor & Francis.

Krzanowski, W.J. 2000. *Principles of Multivariate Analysis: A Users Perspective*. Oxford: Oxford University Press.

Lambert, D. 1982. Qualitative robustness of tests. *Journal of the American Statistical Association* 77: 352–357.

Lasko, T.A., Bhagwat, J.G., Zou, K.H. et al. 2005. The use of receiver operating characteristic curves in biomedical informatics. *Journal of Biomedical Informatics* 38: 404–415.

Lehmann, E.L. 2006. *Nonparametrics: Statistical Methods Based on Ranks*. New York: Springer.

Lehmann, E.L. 1986. *Testing Statistical Hypotheses*. New York: Wiley.

Li, J. and Zhou, X.H. 2009. Nonparametric and semiparametric estimation of the three way receiver operating characteristic surface. *Journal of Statistical Planning and Inference* 139: 4133–4142.

Lin, C.C. and Mudholkar, G.S. 1980. A simple test for normality against asymmetric alternatives. *Biometrika* 67: 455–461.

Lloyd, C.J. 1988. Using smoothed ROC curves to summarize and compare diagnostic systems. *Journal of the American Statistical Association* 93: 1356–1364.

Madansky, A. 1988. *Prescriptions for Working Statisticians*. New York: Springer.

Mann, H.B. and Whitney, D.R. 1947. On a test of whether one of two random variables is stochastically larger than the other. *Annals of Mathematical Statistics* 18: 50–60.

Maritz, J.S. 1981. *Distribution-Free Statistical Methods*. London: Chapman & Hall.

McClish, D.K. 1989. Analyzing a portion of the ROC curve. *Medical Decision Making* 9: 190–195.

Metz, C.E., Herman, B.A., and Shen, J.H. 1998. Maximum likelihood estimation of receiver operating characteristic (ROC) curves from continuously distributed data. *Statistics in Medicine* 17: 1033–1053.

Nair, V.N. 1982. Some extensions of ANOVA techniques to location-scale models. *Communications in Statistics A* 11: 1551–1570.

O'Malley, A.J., Zou, K.H., Fielding, J.R. et al. 2001. Bayesian regression methodology for estimating a receiver operating characteristic curve with two radiologic applications: prostate biopsy and spiral CT of ureteral stones. *Academic Radiology* 8: 713–725.

Obuchowski, N.A. 2005. Estimating and comparing diagnostic test accuracy when the gold standard is not binary. *Academic Radiology* 12: 1198–1204.

O'Malley, A.J. and Zou, K.H. 2006. Bayesian multivariate hierarchical transformation models for ROC analysis. *Statistics in Medicine* 25: 459–479.

Pearson, K. 1896. Mathematical contributions to the theory of evolution III. Regression, heredity and panmixia. *Philosophical Transactions of the Royal Society of London Series A* 187: 253–318.

Pearson, K. 1900. On the criterion that a given system of deviations from the probable in the case of correlated system of variables is such that it can be reasonably supposed to have arisen from random sampling. *Philosophical Magazine* 50: 157–175.

Pepe, M.S. 1998. Three approaches to regression analysis of receiver operating characteristic curves for continuous test results. *Biometrics* 54: 124–135.

Pepe, M.S. 2000. An interpretation for the ROC curve and inference using GLM procedures. *Biometrics* 56:352–359.

Pepe, M.S. 2003. *The Statistical Evaluation of Medical Tests for Classification and Prediction*. Oxford: Oxford University Press.

Pesarin, F. 2001. *Multivariate Permutation Tests: Applications in Biostatistics*. Chichester: Wiley.

Rajaratnam, N. 1960. Reliability formulas for independent decision data when reliability data are matched. *Psychometrika* 25: 261–271.

Ramasundarahettige, C.F., Donner, A., and Zou, G.Y. 2009. Confidence interval construction for a difference between two dependent intraclass correlation coefficients. *Statistics in Medicine* 28: 1041–1053.

Rao, C.R. 1973. *Linear Statistical Inference and Its Applications*, 2nd ed. New York: Wiley.

Rieder, H. 1982. Qualitative robustness of rank tests. *Annals of Statistics* 10: 205–211.

Satterthwaite, F.E. 1946. An approximate distribution of estimates of variance components. *Biometrics* 2: 110–114.
Shapiro, S.S. and Wilk, M.B. 1968. Approximations for the null distribution of the W statistic. *Technometrics* 10: 861–866.
Spearman, C. 1904. The proof and measurement of association between two things. *American Journal of Psychology* 15: 72–101.
Tijms, H. 2007. *Understanding Probability: Chance Rules in Everyday Life*. Cambridge: Cambridge University Press.
van der Waerden, B.L. 1952. Order tests for the two-sample problem and their power. *Proceedings Koninklijke Nederlandse Akademie van Wetenschappen Series A* 55: 453–458.
Corrigenda, J. 1953. *Proceedings Koninklijke Nederlandse Akademie van Wetenschappen Series A* 56: 80.
Venkatraman, E.S. 2000. A permutation test to compare receiver operating characteristic curves. *Biometrics* 56: 1134–1138.
Wald, A. 1943. Tests of statistical hypotheses concerning several parameters when the number of observations is large. *Transactions of the American Mathematical Society* 54: 426–482.
Wieand, S., Gail, M,H., James, B,R. et al. 1989. A family of nonparametric statistics for comparing diagnostic markers with paired or unpaired data. *Biometrika* 76: 585.
Wilcoxon, F. 1945. Individual comparisons by ranking methods. *Biometrics Bulletin* 1: 80–83.
Wilk, M.B. and Gnanadesikan, R. 1968. Probability plotting methods for the analysis of data. *Biometrika* 55: 1–17.
Wilson, E.B. 1927. Probable inference, the law of succession, and statistical inference. *Journal of the American Statistical Association* 22: 209–212.
Zhou, X.H. and Harezlak, J. 2002. Comparison of bandwidth selection methods for kernel smoothing of ROC curves. *Statistics in Medicine* 21: 2045–2055.
Zou, K.H, Hall, W.J., and Shapiro, D.E. 1997. Smooth nonparametric receiver operating characteristic (ROC) curves for continuous diagnostic tests. *Statistics in Medicine* 16: 2143–2156.
Zou, K.H. and McDermott, M.P. 1999. Higher-moment approaches to approximate interval estimation for a certain intraclass correlation coefficient. *Statistics in Medicine* 18: 2051–2061.
Zou, K.H., Wells, W.M., III, Kikinis, R. et al. 2004. Three validation metrics for automated probabilistic image segmentation of brain tumours. *Statistics in Medicine* 23: 1259–1282.
Zou, K.H., Carlsson, M.O., and Quinn, S.A. 2010. Beta-mapping and beta-regression for changes of ordinal-rating measurements on Likert scales: comparison of the change scores among multiple treatment groups. *Statistics in Medicine.*

4

Combination and Pooling of Biomarkers

4.1 Introduction

In the area of biomedical research, a biomarker is generally defined as a distinctive biological or biologically derived indicator of a health condition. Hence, a biomarker can be a substance found in the blood, urine, or other body fluid, an imaging technique, a hormone, or a gene or protein whose change in expression levels indicates the development or presence of a disease. For many diseases, predictive biomarkers are well known. For example, prostate-specific antigen (PSA) is used to diagnose prostate cancer, hemoglobin A1c (HbA1c) for diabetes, cholesterol for coronary and vascular disease, C-reactive protein (CRP) for inflammation, and estrogen receptors for breast cancer, to name a few.

In diagnostic medicine, the effectiveness of even the best known and commonly used biomarkers in diagnosis of a disease is not perfect. New biomarkers are constantly developed in laboratories in efforts to improve diagnostic accuracy. Sensitivity, specificity, and receiver operating characteristic (ROC) curves play an important role in the evaluation of biomarkers. Unlike diagnostic medical devices, biomarkers that have potential diagnostic value for a disease may be abundant, ranging from a few (e.g., growth hormones) to hundreds of thousands (e.g., genes from a DNA microarray experiment). While a single biomarker rarely provides satisfactory diagnostic accuracy, a proper combination of some or all of them may well do so.

Measuring the level of a biomarker may be very costly and developing methodologies that reduce study costs while maintaining the integrity and validity of the study findings thus becomes a major concern in biomedical research. One way to address this concern is to pool individual biosamples and then measure the levels of the biomarker from the pooled samples. While attractive in saving study cost, pooling biospecimens poses many statistical challenges, mainly because pooling blinds individual information. Developing feasible and effective methods for analysis of pooled data has thus become an important research area, particularly in diagnostic medicine.

This chapter intends to address these issues in the context of evaluating the diagnostic accuracy of biomarkers when used as diagnostic tools for diseases. We will first discuss several ways of combining multiple biomarkers, focusing on linear combinations, to achieve larger area under the curve (AUC). We will then present methods to estimate ROC curves when biomarker values are measured from pooled samples.

4.2 Combining Biomarkers to Improve Diagnostic Accuracy

Let us assume that a number of K biomarkers are available and denoted $M_1, \ldots, M_K$. Without confusion, each M_k, $k = 1, \ldots, K$ can be viewed as simply a notation of a biomarker or its level that can be measured in a laboratory from blood or other biosamples. The random (column) vector $M = (M_1, \ldots, M_K)^T$ represents the levels of the K biomarkers; the superscript T indicates the transpose of a vector or a matrix. Biomarker levels are usually measured on a continuous scale. We are interested in combining the K biomarkers to improve diagnostic accuracy. Two questions arise to as how these markers should be combined and what criteria should be used to evaluate the combination.

Mathematically speaking, a combination can be any mapping that transforms M from the K-dimensional Euclidian space to another Euclidian space, usually of lower dimension K'. The disease status D (1 if diseased, 0 if not diseased) is then determined based on the transformed values in the new space. By doing so we expect that higher diagnostic accuracy can be achieved in comparison with any single biomarker or other combinations of biomarkers.

Attention is usually confined to combinations that are scalar-valued functions (i.e., $K' = 1$), whose performance can be evaluated the same way as a single biomarker is evaluated. Commonly used criteria include achieving highest sensitivity at a given specificity, highest sensitivity at all levels of specificity (highest ROC curve), largest AUC, and largest partial AUC (pAUC), among which maximizing the AUC is the most common.

The level of biomarkers is denoted by $X = (X_1, \ldots, X_K)^T$ if $D = 0$, and $Y = (Y_1, \ldots, Y_K)^T$ if $D = 1$, with density functions $f_X = f_X(x_1, \ldots, x_K)$ and $f_Y = f_Y(y_1, \ldots, y_K)$, respectively. The corresponding marginal density functions are denoted by f_{Xk} and f_{Yk} for the kth biomarker. Measured biomarker levels are denoted by $X_i = (X_{1i}, \ldots, X_{Ki})^T$ for the ith healthy subject ($i = 1, \ldots, n^0$), and by $Y_j = (Y_{1j}, \ldots, Y_{Kj})^T$ for the jth diseased subject ($j = 1, \ldots, n^1$). Therefore, the density functions of X_i, Y_j, X_{ki}, *and* Y_{kj} are f_X, f_Y, f_{Xk}, and f_{Yk}, respectively. Their corresponding distribution functions are denoted by F_X, F_Y, F_{Xk}, and F_{Yk}, respectively.

4.2.1 Likelihood Ratio Approach

According to the Neyman–Pearson lemma (1933), a well known fundamental result in statistical hypothesis testing, the likelihood ratio of the density of M|D = 1 to the density of M|D = 0 provides the most powerful result of all tests with the same level of significance (Type I error rate). To elaborate a bit, consider testing the simple null hypothesis H_0: M ~ F_X against a simple alternative hypothesis H_1: M ~ F_Y, at a given level of significance. Define

$$R(M) = \frac{f_Y(M_1,\ldots,M_K)}{f_X(M_1,\ldots,M_K)}. \tag{4-1}$$

The test that rejects H_0 for larger values of $R(M)$ has highest power among other forms of tests. Now consider the diagnostic rule that classifies a subject as diseased if R(M) > c. Its false positive rate is $P(R(\text{M}) > c|D = 0)$—the Type I error of the Neyman–Pearson test. Its true positive rate (sensitivity) is $P(R(\text{M}) > c|D = 1)$—the power of the Neyman–Pearson test. This leads to the conclusion that at any given false positive rate, the likelihood ratio has higher sensitivity than any other functions of M. See Baker (2000, 2003), Eguchi and Copas (2002), and Pepe et al. (2006).

This is an important property of the likelihood ratio function when used as a diagnostic rule. Its optimality is global in the sense that its ROC curve is above ROC curves of other combinations. Therefore the AUC and any pAUC are the largest.

One drawback with the likelihood ratio approach is that the ratio is uniformly optimal (achieving highest sensitivity at any level of specificity) only if the joint conditional distribution function (F_X or F_Y) of the K biomarkers given the disease status is correctly specified. However, specifying the joint distribution of multiple biomarkers may be a difficult task. If the true joint distribution functions depart substantially from the specified, the likelihood ratio approach may lead to an inferior combination rather than its claimed optimality/and the results can be misleading. Another drawback is that the ratio function may lack practical interpretation, and any efforts to do so can become difficult for physicians to understand, which in turn may hinder its use in practice.

4.2.2 Uniformly Optimal Linear Combinations

Combining multiple biomarkers using linear functions has drawn much attention. Besides their simplicity, one motivation for considering linear combinations is that they may often be interpreted in a way that makes sense and is acceptable to physicians. For example, a linear combination with positive coefficients summing up to 1 is simply a weighted average of the biomarkers.

A linear combination is said to be uniformly optimal if its ROC curve is above the ROC curves of other combinations, both linear and nonlinear. Understandably, such a linear combination generally does not exist. However, if the likelihood ratio R(M) is a monotone function of l(M), where l(M) is a linear function of the biomarkers, then the uniformly optimal linear combinations exist and, apart from a scalar, are identical to l(M). In practice, the relationship between the binary outcome D and the biomarkers M is usually achieved by a generalized linear model $g^{-1}(P(D=1|M))=\beta_0+\beta^T M$, where $\beta^T = (\beta_1, \ldots, \beta_K)$ are the regression parameters and g is the link function assumed to be monotone. Following McIntosh and Pepe (2002) and Pepe et al. (2006), we have, using the Bayes rule:

$$R(M)=\frac{P(M|D=1)}{P(M|D=0)}$$

$$=\frac{P(D=1|M)P(M)/P)(D=1)}{P(D=0|M)P(M)/P(D=0)}$$

$$=\frac{g(\beta_0+\beta^T M)\quad P(D=0)}{(1-g(\beta_0+\beta^T M)P(D=1)}.$$

Therefore, the likelihood ratio R(M) is a monotone function of β^TM. This, implies that β^TM is uniformly optimal and moreover, any other uniformly optimal linear combinations are proportional to β^TM. The combination parameters β can be estimated using the standard estimation procedures for generalized linear models. To give an example, let us consider the popular logistic regression model with $g(\cdot) = \exp(\cdot)/(1 + \exp(\cdot))$. It follows that $R(M)=\exp(\beta_0'+\beta^T M)$, where $\beta_0'=\beta_0+\log(P(D=0)/P(D=1))$. Thus R(M) is strictly increasing in β^TM, a uniformly optimal linear combination of M.

4.2.3 Normal Linear Combinations Maximizing AUC

Uniform optimality is the strictest criterion to compare ROC curves; it requires the desirable ROC curve be higher at any point than any other curves. In reality, it may be infeasible to find the uniformly optimal combinations (linear or nonlinear). To deal with this, we usually relax the criterion for comparison and/or consider combinations that have special forms. To this end, linear combinations that maximize the AUC appear most appealing. Note that the AUC of a linear combination remains unchanged when multiplied by a scalar. It suffices to confine the consideration to linear combinations with the first coefficient fixed to be 1; that is, linear combinations of the form $l(\lambda;M)=(1,\lambda^T)M=M_1+\lambda_2M_2+\ldots+\lambda_KM_K$, where the combination coefficients $\lambda = (\lambda_2, \ldots, \lambda_k)^T$ is of $K-1$ dimension. The AUC of the combination is given by $\text{AUC}(\lambda)=P((1,\lambda^T)(\mathcal{Y}-\mathcal{X})>0)$.

The optimal linear combination is defined as the one that maximizes the AUC among all linear combinations. That is, the optimal linear combination λ_{opt} is such that $\text{AUC}(\lambda_{opt}) = \sup_\lambda \text{AUC}(\lambda)$, or equivalently

$$\lambda_{opt}=\text{argmax}\{\text{AUC}(\lambda)\}=\text{argmax}\{P((1,\lambda^T)(\mathcal{Y}-\mathcal{X})>0)\}. \qquad (4\text{-}2)$$

Assuming that the biomarkers' values follow normal distributions, the issue of finding the optimal linear combinations to maximize the AUC was completely solved by Su and Liu (1993). Suppose that X follows a multivariate normal distribution with mean vector μ_X and variance–covariance matrix Σ_X, and that Y follows a multivariate normal distribution with mean vector μ_Y and variance–covariance matrix Σ_Y. For a given combination λ, $l(\lambda; X)$ follows a normal distribution with mean $(1, \lambda^T)\mu_X$ and variance $(1, \lambda^T)\Sigma_X(1, \lambda^T)^T$, and $l(\lambda; Y)$ follows a normal distribution with mean $(1, \lambda^T)\mu_Y$ and variance $(1, \lambda^T)\Sigma_Y(1, \lambda^T)^T$. From this binormal model the AUC of the combination is thus given by

$$\mathrm{AUC}(\lambda) = \Phi\left(\frac{(1,\lambda^T)(\mu_Y - \mu_X)}{\sqrt{(1,\lambda^T)(\Sigma_X + \Sigma_Y)(1,\lambda^T)^T}}\right),$$

where Φ and ϕ denote the standard normal distribution and density function, respectively. Su and Liu (1993) showed that the optimal linear combination is of the form

$$(1,\lambda_{opt}^T) = c \times (\mu_Y - \mu_X)^T(\Sigma_X + \Sigma_Y)^{-1}, \tag{4-3}$$

where c is the reciprocal of the first element of $(\mu_Y - \mu_X)^T(\Sigma_X + \Sigma_Y)^{-1}$. The AUC of the optimal linear combination is given by

$$\mathrm{AUC}_{max} = \mathrm{AUC}(\lambda_{opt}) = \Phi\left(\{(\mu_Y - \mu_X)^T(\Sigma_X + \Sigma_Y)^{-1}(\mu_Y - \mu_X)\}^{1/2}\right). \tag{4-4}$$

Liu et al. (2003) provided a simpler proof for the results using matrix theory. With observations of the biomarkers' levels, X_i and Y_j, $i = 1, \ldots, n^0$, $j = 1, \ldots, n^1$, the maximum likelihood estimates of λ_{opt} and AUC_{max} can be obtained by replacing the mean vectors and variance–covariance matrices by their sample mean vectors and sample variance–covariance matrices. Reiser and Faraggi (1997) derived confidence intervals for the maximum AUC. Under the normality assumption, the log likelihood ratio is given by

$$\log R(M) = (\Sigma_Y^{-1}\mu_Y - \Sigma_X^{-1}\mu_X)^T M + \frac{1}{2}M^T(\Sigma_X^{-1} - \Sigma_Y^{-1})M + const.,$$

where *const.* represents the terms that do not involve M. Note that with equal variance $\Sigma_X = \Sigma_Y$, the likelihood ratio approach yields a linear combination identical to Su and Liu's linear combination. In this case, the optimal linear combination is uniformly optimal and possesses the largest AUC among all scalar-valued functions. However, with unequal variance $\Sigma_X \neq \Sigma_Y$, the optimal combination is a quadratic function of the biomarkers, and hence the optimal linear combination is not the best among scalar-valued functions.

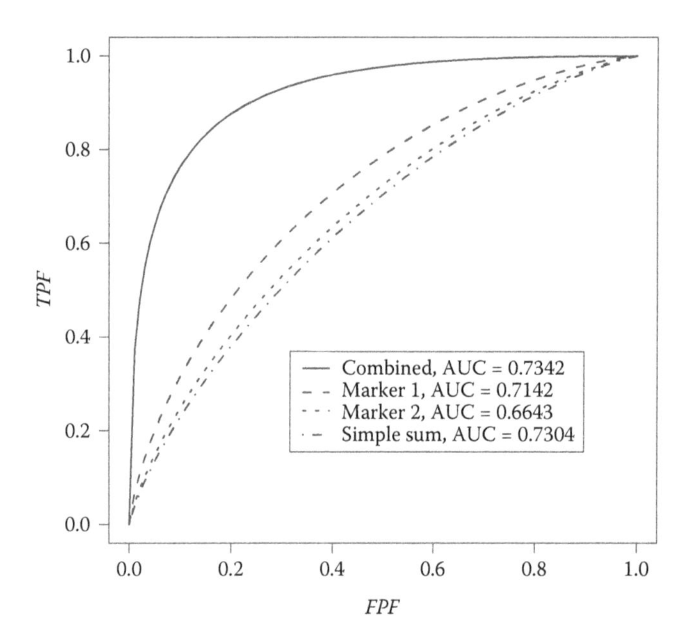

FIGURE 4.1
ROC curves of linear combinations.

The performance of the optimal linear combination is demonstrated in Figure 4.1 for two normally distributed biomarkers with

$$\begin{pmatrix} X_1 \\ X_2 \end{pmatrix} \sim N\left(\begin{pmatrix} 0 \\ 0 \end{pmatrix}, \begin{pmatrix} 1 & 0.3 \\ 0.3 & 1 \end{pmatrix}\right), \begin{pmatrix} Y_1 \\ Y_2 \end{pmatrix} \sim N\left(\begin{pmatrix} 0.8 \\ 0.6 \end{pmatrix}, \begin{pmatrix} 1 & 0.3 \\ 0.3 & 1 \end{pmatrix}\right).$$

Following some algebraic manipulations, we find that the linear combination is $X_1 + 0.5806X_2$ and $Y_1 + 0.5806Y_2$. The ROC curves of this linear combination and of the individual biomarkers are plotted in Figure 4.1. For comparison, the ROC curve of the simple sum $X_1 + X_2$ and $Y_1 + Y_2$ is also plotted. The ROC curve of the optimal linear combination is above the other three curves with the largest AUC of 0.7342. Interestingly, the simple sum also performs better than the individual curves and has an AUC of 0.7304.

4.2.4 Distribution-Free Approach for Linear Combinations

The multivariate normality is the only case found in the literature that has closed forms for λ_{opt} and AUC_{max}, whose maximum likelihood estimates are also available. For other joint distributions, whether a solution to Equation (4-2) exists, and if it does, how the optimal linear combination and its AUC can be estimated have not been well addressed. Several authors (Pepe and Thompson 2000; Pepe at al., 2006; Vexler et al., 2006; Ma and Huang 2007) have considered empirical solutions to the optimal linear combination and its AUC. For each linear combination $l(\lambda; \mathrm{M})$, its empirical AUC is given by:

$$\begin{aligned} \mathrm{AUC}_e(\lambda) &= \frac{1}{n^0 n^1} \sum_{i=1}^{n^0} \sum_{j=1}^{n^1} I(l(\lambda; \mathcal{Y}_j) > l(\lambda; \mathcal{X}_i)) \\ &= \frac{1}{n^0 n^1} \sum_{i=1}^{n^0} \sum_{j=1}^{n^1} I((1, \lambda^T)(\mathcal{Y}_j - \mathcal{X}_i) > 0), \end{aligned} \tag{4-5}$$

where I is the indicator function. The empirical optimal linear combination λ_e is then obtained by maximizing $\mathrm{AUC}_e(\lambda)$, that is:

$$\lambda_e = \operatorname{argmax}\{\mathrm{AUC}_e(\lambda)\} = \operatorname{argmax}\left\{ \frac{1}{n^0 n^1} \sum_{i=1}^{n^0} \sum_{j=1}^{n^1} I((1, \lambda^T)(\mathcal{Y}_j - \mathcal{X}_i) > 0) \right\}. \tag{4-6}$$

Pepe and Thompson (2000), focusing on combining two biomarkers ($K = 2$), commented that $\mathrm{AUC}_e(\lambda)$ is not a continuous function of λ and suggested using global search to numerically find λ_e; see also Pepe et al. (2006). Also for the case of two biomarkers, Vexler et al. (2006) showed that under mild regularity conditions, the maximization problem has a unique solution λ_{opt}, and the empirical estimator λ_e is a consistent estimate of λ_{opt}. They further presented an upper confidence limit for the maximum AUC.

Ma and Huang (2005, 2007) noticed the computational complexity of the maximization problem of Equation (4-6) when either the sample size or the number of biomarkers is relatively large. Arguing that the sigmoid function $s(x) = 1/(1 + \exp(x))$ provides good approximation to the step function, they propose to maximize

$$\mathrm{AUC}_s(\lambda) = \frac{1}{n^0 n^1} \sum_{i=1}^{n^0} \sum_{j=1}^{n^1} s_n((1, \lambda^T)(\mathcal{Y}_j - \mathcal{X}_i)), \tag{4-7}$$

where $s_n(x) = s(x/\sigma_n)$ with $\sigma_n > 0$ and $\lim_{n \to \infty} \sigma_n = 0$.

Under the assumption that the disease status D and the biomarkers' levels M satisfy a generalized linear monotone model, Pepe et al. (2006) noticed that the solution λ_e to the maximization problem (4-6) yields a consistent estimator of λ_{opt}. Similarly, Ma and Huang (2007) showed that the solution to the maximization problem (4-7) also yields a consistent estimator of λ_{opt}, and the estimator is asymptotically normally distributed. These estimators are robust for the parameters in the generalized linear model in the sense that the link function does not need to be specified.

4.3 ROC Curve Analysis with Pooled Samples

The conventional approach to evaluating the accuracy of a diagnostic biomarker is to collect measurements on the level of the biomarker from individual diseased and healthy subjects. Using these individually observed measurements, the sensitivity, specificity, and ROC curve of the biomarker can then be estimated. In practice, however, high cost may prohibit measuring biomarkers from each individual sample available for a study. In other cases, a blood sample collected from an individual such as an infant may not have enough volume to be measured by the instrument. To deal with these issues, individual blood samples are often randomly divided into groups (pools), and the level of the biomarker is then measured from the samples in each pool. The measured level from a pooled sample is usually taken as the average of the levels of the biomarker of the individual samples in that pool.

Pooling provides an effective strategy to reduce study costs. For example, if measuring a biomarker costs $50 per subject per assay, then the cost for assaying 20 subjects is $1000. In a simple pooling design, suppose the 20 subjects are randomly divided into 10 pools with 2 subjects in each group. Then the cost of the study will be reduced by half to $500.

Group testing by searching for a microorganism in pooled biospecimens appeared initially in the context of screening with dichotomous outcomes (Dorfman 1943; Sobel and Groll 1959). This method was further developed by Gastwirth and Johnson (1994) and Litvak et al. (1994) to investigate HIV contamination. Sobel and Elashoff (1975), Chen and Swallow (1990), Farrington (1992), Hughes-Oliver and Swallow (1994), and Tu et al. (1995) estimated population prevalence; Barcellos et al. (1997) localized disease genes. Weinberg and Umbach (1999) proposed a set-based logistic model to explore the association between a disease and exposures when only the pooled exposure values were available. Pooling DNA samples is also common in genetic studies (Jin et al. 2001; Enard et al. 2002; Kendziorski et al. 2003).

Consider a case-control study to investigate the diagnostic accuracy of a biomarker. Suppose the biomarker under investigation is measured on a continuous scale. Let $X_1,\ldots,X_{n^0k}$ be the biomarker levels from n^0k healthy subjects, with distribution F_X. Let $Y_1,\ldots,Y_{n^1k}$ be the biomarker levels from n^1k diseased subjects, with distribution F_Y. If each X_i, $i = 1, \ldots, n^0k$, and Y_j, $j = 1, \ldots, n^1k$, can be observed, then parametric or nonparametric estimation of the distributions F_X and F_Y can be derived and the results used to construct the ROC curve and its AUC of the biomarker. Suppose the pooling strategy is carried out with healthy subjects randomly grouped into n^0 sets and the diseased subjects into n^1 sets, each of size k. Subsequently, without loss of generality, we can assume that instead of observing each individual

X and Y, the average of the Xs and the Ys in each set is observed, yielding n^0 observations, $X_i^* = \sum_{l=k(i-1)+1}^{ik} X_i/k, i = 1,\ldots,n^0$, and n^1 observations $Y_j^* = \sum_{l=k(j-1)+1}^{jk} X_l/k, j = 1,\ldots,n^1$, often called set-based observations. The X^*s are also independent and identically distributed, following the distribution F_X^* of the average of k random draws from F_X. Similarly the Y^*s are independent and identically distributed, following the distribution F_Y^* of the average of k random draws from F_Y. In ROC curve analysis, we are interested in estimating biomarkers' ROC curves based on the set-based data:

$$\mathrm{ROC(FPF)} = 1 - F_Y^{-1}(F_X^{-1}(1 - FPF)) \tag{4-8}$$

and its summary indices such as the AUC:

$$\mathrm{AUC} = P(X_1 > Y_1) = \int_0^1 \mathrm{ROC}(t)dt. \tag{4-9}$$

Because biomarker levels from individual subjects are intractable, estimating the ROC curve and its indexes can be challenging, mainly because for a general distribution F_X or F_Y, the likelihood methods based on set-based data may not be feasible, since the distribution of the averages involves convolution of k random variables of F_X or F_Y. Clearly, for a given cut point c, the sensitivity of the biomarker is $Se(c) = P(Y_1 > c) = 1 - F_Y(c)$, which is not the same as $Se^* = P(Y_1^* > c) = 1 - F_Y^*(c)$. Moreover the ROC curve of the set-based average

$$\mathrm{ROC}^*(FPF) = 1 - F_Y^{*-1}(F_X^{*-1}(1 - FPF)) \tag{4-10}$$

is not the same as the ROC(FPF). Indeed, effective statistical methods, especially nonparametric approaches, still need to be developed to estimate ROC curves using set-based pooled data.

4.3.1 Normal Distributions

For certain distributional forms of F_X and F_Y, the maximum likelihood estimation of the ROC curve and its indices may be derived conveniently based on the pooled data. The method requires that the density functions of the pooled average X_1^* or Y_1^* be workable. Faraggi et al. (2003) and Liu and Schisterman (2003) considered evaluation of diagnostic biomarkers based on pooled specimens whose measurements are assumed to follow normal or gamma distributions. Here we assume that the biomarker levels follow normal distributions, $X_1 \sim N(\mu_X, \sigma_X^2)$, $Y_1 \sim N(\mu_Y, \sigma_Y^2)$. The ROC curve and its AUC are given by:

$$\text{ROC}(FPF) = \Phi(a + b\Phi(FPF)), \ \text{AUC} = \Phi\left(\frac{a}{\sqrt{1+b^2}}\right), \tag{4-11}$$

respectively, where $a = \frac{\mu_Y - \mu_X}{\sigma_Y}$, $b = \frac{\sigma_X}{\sigma_Y}$.

Estimates of the ROC curve and its AUC are then obtained by replacing the mean and variance parameters with their meaningful estimates. Because linear functions of normal variables also have normal distributions, it follows that:

$$X_i^* \sim N(\mu_X, \frac{1}{k}\sigma_X^2),\ i = 1,\ldots,n^0,\ Y_j^* \sim N(\mu_Y, \frac{1}{k}\sigma_Y^2),\ j = 1,\ldots,n^1.$$

The log-likelihood functions of the pooled data are given by, respectively,

$$l_X = -\frac{1}{2}\log\sigma_X^2 - \frac{k}{2\sigma_X^2}\sum_{i=1}^{n^0}(X_i^* - \mu_X)^2 + const.,$$

and

$$l_Y = -\frac{1}{2}\log\sigma_Y^2 - \frac{k}{2\sigma_Y^2}\sum_{j=1}^{n^1}(Y_j^* - \mu_Y)^2 + const.$$

Maximizing these functions then yields the maximum likelihood estimation of the means and variances:

$$\hat{\mu}_X = \frac{1}{n^0}\sum_{i=1}^{n^0} X_i^*,\ \hat{\sigma}_X^2 = k\frac{1}{n^0}\sum_{i=1}^{n^0}(X_i^* - \hat{\mu}_X)^2,$$

$$\hat{\mu}_Y = \frac{1}{n^1}\sum_{j=1}^{n^1} Y_j^*,\ \hat{\sigma}_Y^2 = k\frac{1}{n^1}\sum_{j=1}^{n^1}(Y_j^* - \hat{\mu}_Y)^2.$$

Thus, pooling individual biomarker levels does not change estimation of the mean parameters, but yields estimation of the variance parameters with less precision. Plugging these estimates into Equation (4-11) then yields the maximum likelihood estimates of the ROC curve and its AUC. These maximum likelihood estimates are asymptotically normally distributed. Liu and Schisterman (2003) derived asymptotic variance of the estimated AUC:

$$V(\widehat{\text{AUC}}) = \frac{1}{\sigma_X^2 + \sigma_Y^2} \phi^2\left(\frac{\mu_Y - \mu_X}{\sqrt{\sigma_X^2 + \sigma_Y^2}}\right)\left\{\frac{1}{n^0 k}\sigma_X^2 + \frac{1}{n^1 k}\sigma_Y^2 + \frac{(\mu_Y - \mu_X)^2}{2(\sigma_X^2 + \sigma_Y^2)}\left(\frac{1}{n^0}\sigma_X^4 + \frac{1}{n^1}\sigma_Y^4\right)\right\}.$$

They also obtained statistics for testing the equality of two AUCs with pooled data.

Remark 4.1. For the binormal model, the AUC of the set-based average is given by

$$\text{AUC}^* = P(Y_1^* > X_1^*) = \Phi\left(\frac{\sqrt{k}(\mu_Y - \mu_X)}{\sqrt{\sigma_X^2 + \sigma_Y^2}}\right).$$

If $\mu_Y > \mu_X$, that is, the biomarker levels are on average higher among diseased subjects than among healthy subjects, then AUC* is larger than AUC. Furthermore $\Phi^{-1}(\text{AUC}^*)/\Phi^{-1}(\text{AUC}) = \sqrt{k}$. Therefore, the set-based empirical AUC

$$\widehat{\text{AUC}}^* = \frac{1}{n^0 n^1} \sum_{i=1}^{n^0} \sum_{j=1}^{n^1} I(Y_j^* > X_i^*)$$

overestimates the biomarker's AUC = $P(Y_1 > X_1)$.

To illustrate, consider the ROC curve of (X, Y) with $X \sim N(0, 1)$ and $Y \sim N(0.5, 1)$, and of (X^*, Y^*) with $X^* \sim N(0, 1/k)$ and $Y^* \sim N(0.5, 1/k)$, where k is the pooling size. Figure 4.2 presents the ROC curves of the set-based average for each pooling size. Clearly the ROC curve rises as the pooling size gets bigger. Therefore the ROC curve of the biomarker cannot be estimated using the set-based ROC curves.

4.3.2 Gamma Distributions

A gamma distribution with shape parameter c and scale parameter b has a density function

$$\gamma(x; b, c) = \frac{x^{c-1}\exp(-x/b)}{b^c \Gamma(c)},$$

where $\Gamma(c) = \int_0^\infty \exp(-s) s^{c-1} ds$ is the gamma function; see e.g. Evans et al. (2000, Chapter 19). Because gamma distributions allow various skewed shapes, they are often used to characterize the levels of a biomarker when the normality assumption is not justified. Faraggi et al. (2003) discussed estimation of the

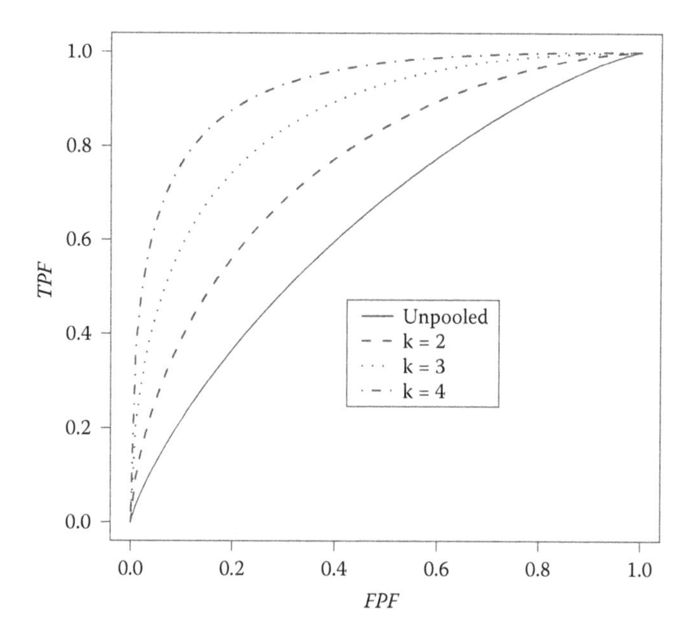

FIGURE 4.2
ROC curves of set-based averages.

AUC with pooled data for a gamma distributed biomarker. Because the sum of gamma variables is also a gamma variable, the maximum likelihood estimation of the ROC curve and its area can be obtained from the set-based averages, similar to normal distributions.

Suppose the biomarker levels $X_1,\ldots,X_{n^0k}$ from the healthy subjects have a common gamma density function $\gamma(x;\, b_X,\, c_X)$ and the biomarker levels $Y_1,\ldots,Y_{n^1k}$ from the diseased subjects have a common gamma density function $\gamma(y;\, b_Y,\, c_Y)$. The set-based sums $kX_1^*,\ldots,kY_{n^0}^*$ have a common density function $\gamma(x;\, b_X,\, kc_X)$ and $kY_1^*,\ldots,kY_{n^0}^*$ have a common density function $\gamma(y;\, b_Y,\, kc_Y)$. Hence, the maximum likelihood estimation of the scale and shape parameters may be derived by maximizing the log-likelihood function:

$$l(b_X, c_X) = kc_X \sum_{i=1}^{n^0} \log X_i^* - \frac{1}{b_X} \sum_{i=1}^{n^0} X_i^* - n^0 kc_X \log b_X - n^0 \log \Gamma(kc_X) + const.$$

and

$$l(b_Y, c_Y) = kc_Y \sum_{j=1}^{n^1} \log Y_j^* - \frac{1}{b_Y} \sum_{j=1}^{n^1} Y_i^* - n^1 kc_Y \log b_Y - n^0 \log \Gamma(kc_Y) + const.$$

Following Evans et al. (2000), the maximum likelihood estimates of the parameters can only be solved numerically from the simultaneous equations:

$$k\hat{b}_X\hat{c}_X = \bar{X}^*,\ \log k + \log \hat{c}_X - \psi(k\hat{c}_X) = \log \bar{X}^* - \frac{1}{n^0}\sum_{i=1}^{n^0} \log X_i^*$$

$$k\hat{b}_Y\hat{c}_Y = \bar{Y}^*,\ \log k + \log \hat{c}_Y - \psi(k\hat{c}_Y) = \log \bar{Y}^* - \frac{1}{n^1}\sum_{j=1}^{n^1} \log Y_i^*,$$

where $\bar{X}^* = \sum_{i=1}^{n^0} X_i^*/n^0, \bar{Y}^* = \sum_{j=1}^{n^1} Y_j^*/n^1$, and $y(c)$ is the derivative of log $\Gamma(c)$ with respect to c. The AUC is shown to be (Constantine et al., 1986; Faraggi et al., 2003):

$$\text{AUC} = \frac{1}{B(c_Y, c_X)} \int_0^{b_Y/(b_X+b_Y)} s^{c_X-1}(1-s)^{c_Y-1} ds,$$

where $B(\nu,\omega) = \int_0^1 t^{\nu-1}(1-t)^{\omega-1}$ is the beta function. Replacing the scale and shape parameters by their maximum likelihood estimates then yields the maximum likelihood estimate of the AUC under the gamma model:

$$\widehat{\text{AUC}} = \frac{1}{B(\hat{c}_Y, \hat{c}_X)} \int_0^{\hat{b}_Y/(\hat{b}_X+\hat{b}_Y)} s^{\hat{c}_X-1}(1-s)^{\hat{c}_Y-1} ds.$$

The asymptotic variance of the AUC estimate can be derived using the conventional large sample theory for maximum likelihood estimation or a resampling technique.

4.3.3 Stable Distributions

The methods described above for normal or gamma distributions apply well to other distributions whenever the density function of the set-specific averages or sums is convenient to work with. As another example, suppose that X and Y both follow an exponential distribution. Then each of the set-specific sums kX^* and kY^* has a gamma distribution. The maximum likelihood estimation of the exponential density parameters can be derived by maximizing the product of these set-specific gamma densities. Estimates of the ROC curve and its AUC can then be derived.

In most cases, working directly with the density of the set-specific sums or averages can be extremely difficult. Vexler et al. (2008) considered a different approach to dealing with stable distributions. A stable distribution is not defined by its density but rather by its characteristic function of a particular form:

$$\omega(t;\theta) = \omega(t;\theta_1,\theta_2,\theta_3,\theta_4) = \exp\{i\theta_1 t - \theta_2 |t|^{\theta_3}(1 + i\theta_4 t h(t,\theta_3)/|t|)\}, \quad (4\text{-}12)$$

where $\theta = (\theta_1, \theta_2, \theta_3, \theta_4)$, $\theta_2 \geq 0$, $\theta_3 \in (0, 2]$, $|\theta_4| \leq 1$, and

$$h(t,\theta_3) = \begin{cases} \tan(\pi\theta_3/2), & \theta_3 \neq 1; \\ 2\log|t|/\pi, & \theta_3 = 1. \end{cases}$$

(See Vexler et al., 2003.) Suppose the biomarker levels follow a stable distribution with characteristic function $\omega_X(t;\theta_X) = \omega(t;\theta_X)$, $\theta_X = (\theta_{1X}, \theta_{2X}, \theta_{3X}, \theta_{4X})$ for the healthy subjects and $\omega_Y(t;\theta_Y) = \omega(t;\theta_Y)$, $\theta_Y = (\theta_{1Y}, \theta_{2Y}, \theta_{3Y}, \theta_{4Y})$ for the diseased subjects. With pooling size k the set-specific sum also follows a stable distribution with characteristic function $\omega_X^*(t;\theta_X) = \{\omega(t;\theta_X)\}^k = \omega(t; k\theta_{1X}, k\theta_{2X}, \theta_{3X}, \theta_{4X})$ for kX^* and $\omega_Y^*(t;\theta_Y) = \{\omega(t;\theta_Y)\}^k = \omega(t; k\theta_{1Y}, k\theta_{2Y}, \theta_{3Y}, \theta_{4Y})$ for kY^*. The density function of the set-specific sum can then be derived using the popular conversion theorem. We have $f_X^*(x) = 1/2\pi\int_{-\infty}^{\infty}\exp(-itx)\omega_X^*(t;\theta_X)dt$ and $f_Y^*(y) = 1/2\pi\int_{-\infty}^{\infty}\exp(-ity)\omega_Y^*(t;\theta_Y)dt$, where i is the imaginary number, that is, $i^2 = -1$. Thus the log-likelihood function based on the observed set-specific sums is given by $l_X = \sum_{i=1}^{n0} \log f^*(kX_i^*)$, $l_Y = \sum_{j=1}^{n1} \log f_Y^*(kY_j^*)$.

Maximizing the log-likelihood functions leads to the maximum likelihood estimates $\hat{\theta}_X$ and $\hat{\theta}_Y$ of the distributional parameters that in turn yield estimates of the characteristic functions $w(t;\theta_X)$ and $w(t;\theta_Y)$. Converting the estimated characteristic functions to their corresponding density and distribution functions yields estimates of the ROC curves and their AUC; see Vexler et al. (2003) for more details.

4.3.4 Distribution-Free Approach

The methods described above for stable distributions were further extended by Vexler et al. (2010) to obtain nonparametric estimations of the ROC curve and its AUC. Using the observed set-specific sums, we can construct the empirical estimate $\hat{\omega}^*(t)$ of the characteristic function $\omega^*(t)$ of the set-specific sum:

$$\hat{\omega}_X^*(t) = \frac{1}{n^0}\sum_{i=1}^{n^0}\exp(itkX_i^*), \quad \hat{\omega}_Y^*(t) = \frac{1}{n^1}\sum_{j=1}^{n^1}\exp(itkY_j^*).$$

Note that $w^*(t) = \{w(t)\}^k$ because the characteristic function of the sum of independent variables is the product of the characteristic functions of the individual variables. Hence, under certain conditions (Vexler et al., 2010), we may use $\hat{\omega}(t) = \{\hat{\omega}(t)\}^{1/k}$ as an estimate of w. Estimates of the density and distribution functions are again obtained by converting the estimated characteristic functions. The estimates are then used to construct the ROC curve and its AUC.

4.4 Remarks and Further Reading

4.4.1 Combination of Biomarkers

Pfeiffer and Bura (2008) proposed a model-free approach to combining biomarkers. The idea is to use sufficient dimension reduction methods to find an orthogonal projection matrix P_S of dimension $K' \times K$ with $K' < K$ such that the conditional probability of D given M is identical to the conditional probability of D given $P_S M$. One or a few linear combinations of $P_S M$ can then be combined using approximate normality via the likelihood ratio statistic for diagnosis. This approach requires only the first two moments of the biomarkers be specified. Pfeiffer and Bura (2008) investigated two methods for sufficient dimension reduction—sliced inverse regression (SIR; Li, 1991) and sliced average variance estimation (SAVE; Cook and Weisberg, 1991)—to construct the projection matrix. Under multivariate normality, the two methods led, respectively, to Su and Liu's (1993) linear combination and the likelihood ratio combination.

Zou and O'Malley (2006) proposed a Bayesian multivariate hierarchical transformation model that assumes the Box–Cox transformed test outcomes, along with covariates, satisfy a random effect regression model. The authors examined combinations using Markov chain Monte Carlo (MCMC). They compared their discriminant function approach and the popular logistic regression analysis, illustrated by using two classifiers, prostate-specific antigen and Gleason score, as predictors for prostate cancer stages. The authors concluded that logistic regression analysis would produce a more sensitive classification rule. Further analytic and numerical work is needed to compare with other methods for combing such markers using the Bayesian multivariate hierarchical transformation model.

Relatively less attention has been given to obtaining the variance and confidence intervals for the optimal combinations and their resulting AUCs. Under multivariate normality, Reiser and Faraggi (1997) constructed confidence intervals for the AUCs of Su and Liu's (1993) optimal linear combinations. Their method is essentially based on likelihood and can be extended as follows. Suppose the distributions of the biomarkers are known up to some parameters, say, θ_X for healthy and θ_Y for diseased. Then the AUC of the likelihood ratio combination AUC = $P(R(\mathcal{Y}) > R(\mathcal{X}))$ is a function of θ_X and θ_Y. With observed levels of the biomarkers, the maximum likelihood estimates of θ_X and θ_Y can be obtained, which in turn result in the maximum likelihood estimate of the AUC. The (asymptotic) variance of the estimated AUC can then be derived using the delta method (Rao, 1972). Alternatively, the variance of the optimal AUC, either from a parametric or a nonparametric model, can be estimated using the bootstrap method (Efron and Tibshirani 1993).

4.4.2 Pooling of Biomarkers

Estimation of an ROC curve based on pooled data appears relatively easy for certain distributions such as normal, gamma, or exponential types. Further research is needed to (1) obtain the maximum likelihood estimation of the ROC curve and its AUC for other popular distributions such as the lognormal; and (2) develop nonparametric and semiparametric estimations of the ROC curve and its AUC.

In practice, assays measuring the levels of biomarkers from blood, urine, and other biospecimens are often subject to a detection limit—an important issue that must be dealt with when evaluating the diagnostic accuracies of biomarkers. For an assay with a detection limit, the level of a biomarker cannot be quantified accurately if the biomarker level is below the limit. Methods have been proposed in the literature to estimate the ROC curve and its AUC from pooled data when the level of a biomarker is subject to a limit of detection; see Mumford et al. (2006), Vexler et al. (2006), and Vexler et al. (2008).

References

Baker, S. 2000. Identifying combinations of cancer markers for further study as triggers of early intervention. *Biometrics* 56: 1082–1087.

Baker, S. 2003. The central role of receiver operating characteristic (ROC) curves in evaluating tests for the early detection of cancer. *Journal of the National Cancer Institute* 95: 511–515.

Barcellos, L.F., Klitz, W., Field, L.L. et al. 1997. Association mapping of disease loci by use of a pooled DNA genomic screen. *American Journal of Human Genetics* 61: 734–747.

Chen, C.L. and Swallow, W.H. 1990. Using group testing to estimate a proportion and to test the binomial model. *Biometrics* 46: 1035–1046.

Constantine, K., Karson, M. et al. 1986. Estimation of P(Y < X) in the gamma case. *Communication Statistics Simulation* 15: 365–388.

Cook, R.D. and Weisberg, S. 1991. Discussion of Li. *Journal of the American Statistical Association* 86: 328–332.

Dorfman, R. 1943. The detection of defective members of large populations. *Annals of Mathematical Statistics* 14: 436–440.

Efron, B. and Tibshirani, R. 1993. *An Introduction to the Bootstrap*. Boca Raton: Chapman & Hall.

Eguchi, S. and Copas, J.B. 2002. A class of logistic-type discriminant functions. *Biometrika* 89: 1–22.

Enard, W., Khaitovich, P., Klose, J. et al. 2002. Intra- and inter-specific variation in primate gene expression patterns. *Science* 296: 340–343.

Evans, M., Hastings, N., and Peacock, B. 2000. *Statistical Distributions*. 3rd Ed. New York: Wiley.

Faraggi, D., Reiser, B., and Schisterman, E.F. 2003. ROC curve analysis for biomarkers based on pooled assessments. *Statistics in Medicine* 22: 2515–2527.

Farrington, C. (1992). Estimation prevalence by group testing using generalized linear models. *Statistics in Medicine* 11: 1591–1597.

Gastwirth, J. and Johnson, W. 1994. Screening with cost-effective quality control: potential applications to HIV and drug testing. *Journal of the American Statistical Association* 89: 972–981.

Green, D.M. and Swets, J.A. 1966. *Signal Detection Theory and Psychophysics*. New York: Wiley.

Hughes-Oliver, J.M. and Swallow, W.H. 1994. A two-stage adaptive group-testing procedure for estimating small proportions. *Journal of the American Statistical Association* 89: 982–993.

Jin, W., Riley, R.M., Wolfinger, R.D. et al. 2001. The contributions of sex: genotype and age to transcriptional variance in *Drosophila melanogaster*. *Nature Genetics* 29: 389–395.

Kendziorski, C.M., Zhang, Y., Lan, H. et al. 2003. The efficiency of pooling mRNA in microarray experiments. *Biostatistics* 4: 465–477.

Li, K.C. 1991. Sliced inverse regression for dimension reduction. *Journal of the American Statistical Association* 86: 316–342.

Liu, A. and Schisterman, E.F. 2003. Comparison of diagnostic accuracy of biomarkers with pooled assessments. *Biometrical Journal* 45: 631–644.

Liu, A., Schisterman, E.F., and Zhu, Y. 2005. On linear combinations of biomarkers to improve diagnostic accuracy. *Statistics in Medicine* 24: 37–47.

Litvak, E., Tu, X.M., and Pagano, M. 1994. Screening for the presence of a disease by pooling sera samples. *Journal of the American Statistical Association* 89: 424–434.

Ma, S. and Huang, J. 2005. Regularized ROC method for disease classification and biomarker selection with microarray data. *Bioinformatics* 21: 4356–4362.

Ma, S. and Huang, J. 2007. Combining multiple markers for classification using ROC. *Biometrics* 63: 751–757.

Mumford, S.L., Schisterman, E.F., Vexler, A. et al. 2006. Pooling biospecimens and limits of detection: effects on ROC curve analysis. *Biostatistics* 7: 585–598.

Neyman, J. and Pearson, E.S. 1933. On the problem of the most efficient tests of statistical hypothesis. *Philosophical Transactions of the Royal Society of London Series A* 231: 289–337.

O'Malley, A.J. and Zou, K.H. 2006. Bayesian multivariate hierarchical transformation models for ROC analysis. *Statistics in Medicine* 25: 459–479.

Pepe, M.S., Cai, T., and Longton, G. 2006. Combining predictors for classification using the area under the receiver operating characteristic curve. *Biometrics* 62: 221–229.

Pepe, M.S. and Thompson, M.L. 2000. Combining diagnostic test results to increase accuracy. *Biostatistics* 1: 123–140.

Pfeiffer, R.M. and Bura, E. 2008. A model free approach to combining biomarkers. *Biometrical Journal* 50: 558–570.

Rao, C.R. 1972. *Linear Statistical Inference and Its Applications*. New York: Wiley.

Reiser, B. and Faraggi, D. 1997. Confidence intervals for the generalized ROC criterion. *Biometrics* 53: 644–652.

Sobel, M. and Elashoff, R. 1975. Group testing with a new goal: estimation. *Biometrika* 62: 181–193.

Su, J.Q. and Liu, J.S. 1993. Linear combinations of multiple diagnostic markers. *Journal of the American Statistical Association* 88: 1350–1355.

Tu, X.M., Litvak, E., and Pagano, M. 1995. On the informativeness and accuracy of pooled testing in estimating prevalence of a rare disease: application to HIV screening. *Biometrika* 82: 287–297.

Vexler, A., Liu, A., and Schisterman, E.F. 2006. Efficient design and analysis of biospecimens with measurements subject to detection limit. *Biometrical Journal* 48: 780–791.

Vexler, A., Liu, A., and Schisterman, E.F. 2010. Nonparametric deconvolution of density estimation based on observed sums. *Journal of Nonparametric Statistics* 22: 23–29.

Vexler, A., Schisterman, E.F., and Liu, A. 2008. Estimation of ROC based on stably distributed biomarkers subject to measurement error and pooling mixtures. *Statistics in Medicine* 27: 280–296.

Vexler, A., Liu, A., Schisterman, E.F. et al. 2006. Note on distribution-free estimation of maximum linear separation of two multivariate distributions. *Journal of Nonparametric Statistics* 18: 145–158.

Weinberg, C.R. and Umbach, D.M. 1999. Using pooled exposure assessment to improve efficiency in case-control studies. *Biometrics* 55: 718–726.

5

Bayesian ROC Methods

5.1 Introduction

Bayesian approaches are different from the more conventional non-Bayesian approaches. In essence, given the observed data, after the prior distribution and the statistical model are specified, probability methods are applied to derive posterior distributions of the parameters in the model or the functions of these parameters. In multicenter trials and medical image analyses, Bayesian methods may be more natural for dealing with complex data structures. Expensive imaging studies are usually conducted with very limited sample sizes due to the high cost of each study. Consequently, several challenges surround the analysis of diagnostic and radiological data from complex multicenter clinical trials for a number of reasons.

First, the effect of cluster: patients enrolled from different clusters, such as clinical centers, may exhibit different characteristics. They may be more similar within one participating center than another. A pooled analysis may be too liberal, while a stratified analysis that does not consider the correlations of different clusters may be too conservative. If the distribution of unmeasured confounding variables varies by cluster, an apparent effect of the clusters will result. If such effects of clustering are not accounted for, pooled analysis can lead to biased results. A simpler method may be to conduct subgroup analysis via stratification.

The next factor is the effect of covariates: a large number of variables are available in a large clinical trial by hierarchical multireader multimodality studies (Wang and Gatsonis, 2008). Third is the availability of prior information: existing data from pilot studies or prior knowledge may be utilized and incorporated in a current study, particularly in more costly imaging studies. Finally, the need for a flexible model to accomodate assumptions such as transformation to normality: when dealing with continuous diagnostic outcome data such as PSA values, the binormal model assumes that the outcome data have normal distributions with different means and variances. It is useful to perform a normality transformation before applying this model (Metz et al., 1998; O'Malley et al., 2001; Zou and O'Malley, 2005; O'Malley and Zou, 2006; Fluss, 2005). For example, O'Malley and Zou (2006) embedded transformation in the model so that the uncertainty in the value of the transformation parameter (exponent lambda) can propagate through the analysis.

By employing Bayesian methodology, one may better utilize prior information from a pilot study to design a more compact study. For small sample sizes or small numbers of clusters, Bayesian methods can be more efficient based on reductions in sample size and utilization of prior knowledge. Bayesian methodology may be applicable to study designs in a variety of other clinical domains. Estimation methods for complex functions of parameters or hyperparameters are also applicable to the analysis of data from such studies. Following Parmigiani (2002), the Bayesian framework is useful for the analysis of data by borrowing strength when multiple clusters are present. The parameters or hyperparameters are then estimated among clusters.

One may compute the highest posterior density (HPD) region and, alternatively but more simply, the average coverage or average length criterion of Joseph and Wolfson (1997), Zou and Normand (2001), Normand and Zou (2002), and Cao et al. (2009) due to the complex hierarchical structure of a study. In the Bayesian framework, the average length criteria can be viewed as analogous to those based on the confidence intervals in frequentist methods, and are therefore practical for computations.

We address all of the above issues in analyzing multicenter diagnostic clinical trial data by extending the Bayesian regression approaches using the BUGS software such as winBUGS or Open BUGs (Lunn et al., 2009; http://www.mrc-bsu.cam.ac.uk/bugs), as well as the R2WinBUGS package by Gelman et al. (http://www.stat.columbia.edu/~gelman/bugsR).

5.2 Methods for Sensitivity, Specificity, and Prevalence

Multi-institutional classification studies often rely on complex designs and analyses, with data having multilevel structures; individual patients at the first level, with physicians, hospitals, and geographic regions forming the higher level clusters. Donner et al. (2004) and Zou et al. (2005) demonstrated that clusters may have different sizes at each level of a hierarchy, and thus it is important to consider cluster randomization in study design. Besides data clustered according to provider types or geographical regions, many individual and cluster level covariates are present. Disease status or severity, comorbidity conditions, and organizational characteristics of a particular center may vary at cluster level where diagnostic tests are conducted.

Consider two random samples, X_i ($I = 1, \ldots, m$) and Y_j ($j = 1, \ldots, n$), drawn from the H and D populations, respectively. At a given decision threshold, the resulting binary decision variable generates a 0 or 1 value while the gold standard (GS) determines the true individual classes. We assume that the GS has a Bernoulli distribution; the prevalence $P(D = 1) = 1 - p = n^1/N$; the fractional sample size for class C_1; and similarly for the fractional sample size for class C_0 with a probability of $P(D = 0) = 1 - p = n^0/N$, where $N = n^0 + n^1$. Using the Bayes theorem, the marginal distribution of the observed continuous random variable Z consists of a mixture of F_X and F_Y, with mixing proportions $1 - p$ and p. The CDF of $H(z) = (1-\pi)F_X(z) + \pi F_Y(z)$, with the corresponding PDF, $h(z)$, is calculated by:

$$h(z) = (1-\pi) f_X(z) + \pi f_Y(z), \ \forall z \in R. \tag{5-1}$$

By specifying any arbitrary positive threshold (*a priori* cutoff value), ξ, a dichotomized form of the decision random variable T_ξ, is generated. This implies the equivalence of $\{T_\xi = 1\} \equiv \{Z > \xi\}$. Consequently, a 2 × 2 contingency table may be formed (Table 5.1).

$$\begin{aligned}
p^{00} &= P(T_\xi = 0, GS = 0) = P(Z \le \xi \mid D = 0) = (1-p)F_X(\xi),\\
p^{10} &= P(T_\xi = 1, GS = 0) = P(Z > \xi \mid D = 0) = (1-p)[1 - F_X(\xi)],\\
p^{01} &= P(T_\xi = 0, GS = 1) = P(Z \le \xi \mid D = 1) = p[1 - F_Y(\xi)],\\
p^{11} &= P(T_\xi = 1, GS = 1) = P(Z > \xi \mid D = 1) = pF_Y(\xi).
\end{aligned} \tag{5-2}$$

Based on Table 5.1, the accuracy measures may be derived using the Bayes theorem.

$$\begin{aligned}
&\text{Prevalence} = P(D = 1) = p = p^{01} + p^{11},\\
&FPF = 1 - Sp = P(T_\xi = 1 \mid D = 0) = p^{10}/(p^{00} + p^{10}),\\
&TPF = Se = P(T_\xi = 1 \mid D = 1) = p^{11}/(p^{01} + p^{11}),\\
&PV^- = P(D = 0 \mid T_\xi = 0) = p^{00}/(p^{00} + p^{01}),\\
&PV^+ = P(D = 1 \mid T_\xi = 1) = p^{11}/(p^{10} + p^{10}).
\end{aligned} \tag{5-3}$$

TABLE 5.1

2 × 2 Table of Counts and Joint Probabilities of Gold Standard versus Corresponding Dichotomized Decision (T_ξ) at Each Possible Threshold ξ

Dichotomized Decision versus Gold Standard	*D = 0* (Healthy)	*D = 1* (Diseased)
T_ξ=0	(n^{00}, p^{00})	(n^{01}, p^{01})
T_ξ=1	(n^{10}, p^{10})	(n^{11}, p^{11})
Marginal Total	(n^0, 1 − p)	(n^1, p)

TABLE 5.2

2 × 2 Table of Prior Information

Dichotomized Decision versus Gold Standard	$D = 0$ (Healthy)	$D = 1$ (Diseased
T_ξ=0	(m^{00}, p^{00})	(m^{01}, p^{01})
T_ξ=1	(m^{10}, p^{10})	(m^{11}, p^{11})
Marginal Total	(m^0, 1 – p)	(m^1, p)

Assume that the same diagnostic threshold ξ was applied to elicit prior information, with the corresponding 2 × 2 table (Table 5.2). Broemeling (2007) specified a multinomial prior distribution as follows, with the total count M in the pilot data:

$$f(\mathbf{m},\mathbf{p}) = f(m^{00},m^{01},m^{10},m^{11};m,p^{00},p^{01},p^{10},p^{11})$$

$$= \begin{cases} \dfrac{m!}{m^{00}!m^{01}!m^{10}!m^{11}!}\left(p^{00}\right)^{m^{00}}\left(p^{01}\right)^{m^{01}}\left(p^{10}\right)^{m^{10}}\left(p^{11}\right)^{m^{11}}, \end{cases} \tag{5-4}$$

$$\text{where} \sum_{k'=0}^{1}\sum_{k=0}^{1} m^{kk'} = M, 0, \text{ otherwise.}$$

Similarly, the joint likelihood function $\mathbf{P}$ = (p^{00}, p^{01}, p^{10}, p^{11}) is given below, with the total count N in the current data:

$$L(\mathbf{p} \mid \mathbf{n}) = \begin{cases} \dfrac{n!}{n^{00}!n^{01}!n^{10}!n^{11}!}\left(p^{00}\right)^{n^{00}}\left(p^{01}\right)^{n^{01}}\left(p^{10}\right)^{n^{10}}\left(p^{11}\right)^{n^{11}} & \text{where} \displaystyle\sum_{k'=0}^{1}\sum_{k=0}^{1} n^{kk'} = N, \\ 0, \text{ otherwise.} \end{cases} \tag{5-5}$$

It can be shown that the posterior distribution for $\mathbf{p}$ is a Dirichlet distribution:

$$\mathbf{p} \mid \mathbf{m},\mathbf{n} \sim Dir(m^{00}+n^{00}+1, m^{01}+n^{01}+1, m^{10}+n^{10}+1, m^{11}+n^{11}+1),$$

where

$$f(\mathbf{p} \mid \mathbf{m},\mathbf{n}) = \frac{1}{Z(\mathbf{m},\mathbf{n})}\prod_{k'=0}^{1}\prod_{k=0}^{1}\left(p^{kk'}\right)^{\left(m^{kk'}+n^{kk'}-1\right)}, \tag{5-6}$$

with a normalizing constant:

$$\frac{1}{Z(\mathbf{m},\mathbf{n})} = \frac{\prod_{k'=0}^{1}\prod_{k=0}^{1}\Gamma\left(m^{kk'}+n^{kk'}\right)}{\Gamma\left[\sum_{k'=0}^{1}\sum_{k=0}^{1}\left(m^{kk'}+n^{kk'}\right)\right]}.$$

TABLE 5.3

2 × 2 Table of Dichotomized Prostate-Specific Antigen Values for Local and Advanced Prostate Cancer Stages Using Decision Threshold Levels $\xi \leq 10$ versus $\xi > 10$

Dichotomized Decision versus Gold Standard	$D = 0$ (Local Disease State)	$D = 1$ (Advanced Disease Stage)
$T_{10} = 0$	(58, 0.32)	(54, 0.30)
$T_{10} = 1$	(8, 0.04)	(60, 0.33)
Marginal Total	(66, 0.37)	(114, 0.63)

The parameter $(m^{kk'} + n^{kk'})$is interpreted as a prior observation count for events governed by **p**; $\Gamma(\bullet)$ is the gamma function. To sample the function (rdiric) from the Direchlet, the R software VGAM package of Yee (2010) may be used. http://www.stat.auckland.ac.nz/~yee/VGAM/index.html.

Example: prostate-specific antigen in staging local versus advanced prostate cancer — This example was illustrated in Chapter 3. O'Malley and Zou (2006) analyzed the data covering radical prostatectomies performed in all cases to provide a binary gold standard; patients were classified into two groups. Among 180 subjects, 66 patients had local disease (Stage A or B) and 114 patients had advanced disease (Stage C1, C2, or D). The PSA level was treated as the outcome variable. A dichotomizing threshold [ξ £ 10 versus $\xi > 10$] was considered with resulting frequency counts under the two classes presented in Table 5.3. The resulting sample estimates were prevalence = 0.63; specificity = 0.88; sensitivity = 0.53; $PV^- =$ 0.52; and $PV^+ = 0.88$.

We assume a lack of prior information, with $\mathbf{m} = (m^{00}, m^{01}, m^{10}, m^{11}) =$ (0,0,0,0), which is equivalent to a uniform prior distribution for the various underlying proportions. We then assume a hypothetical informative prior distribution, with $\mathbf{m} = (m^{00}, m^{01}, m^{10}, m^{11}) = (50, 50, 50, 50)$. Such prior knowledge is derived using prevalence = 0.50; specificity = 0.50; sensitivity = 0.50; $PV^- = 0.50$; and $PV^+ = 0.50$, implying low sensitivity and specificity values with substantial masses at high and low values.

Direct sampling with 1000 samples was performed from the posterior distribution using a Dirichlet distribution from Equation (5-6) and the VGAM package in R. The HPD regions were formed for each of these prior distributions (Figure 5.1). Summary statistics from the posterior distributions are shown in Table 5.4. Note that the uniform prior led to the posterior medians similar to those observed in the current data, while the sharp informative prior yielded a compromise between it and the current observed data (Figure 5.2).

In the absence of a GS and with correlated tests, Joseph et al. (1995), Black and Craig (2002), and Dendukuri et al. (2001) specified conditional dependence of multiple diagnostic tests and developed Bayesian methods for estimating prevalence. Dendukuri et al. (2004) used the Bayesian average coverage,

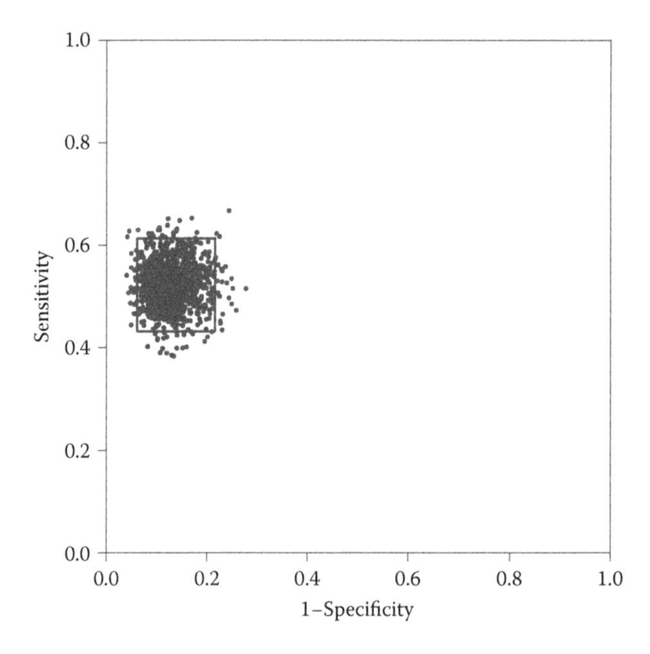

FIGURE 5.1
Posterior samples and 95% HPD regions using uniform prior information by drawing 1000 samples from corresponding Dirichlet distributions.

TABLE 5.4
Estimated Functions of Parameters Based on Corresponding Dirichlet Distributions for Posterior Distributions

Prior Information for m	Function	Median	HPD Region 2.5-th Percentile	HPD Region 97.5-th Percentile
$(m^{00}, m^{01}, m^{10}, m^{11})$	Prevalence	0.63	0.56	0.68
$= (0, 0, 0, 0)$	Specificity	0.87	0.78	0.92
	Sensitivity	0.53	0.43	0.59
	PV^-	0.52	0.42	0.58
	PV^+	0.88	0.79	0.92
$(m^{00}, m^{01}, m^{10}, m^{11})$	Prevalence	0.56	0.51	0.60
$= (50, 50, 50, 50)$	Specificity	0.65	0.58	0.70
	Sensitivity	0.51	0.45	0.56
	PV^-	0.51	0.45	0.56
	PV+	0.65	0.59	0.70

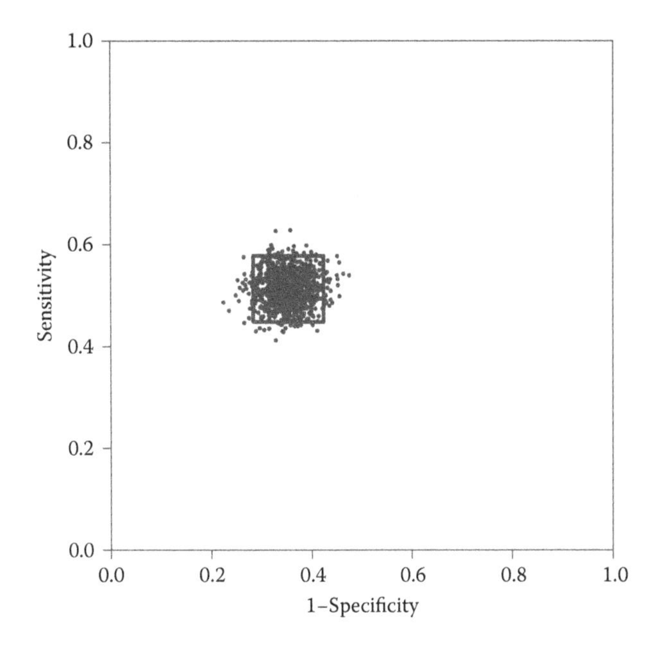

FIGURE 5.2
Posterior samples and 95% HPD regions using informative prior information by drawing 1000 samples from corresponding Dirichlet distributions.

average length, and worst outcome criteria for sample size calculations for designing prevalence studies. Choi et al. (2006) compared AUCs to quantify several tests. The kappa statistic based on two binary diagnostic tests may be computed using the joint posterior Dirichlet distribution (Broemeling, 2007). Additional agreement indices in reliability analysis may be found in Fleiss (1986) and Shoukri (2004).

5.3 Clustered Data Structures and Hierarchical Methods

Several authors evaluated various functions other than mean prevalence rates over different clusters. Joseph et al. (1995; 1997) and Dendukuri et al. (2004) studied the difference between two proportions. Functions such as the range of prevalence under fully exchangeable or partially exchangeable assumptions were studied by Zou and Normand (1999) and Normand and Zou (2001).

Example: designing predictive study of complications following angioplasty — Zou et al. (2006) illustrated Bayesian hierarchical methods to design a hypothetical study of in-hospital complications following angioplasty. Computerized models were used by clinical providers to predict major complications using an algorithm based on preprocedural variables. A multilevel model may be assumed using the following data structure.

Strata: There are $k = 1,\ldots s$, with $s = 3$ strata (postgraduate years = PGY4 and PGY7; physician assistant = PA) indicating category of provider experience.

Clusters: For the k-th strata, there are a total of c_k clusters (providers). Specifically, $c_1 = 28$ PGY4s, $c_2 = 10$ PGY7s, and $c_3 = 12$ PAs.

Individuals: The number of cluster-specific individuals n_k is assumed to be balanced: n_1 individuals per PGY4, n_2 individuals per PGY7, and n_3 individuals per PA, with a total $N = \Sigma_{k=1}^{s} n_k c_k$ during the length of study.

The mean risk of death was based on pilot data provided by Resnic et al. (2001). The sample size was computed for a target length Δ of a $(1 - \delta)\%$ confidence interval. For each stratum k, the estimated number of event Y_{ki} for provider i, $I = 1,\ldots,c_k$, is assumed to have an independent binomial distribution with an event rate θ_{ki},

$$(Y_{ki} \mid n_k, \theta_{ki}) \sim Binormial(n_k, \theta_{ki}). \tag{5-7}$$

For simplicity, all of the above θ_k share a common θ, i.e., $\theta_k = \theta$, $\forall_k$. The lower and upper bounds of an approximate $100(1-\delta)\%$ posterior credible region constructed for $\bar{\theta} = 1/c_k \Sigma_{i=1}^{c_k} \theta_{ki}$ is defined by:

$$\pm\Phi^{-1}\left(1 - \frac{\delta}{2}\right)\left\{\frac{\theta(1-\theta)}{n_k c_k}\right\}^{1/2}, \tag{5-8}$$

where the first term $\Phi^{-1}(1 - \delta/2)$ is the inverse standard normal quantile with a tail probability of $\delta/2$. The sample size per cluster is given by:

$$n_s = \frac{2\left\{\Phi^{-1}\left(1 - \frac{\delta}{2}\right)\right\}^2 \theta(1-\theta)}{c_k \Delta^2}. \tag{5-9}$$

Assume $\Delta = 1\%$ and the underlying event rate such as death is typically low ($\theta = 2\%$). Based on the pilot data provided by Resnic et al. (2001), we assume that for each stratum, k the event rate θ_{ki} has a common beta distribution with hyperparameters (a_k, b_k).

$$(\theta_{ki} \mid a_k, b_k) \sim beta(a_k, b_k) \tag{5-10}$$

Several methods can elicit the hyperparameters. A uniform flat prior gives [1,1]. When a and b are equal, the density function is symmetric at 0.5. However, when $a > b$, the function is right skewed with the tail pointing toward 1. Conversely, when $a < b$, it is left skewed with tail toward 0. Jeffery's prior is $(a, b) = (0.5, 0.5)$. Realistic values for the hyperparameters (a_k, b_k) are specified using the method-of-moments estimation:

$$\mu_{ki} = E(\theta_{ki} \mid a_k, b_k) = \frac{a_k}{a_k + b_k} \text{ and } Var(\theta_{ki} \mid a_k, b_k) = \frac{1}{(a_k + b_k + 1)} \mu_{ki}(1 - \mu_{ki}). \quad (5\text{-}11)$$

Because the mean rate is at 2%, under Equation (5-11), the hyperparameters at $(a_k, b_k) = (1.0, 49.0)$ for PGY4s with a prior SD of 1.96%; (1.1, 55.0) for PGY7s with SD of 1.83%; and (1.2, 59.0) for PAs with SD of 1.79%, suggesting less variability among the PAs since they have greater clinical experience in subjective risk assessment. The posterior distribution of the rate parameter also has a beta distribution:

$$(\theta_{ki} \mid y_{ki}, a_k, b_k) \sim beta(u_{ki}, v_{ki}), \quad (5\text{-}12)$$

where $u_{ki} = y_{ki} + a_k$ and $v_{ki} = n_k - y_{ki} + b_k$. The posterior mean and variance of the mean rate in each stratum, $\bar{\theta} = 1/k_k \Sigma_{i=1}^{c_k} \theta_{ki}$, are derived using the beta distribution:

$$\mu_k = E(\bar{\theta} \mid y_k, a_k, b_k) = \frac{1}{c_k} \sum_{i=1}^{c_k} \frac{u_{ki}}{u_{ki} + v_{ki}},$$

$$\sigma_k^2 = \text{var}(\bar{\theta} \mid y_k, a_k, b_k) = \frac{1}{c_k^2} \sum_{i=1}^{c_k} \frac{u_{ki} v_{ki}}{(u_{ki} + v_{ki})^2 (u_{ki} + v_{ki} + 1)}. \quad (5\text{-}13)$$

The priors u_{sj} and v_{sj} are given in Equation (5-12). The lower and upper bounds of a $100(1 - \delta)\%$ HPD region for estimating $\bar{\theta} = 1/c_k \Sigma_{i=1}^{c_k} \theta_{ki}$ are constructed by approximating the posterior beta distribution by a normal distribution:

$$\pm \Phi^{-1}\left(1 - \frac{\delta}{2}\right)\left(\sigma_k^2\right)^{1/2}, \quad (5\text{-}14)$$

with σ_k^2 given in Equation (5-13).

To compute the necessary sample size for each stratum, y_{ki} values are simulated and the optimal sample sizes are computed using Markov chain Monte Carlo (MCMC) (Chen et al., 2000). Numerical methods and enhanced Bayesian software programs such as OpenBUGS or WinBugs allow faster and more complex computations (Lunn and Spiegelhalter, 2009).

During each l Monte Carlo iteration, $\forall l = 1, \ldots, L$, with a guess of the target sample size n_k, the length of an HPD region is computed by $\hat{\Delta}_{kl} = 2\Phi^{-1}(1 - \delta/2)\sigma_{kl}$. Over L iterations, the corresponding average estimated length is then $\hat{\Delta}_k = 1/L \Sigma_{l=1}^{L} \hat{\Delta}_{kl}$. The optimal sample size n_1 is the largest integer such that the average HPD region stays within the specified target length $\hat{\Delta}_{kl} \leq \Delta_k$. For example, the target interval length Δ is fixed at 1% for all strata. A reasonable initial guess of the sample size n_s is to subtract the

TABLE 5.5

Estimated Sample Sizes for Design of Hypothetical Predictive Study (Bayesian Method) of Complications Following Angioplasty

Provider Type (s)	Number of Clusters (k_s)	Beta Priors (a_s, b_s)	Optimal Cluster Size (n_s)	Total Stratum Size ($N_s = n_s k_s$)
PGY4	28	(1.0, 49.0)	51	1428
PGY7	10	(1.1, 55.0)	199	1990
PA	12	(1.2, 59.0)	170	2040

precision parameter from the non-Bayesian solution presented in Equation (5-9), i.e., $n_{k[\text{Initial}]} = n_{k[\text{Non-Bayesian}]} - (a_s + b_s)$. See Zou and Normand, 2001.

At the significance level, $\delta = 5\%$, the target average length is $\Delta = 1\%$ and the underlying predicted mortality rate is $\theta = 2\%$. The sample sizes required in the cardiovascular clinical example by the Bayesian method are presented in Table 5.5. Total stratum size = 5458 patients. In contrast, the non-Bayesian solution requires $N = 9056$ patients: for a total of 50 providers (108 patients each for 28 PGY4s, 302 patients each for 10 PGY7s, and 251 patients each for 12 PAs) were required.

5.4 Assumptions and Models for ROC Analysis

Let **Y** be the vector of outcomes, **X** be the design matrix, and **è** a set of associated regression parameters. The number of observations is denoted by N and the number of regression parameters by k. Define $\mathbf{I}(\sigma_1^2, \sigma_2^2)$ as an n -dimensional diagonal matrix with the i-th diagonal element σ_1^2 if Subject i is nondiseased and σ_2^2 if this subject is diseased.

For simplicity, examine two diagnostic variables, x_1 and x_2, along with disease status D. The design matrix contains rows of the form $(1, D, x_1, x_2)$ and $(1, D, x_1, x_2, x_1 x_2)$, respectively. An essential feature of this model is that besides disease status, the regression effects are the same for diseased and nondiseased patients. Two regression models relate the expected value of the outcome to the GS and covariates. First, in the "full" model, all terms are considered, including interactions between disease status and covariates and interactions among covariates. Second, in the "partial" model, the disease–covariate interaction terms are omitted. For the prostate example, the regression equations are given by:

$$\text{Partial Model: } \mu_{D,X} = \theta^* + \theta_0 D + \theta_1 x_1 + \theta_2 x_2,$$
$$\text{Full Model: } \mu_{D,X} = \theta^* + \theta_0 D + \theta_1 x_1 + \theta_2 x_2 + \theta_3 D x_1 + \theta_4 D x_2. \tag{5-15}$$

If interactions between the covariates are included, these models may be expanded. In this case, the design matrix for the full model contains rows of the forms (1, D, x_1, x_2, Dx_1, Dx_2) and (1, D, x_1, x_2, $x_1 x_2$, Dx_1, Dx_2, $Dx_1 x_2$), respectively.

$$\text{Partial Model: } \mu_{D,X} = \theta^* + \theta_0 D + \theta_1 x_1 + \theta_2 x_2 + \theta_3 x_1 x_2,$$

$$\text{Full Model: } \mu_{D,X} = \theta^* + \theta_0 D + \theta_1 x_1 + \theta_2 x_2 + \theta_3 x_1 x_2 + \theta_4 D x_1 + \theta_5 D x_2 + \theta_6 D x_1 x_2. \tag{5-16}$$

To generalize, consider diagnostic data in the form of a triplet (Y,D,X). Let f denote the joint probability distribution function of any random variables. The statistical model is expressed as:

$$\begin{aligned} &\mathbf{Y} \mid \mathbf{X}, \theta, \sigma_1^2, \sigma_2^2 \sim N\{\mathbf{X}\theta, \mathbf{I}(\sigma_1^2, \sigma_2^2)\}, \\ &\theta_j \sim N(\mu_j, \tau_j^2), \\ &\sigma_s^2 \sim IG(\upsilon_{s1}, \upsilon_{s2}), \end{aligned} \tag{5-17}$$

where (μ_j, τ_j^2), ($j = 1,\ldots,k$), and $\upsilon_{s1}, \upsilon_{s2}$ ($s = 1,2$) are prior parameters. The posterior distribution of θ is expressed as:

$$f(\theta, \theta^2 \mid \mathbf{Y}, D, \mathbf{X}) = \frac{f(\mathbf{Y} \mid D, \mathbf{X}, \theta, \sigma^2) f(\theta, \sigma^2)}{f(\mathbf{Y} \mid D, \mathbf{X})}, \tag{5-18}$$

where $\theta = (\theta^*, \theta_0, \theta_1, \ldots, \theta_k)$, $\sigma^2 = (\sigma_1^2, \sigma_2^2)$, and $f(\mathbf{Y} \mid D, \mathbf{X}) = \int f(\mathbf{Y} \mid D, \mathbf{X}, \theta, \sigma^2) f(\theta, \sigma^2)$ $d\theta$ as the marginal distribution of the data. The posterior expectation of any function of the parameters, say, $g(\theta)$, is given by:

$$E[g(\theta) \mid \mathbf{Y}, d, \mathbf{X}] = \int g(\theta) p(\theta \mid \mathbf{Y}, D, \mathbf{X})\, d\theta. \tag{5-19}$$

The Gibbs sampler can be used to approximate the posterior distribution (see Gelman et al., 1995; Calin and Louis, 2000; Gamerman and Lopes, 2006). For computations, OpenBUGS or WinBugs software programs (Lunn and Spiegelhalter, 2009; http://www.mrc-bsu.cam.ac.uk/bugs) may be used to directly simulate the posterior distribution or the posterior mean via the Gibbs sampler, Metropolis–Hastings algorithm, or adaptation thereof.

5.5 Normality Transformation

The Box–Cox transformation may improve goodness of fit because the subsequent linear regression analysis more closely satisfies the assumptions of the model. In practice, an ad hoc log transformation of positive data is often employed. However, simply taking a log transformation of positively valued marker data may not yield normally distributed random variables. For each cluster, the Box–Cox transformation is applied to estimate an optimal nonlinear transformation of the positive valued diagnostic outcome data:

$$h_{\lambda_k}(Y_{ki}, \lambda_k) = \begin{cases} \dfrac{Y_i^{\lambda_k} - 1}{\lambda_k}, & if \lambda_k \neq 0, \\ \log(Y_{ki}^{\lambda_k}), & otherwise. \end{cases} \tag{5-20}$$

Besides a flat prior, a useful noninformative one for λ_k is the Jeffreys' prior (Jeffreys 1961; Kass and Wasserman 1996; 1998). The latter is the square root of the determinant of the Fisher information matrix.

Example: prostate-specific antigen in staging local versus advanced prostate cancer — See O'Malley and Zou (2006) and Chapter 3 for a description of this example. The outcome variable is prostate-specific antigen (PSA) level. Using a noninformative prior for the optimal Box–Cox transformation, the estimated coefficients ranged from 0.30 to 0.40 across different clusters. The posterior distributions of the estimated Box–Cox transformation coefficient are displayed in Figure 5.3. The means and standard errors (SEs) of

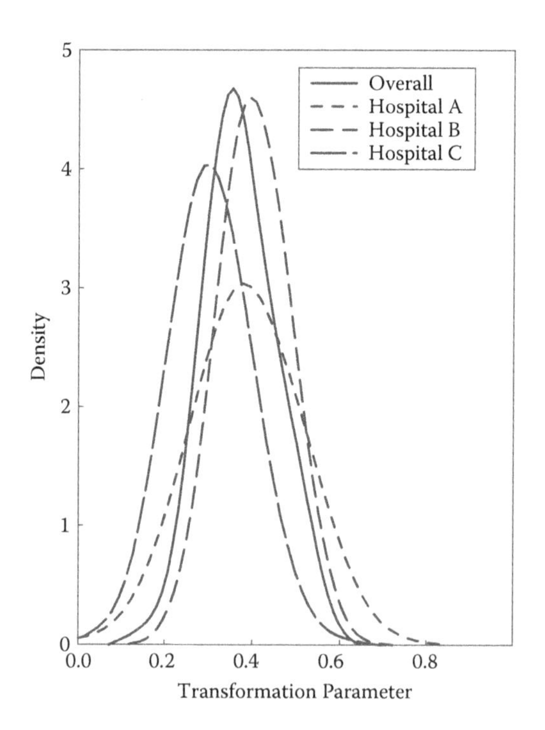

FIGURE 5.3
Estimated optimal Box–Cox transformation coefficient using diffuse prior for PSA example.

the estimated power coefficient of the transformation were 0.39 (SE = 0.12), 0.40 (SE = 0.08), and 0.30 (SE = 0.09) for the three strata (hospitals), respectively. Under pooled analysis, an overall transformation of 0.37 (SE = 0.08) was obtained. Thus, different transformations for each hospital appear necessary.

5.6 Elicitation of Prior Information

In radiology studies, prior information about diagnostic tests may often be extracted from pilot data, meta-analyses of the relevant literature, or existing scientific theory. The incorporation of prior information often results in inferences that are more precise than by the use of frequentist methods, if supported by data. Elicitation of prior distribution was already illustrated. Here we elaborate further on the appropriate choice of prior distribution. Although anticonservative priors may lead to much more precise information, the assumptions should be investigated carefully using pilot data. By adding another stage, the estimation procedure becomes more cumbersome.

Eliciting prior information requires a number of considerations. No prior information or noninformative prior distributions may be available. If pilot data are scarce (no information or vague information), the construction of informative priors may be ad hoc and thus diffuse priors may be considered. This level of knowledge is introduced by specifying prior distributions with very large values for the underlying variance, and is appropriate for analyzing studies based on very little prior knowledge. Bayesian inferences under a diffuse prior are generally indistinguishable from those based on maximum likelihood estimation. This will not be the case when the posterior distribution is asymmetric using a Bayesian estimator, e.g., a posterior mean other than the posterior mode.

Where informative prior distributions are available, the sharper the prior distribution, the more informative the prior becomes, resulting in greater impact on the results based on the posterior distribution. Informative prior distributions are considered for the main regression coefficient of the GS. This parameter is the most important because the estimated diagnostic accuracies are highly sensitive to it. The prior distributions for all regression coefficients may be assumed to have independent normal distributions. The prior distributions for variance terms are assumed to be independent inverse gamma distributions. Other hyperparameters may be determined (Kass and Wasserman, 1996; 1998).

The advantage of incorporating prior information is that the knowledge obtained prior to the analysis may be incorporated. The resulting estimated diagnostic accuracy would show various degrees of sensitivity to the choice of priors. Thus, a conservative or noninformative prior distribution may result in lower estimated diagnostic accuracy. On the other hand, an optimistic or sharper prior distribution is recommended if a test is believed to perform well despite variability in the observed data. Choosing prior distributions should not be arbitrary; it should depend on the pilot data or available prior beliefs. The sensitivity of the choice of prior distributions must be investigated.

If prior information does not agree well with evidence in the data, the posterior distribution will be less precise. The prior for a secondary clinical study may also be quite useful since the posterior distribution of the parameters derived from the current study as its prior construction, or at least the basis of its prior distribution.

5.7 Estimation of ROC Parameters and Characteristics

By designating a specificity value, the corresponding point on the ROC curve for cluster k is (1-specificity, sensitivity) or $[FPF = \Phi\{\mu_k + \nu_k\Phi^{-1}(1 - FPF)\}]$, where Φ is the CDF of $N[0,1]$. For given 1-specificity = FPF, the underlying sensitivity is $TPF_k = \Phi\{\mu_k + \nu_k\Phi^{-1}(FPF)\}$. The AUC is given by $A_k = \Phi(\mu_k/\sqrt{1+\nu_k^2})$. HPD regions may be constructed for both measures.

To obtain the posterior distribution, MCMC may be performed. With a burn-in of 2,000 iterations and a main simulation of 10,000 iterations, MCMC revealed that the accuracy was the highest for Hospital C (AUC = 0.75) and lowest for Hospital A (AUC = 0.63). See both Figure 5.4 and Table 5.6.

The ROC curves did not vary with different choices of prior distributions (Figure 5.5). Thus, the estimation method is not too sensitive to the choice of prior distribution given the sample size of the data available. By increasing the mean of the normal prior distribution for θ_0 while fixing the variance, the curves move from conservative (e.g., smaller AUC) to anticonservative (e.g., larger AUC). When increasing the variance of the normal prior distribution for θ_0 while fixing the mean, they become more conservative.

5.9 Remarks and Further Reading

Data in radiology research are often subject to variability, reflected in the distributions of regression parameters and error variances. Complex data structures typically include individual subjects, healthcare providers, clinical centers, and geographic regions, thereby allowing for several levels in a hierarchical analysis. Cluster sizes may vary substantially. In addition, both individual- and cluster-level covariates are often available for

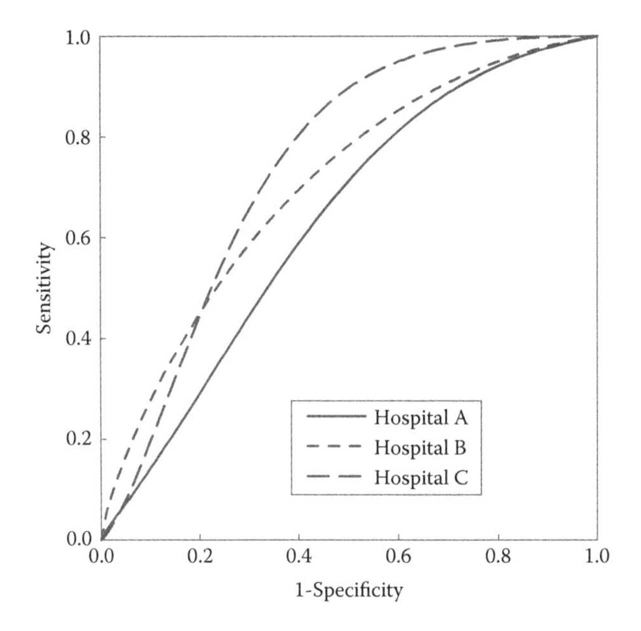

FIGURE 5.4
ROC curves by cluster (hospital) for prostate-specific antigen example.

TABLE 5.6
Estimated AUCs by Cluster and Risk Group

Cluster or Risk Group		Sample Size (%)	AUC (SE)
Hospital	A	25 (14%)	0.63 (0.07)
	B	93 (52%)	0.70 (0.05)
	C	62 (34%)	0.75 (0.06)
Risk Group	Low (L)	88 (49%)	0.67 (0.06)
	Intermediate (I)	51 (28%)	0.77 (0.07)
	High (H)	41 (23%)	0.70 (0.13)

measuring, for example, disease severity and comorbidity for individual patients, and the location, size, and organizational characteristics of a specific clinical center.

Bayesian methods have been used widely in diagnostic medicine and meta-analysis. ROC analysis involves several nonlinearities. The expression for the AUC under the binormal model, the maximum improvement of sensitivity (equivalent to that of the Youden index) over random chance (O'Malley et al., 2001), and Bayesian computational techniques provide natural ways of evaluating inferences without resorting to analytical (closed-form) approximations. Bayesian analysis or computation based on nonlinear problems may be particularly useful.

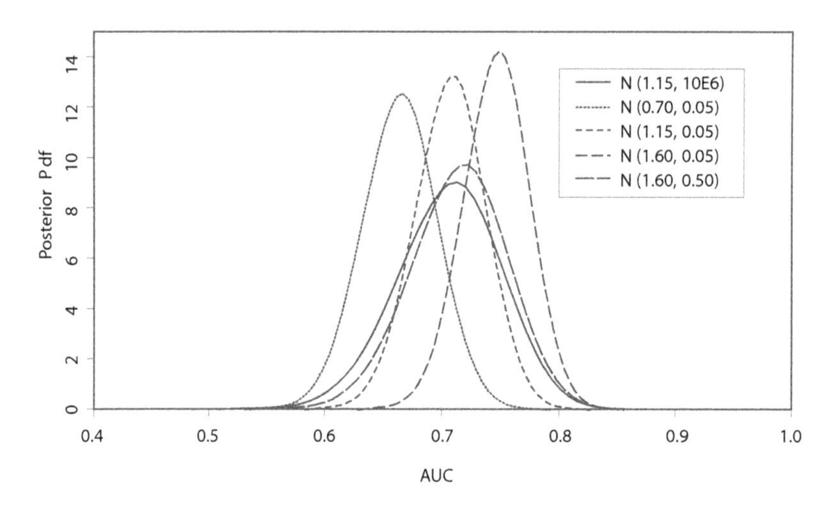

FIGURE 5.5
ROC curves derived under various prior distributions for prostate-specific antigen example.

For further readings, refer to Rutter and Gatsonis (1995; 2001), Peng and Hall (1996), Helmich et al. (1998), Ishwaran and Gatsonis (2000), O'Malley et al. (2001), O'Malley and Zou (2006), Erkani et al. (2006), Gu et al. (2008), Branscum et al. (2008), Wang and Gatsonis (2008), and Miller et al. (2009), among other works. A number of advantages arise from a Bayesian approach. Complex designs may be incorporated using a hierarchical structure. The parameters in the model or their functions, such as summary measures and characteristics, may be simulated directly from posterior distributions. Prior knowledge or pilot information may be incorporated into the models.

References

Black, M.A. and Craig, B.A. 2002. Estimating disease prevalence in the absence of a gold standard. *Statistics in Medicine* 21: 2653–2669.

Branscum, A.J., Johnson, W.O., Hanson, T.E. et al. 2008. Bayesian semiparametric ROC curve estimation and disease diagnosis. *Statistics in Medicine* 27: 2474–2496.

Broemeling, L.D. 2007. *Bayesian Biostatistics and Diagnostic Medicine*. Boca Raton: Chapman & Hall.

Cao, J., Lee, J.J., and Alber, S. 2009. Comparison of Bayesian sample size criteria: ACC, ALC, and WOC. *Journal of Statistical Planning and Inference* 139: 4111–4122.

Carlin, B.P. and Louis, T.A. 2000. *Bayes and Empirical Bayesian Methods for Data Analysis*. London: Chapman & Hall.

Chen, M.H., Shao, Q.M., and Ibrahim, J.G. 2000. *Monte Carlo Methods in Bayesian Computation*. New York: Springer.

Choi, Y.K., Johnson, W.O., Collins, M.T. et al. 2006. Bayesian inferences for receiver operating characteristic curves in the absence of a gold standard. *Journal of Agricultural, Biological, and Environmental Statistics* 11: 210–229.

Dendukuri, N. and Joseph, L. 2001. Bayesian approaches to modeling the conditional dependence between multiple diagnostic tests. *Biometrics* 57: 158–167.

Dendukuri, N., Rahme, E., Bélisle, P. et al. 2004. Bayesian sample size determination for prevalence and diagnostic test studies in the absence of a gold standard. *Biometrics* 60: 388–397.

Donner, A. and Klar, N. 2004. Pitfalls of and controversies in cluster randomization trials. *American Journal of Public Health* 94: 416–422.

Erkanli, A., Sung, M., Costello, E.J. et al. 2006. Bayesian semi-parametric ROC analysis. *Statistics in Medicine* 25: 3905–3928.

Fleiss, J.L. 1986. *The Design and Analysis of Clinical Experiments*. New York: Wiley.

Fluss, R., Faraggi, D., and Reiser, B. 2005. Estimation of the Youden index and its associated cutoff point. *Biometrical Journal* 47: 458–472.

Gammerman, D. and Lopes, H.F. 2006. *Markov Chain Monte Carlo: Stochastic Simulation for Bayesian Inference*. Boca Raton: Chapman & Hall.

Gelman, A., Carlin, J.B., Stern, H.S. et al. 1995. *Bayesian Data Analysis*. London: Chapman & Hall.

Gu, J., Ghosal, S., and Roy, A. 2008. Bayesian bootstrap estimation of ROC curve. *Statistics in Medicine* 27: 5407–5420.

Hellmich, M., Abrams, K.R., Jones, D.R. et al. A Bayesian approach to a general regression model for ROC curves. *Medical Decision Making* 18: 436–443.

Ishwaran, H. and Gatsonis, C.A. 2000. A general class of hierarchical ordinal regression models with applications to correlated ROC analysis. *Canadian Journal of Statistics* 28: 731–775.

Jeffreys, H. 1961. *Theory of Probability*. Oxford: Oxford University Press.

Joseph, L., du Berger, R., and Bélisle, P. 1997. Bayesian and mixed Bayesian likelihood criteria for sample size determination. *Statistics in Medicine* 16: 769–781.

Joseph, L., Gyorkos, T.W., and Coupal, L. 1995. Bayesian estimation of disease prevalence and the parameters of diagnostic tests in the absence of a gold standard. *American Journal of Epidemiology* 141: 263–272.

Joseph, L. and Wolfson, D.B. 1997. Interval-based versus decision theoretic criteria for the choice of sample size. *Statistician* 46: 145–149.

Kass, R.E. and Wasserman, L. 1996. The selection of prior distributions by formal rules. *Journal of the American Statistical Association* 91: 1343–1370.

Kass, R.E. and Wasserman, L. 1998. The selection of prior distributions by formal rules. *Journal of the American Statistical Association* 93: 412.

Lunn, D., Spiegelhalter, D., Thomas, A. et al. 2009. The BUGS project: evolution, critique and future directions. *Statistics in Medicine* 28: 3049–3067.

Metz, C.E., Herman, B.A., and Shen, J.H. 1998. Maximum likelihood estimation of receiver operating characteristic (ROC) curves from continuously distributed data. *Statistics in Medicine* 17: 1033–1053.

Miller, S.W., Sinha, D., Slate, E.H. et al. 2009. Bayesian adaptation of the summary ROC Curve method for meta-analysis of diagnostic test performance. *Journal of Data Science* 7: 349–364.

Normand, S.L. and Zou, K,H. 2002. Sample size considerations in observational health care quality studies. *Statistics in Medicine* 21: 331–345.

O'Malley, A.J., Zou, K.H., Fielding, J.R. et al. C.M. 2001. Bayesian regression methodology for estimating a receiver operating characteristic curve with two radiologic applications: prostate biopsy and spiral CT of ureteral stones. *Academic Radiology* 8: 713–725.

O'Malley, A.J. and Zou, K.H. 2006. Bayesian multivariate hierarchical transformation models for ROC analysis. *Statistics in Medicine* 25: 459–479.

Parmigiani, G. 2002. Measuring uncertainty in complex decision analysis models. *Statistical Methods in Medical Research* 11: 513–537.

Peng, F. and Hall, W. J. 1996. Bayesian analysis of ROC curves using Markov chain Monte Carlo methods. *Medical Decision Making* 16: 404–411.

Resnic, F.S., Ohno-Machado, L., Selwyn et al. 2001. Simplified risk score models accurately predict the risk of major in-hospital complications following percutaneous coronary intervention. *American Journal of Cardiology* 88: 5–9.

Rutter, C.M. and Gatsonis, C.A. 2001. A hierarchical regression approach to meta-analysis of diagnostic test accuracy evaluations. *Statistics in Medicine* 20: 2865–2884.

Shoukri, M.M. 2004. *Measures of Inter-Observer Agreement*. Boca Raton: Chapman & Hall.

Wang, F. and Gatsonis, C.A. 2008. Hierarchical models for ROC curve summary measures: design and analysis of multi-reader, multi-modality studies of medical tests. *Statistics in Medicine* 27: 243–256.

Yee, T.W. 2010. The VGAM package for categorical data analysis. *Journal of Statistical Software* 32: 1–34.

Zou, G.Y., Donner, A., and Klar, N. 2005. Group sequential methods for cluster randomization trials with binary outcomes. *Clinical Trials* 2: 479–487.

Zou, K.H. and Normand, S.L. 2001. On determination of sample size in hierarchical binomial models. *Statistics in Medicine* 20: 2163–2182.

Zou, K.H. and O'Malley, A.J. 2005. A Bayesian hierarchical nonlinear regression model in receiver operating characteristic analysis of clustered continuous diagnostic data. *Biometrical Journal* 47: 417–427.

Zou, K.H., Resnic, F.S., Gogate, A. et al. 2003. Efficient Bayesian sample size calculation for designing a clinical trial with multicluster outcome data. *Biometrical Journal* 45: 826–836.

Section III

Advanced Approaches and Applications

6

Sequential Designs of ROC Experiments

6.1 Introduction

Sequential procedures describe ways to collect data from a target population in conducting a statistical experiment. When a sequential procedure is employed, the data collection process may be terminated based on accumulated data before it reaches the maximum duration. In contrast, a fixed size procedure always continues to its maximum duration that is specified prior to data collection. Therefore a sequential procedure must clearly define when and how the accumulated data are looked at and what criteria are to be used for the sampling process to be terminated.

The origin of sequential methods in design of experiments can be traced back as early as the Second World War in the 1940s, when it was imperative that war-time products produced on a massive scale be inspected in a timely and effective manner. Products that met the standard were to be distributed without delay and the number of products with defects was to be controlled at a reasonable level. These demands subsequently gave birth to certain statistical procedures, now commonly called sequential analysis. Wald's (1945) seminal paper on the sequential probability ratio test (SPRT) procedures provided theoretical justification for the application of sequential methods.

In the past three decades, clinical trials and drug developments have provided much of the motivation for development of new sequential procedures and resulted in a few excellent books summarizing these procedures; see Whitehead (1997), Jennison and Turnbull (2000), and Proschan et al. (2006). Sequential procedures are often cited in the clinical trial literature in the form of *group sequential tests* and include terms such as *early stopping, interim analyses, interim looks, interim monitoring, stopping boundaries,* and *stopping times*. Sequential procedures are utilized mainly to address ethical, administrative, and economic concerns when planning clinical trials. Since clinical trials involve human subjects, it is imperative that unsafe, inferior, and ineffective treatments be avoided, and that effective treatments be administered to patients as early as possible. Such demands can be met by making possible early cessation of a trial when substantial evidence shows superiority of a certain treatment over others. The possible reduction of the number of patients necessary to reach a firm conclusion is also cost effective, reducing both patient costs and administrative burdens.

Accurate diagnosis is the first important step in finding a cure for a disease. Although studies in diagnostic medicine usually concern screening of human subjects for diseases and do not involve life-threatening situations, the needs to employ sequential procedures are parallel. In comparative accuracy trials of diagnostic tests, the main interest is to determine the diagnostic test with the best diagnostic accuracy measured by its sensitivity, specificity, AUC or pAUC (partial AUC), and other plausible measures. Obviously more accurate diagnostic tests should be identified in a timely manner and utilized without delay. Many diagnostic procedures are expensive or inconvenient to patients. Some, such as tumor biopsies for cancer diagnosis, can be very painful to patients and hence should be stopped during a trial if early evidence shows them to be inefficient. Mazumdar (2004) provided a detailed rationale advocating the use of sequential procedures in diagnostic medicine. Various parametric and nonparametric sequential procedures have been developed recently by Mazumdar and Liu (2003), Shu et al. (2007), Liu et al. (2008), Tang et al. (2008) and Zhou et al. (2008).

6.2 Group Sequential Tests Using Large Sample Theory

Implementation of group sequential testing procedures requires evaluation of multiple integration and distribution of a series of correlated test statistics. Except for a few special cases, exact calculation of the operating characteristics (Type I error, power, sample size) of test statistics is usually extensive and difficult, even when the distributions are assumed normal. To further complicate this issue, comparative diagnostic accuracy studies often involve correlated test outcomes resulting from application of a diagnostic test under investigation to the same subjects from diseased and healthy populations. All these factors make exact solutions intractable. Therefore, we often rely on large sample approximations to compute these characteristics when designing a comparative diagnostic accuracy study. To this end, many sequential calculations in clinical trials are based on large sample approximations via the use of Brownian motion, most of which can be straightforwardly extended to diagnostic accuracy studies.

6.2.1 Approximating Test Statistics via Brownian Motion

A Brownian motion $W(t)$ ($t \geq 0$ with $W(0) = 0$) with drift θ is a stochastic process that has many valuable properties. To name a few, for each t, $W(t)$ is normally distributed with mean θt and variance t, i.e., $W(t) \sim N(\theta t, t)$; and for any $0 < t_1 < t_2 < \ldots < t_k < \infty$, $W(t_1)$, $W(t_2) - W(t_1)$, …, $W(t_k) - W(t_{k-1})$ are mutually independent with $W(t_j) - X(t_i) \sim N(\theta(t_j - t_i), t_j - t_i)$ and $COV(W(t_i), W(t_j)) = t_i$, for $i < j$. The Brownian motion framework provides a satisfactory large sample approximation for most test statistics useful in diagnostic medicine whether the test outcomes are continuous, ordinal, or binary. In comparative diagnostic accuracy studies, the θ parameter usually measures the difference in diagnostic accuracy between two tests. For example, when test outcomes are continuous, θ can be defined as the difference between two AUCs or pAUCs. Thus, the null hypothesis of no difference in diagnostic accuracy is set generally to be H_0: $\theta = 0$, versus the two-sided alternative H_1: $\theta \neq 0$.

For a specific diagnostic accuracy study, the t and $W(t)$ statistics may be obtained via a "unified" approach described in Whitehead (1997, 1999) when the likelihood functions are workable. Suppose that $l(\theta, \gamma)$ is the likelihood function of the primary parameter θ under investigation and a nuisance parameter vector γ. Write $l_\theta(\theta, \gamma)$ and $l_\gamma(\theta, \gamma)$ as the first derivatives and $l_{\theta\theta}(\theta, \gamma)$, $l_{\theta\gamma}(\theta, \gamma)$, $l_{\gamma\theta}(\theta, \gamma)$, and $l_{\gamma\gamma}(\theta, \gamma)$ for the second derivatives of the likelihood function with respect to the corresponding parameter(s). Let γ_0^* be the maximum likelihood estimator of γ when $\theta = 0$. Then:

$$t = l_{\theta\theta}(0, \gamma_0^*) - l_{\theta\gamma}(0, \gamma_0^*)\{l_{\gamma\gamma}(0, \gamma_0^*)\}^{-1} l_{\gamma\theta}(0, \gamma_0^*) \tag{6-1}$$

and

$$W(t) = l_\theta(0, \gamma_0^*) \tag{6-2}$$

asymptotically behave like a Brownian motion with drift parameter θ. In these formulas, γ_0^* can be replaced by the maximum likelihood estimator (without assuming $\theta = 0$) or any consistent estimator of γ. An asymptotically equivalent approach is working with maximum likelihood estimation. Let $\hat{\theta}$ be the maximum likelihood estimate of θ, then t is the reciprocal of its estimated variance, and $W(t) = \hat{\theta} t$.

This unified theory cannot be directly extended to nonparametric settings. If nonparametric test statistics are used, special treatment is needed to ensure that the Brownian motion resemblance is appropriate. Fortunately, most nonparametric statistics used in diagnostic medicine are based on U-statistics that may be asymptotically expressed as sums of independent variables (Lehmann, 1999), thus warranting the use of Brownian motion as an approximation. Suppose $\hat{\theta}$ is a nonparametric estimator of θ with variance $V(\hat{\theta})$. Let $\hat{V}$ be a consistent estimator of variance. In general, $\hat{\theta}/\hat{V}$ resembles a Brownian motion with drift θ and $t = 1/\hat{V}$.

It is worth noting that in the formation of a Brownian motion, t is a function of sample sizes—represented in diagnostic accuracy studies as the numbers of diseased and healthy subjects, n^0 and n^1, respectively. This function is often converted to yield the sample sizes needed for the study; see Section 6.6 below.

6.2.2 Group Sequential Testing Procedures

Group sequential procedures for testing a hypothesis are generally based on a fixed size procedure. Within the Brownian motion framework, a fixed sample size procedure tests the null hypothesis based on an observed sample path of the Brownian process over $[0, t]$ where t is fixed. Note that under H_0 $W(t)/\sqrt{t}$ follows a standard normal distribution $N[0, 1]$. Then, with a two-sided alternative $\theta \neq 0$, the null hypothesis H_0: $\theta = 0$ is rejected if $|W(t)| > \sqrt{t}\Phi^{-1}(1-\alpha/2)$, where Φ and φ throughout are, respectively, the cumulative distribution and density function of $N[0, 1]$.

A natural extension of this fixed sample size procedure to a sequential one is as follows. Suppose we wish to conduct up to K interim analyses when t equals to $t_1, t_2, \ldots$, and t_K. The first interim analysis is conducted at $t = t_1$ based on the observed Brownian path on $[0, t_1]$. If $|W(t_1)| > c_1\sqrt{t_1}$, where c_1 is some critical value for the standardized test statistic $W(t_1)/\sqrt{t_1}$, we stop collecting data and reject H_0. If $|W(t_1)| \leq c_1\sqrt{t_1}$, then we continue to the second analysis by observing an additional path on $[t_1, t_2]$.

The second analysis is conducted based on all data collected, that is, $(t_2, W(t_2))$. If $|W(t_2)| > c_2\sqrt{t_2}$, we stop and reject H_0. Otherwise we continue to the next analysis by observing one more additional path on $[t_2, t_3]$. If the test continues to the kth analysis, that is, $|W(t_j)| \leq c_j\sqrt{t_j}$ for each $j \leq k-1$, then the test continues to the kth analysis and H_0 is rejected if $|W(t_k)| > c_k\sqrt{t_k}$. Otherwise the test continues to the $(k + 1)$th stage by observing an additional path from t_k to t_{k+1}. Data collection will be forced to terminate at the last stage, the Kth analysis if $|W(t_k)| \leq c_k\sqrt{t_k}$ for $1 \leq k \leq K-1$, with rejection of the null hypothesis if $|W(t_K)| > c_K\sqrt{t_K}$.

Such a group sequential procedure, often called a symmetric group sequential procedure, is the most popular choice for therapeutic clinical trials. The critical values are often called stopping boundaries (for standardized test statistics). These sequential tests allow early stopping only for rejection of the null hypothesis. A decision not to reject the null hypothesis can be made only at the last stage. Other versions of sequential testing procedures also appear in the literature. For example, asymmetric boundaries $a_k < b_k$ can be used, in which case stopping occurs with rejection of H_0 at the kth stage if $a_j\sqrt{t_j} \leq W(t_j) \leq b_j\sqrt{t_j}$ for $j \leq k-1$ and $W(t_j) < a_j\sqrt{t_j}$ or $W(t_j) > b_j\sqrt{t_j}$ for $j = k$. If early stopping is also imposed for acceptance of the null hypothesis, then some inner-wedge boundaries are needed. For more details on group sequential procedures, see Jennison and Turnbull (2000) and Proschan et al. (2006).

6.2.3 Choosing Stopping Boundaries

To implement a group sequential procedure for a diagnostic accuracy study, we specify K, the total number of interim analysis, t_k, $k = 1, \ldots, K$, the time points at which an interim analysis is performed, and c_k, the stopping boundaries, and rejection region of the null hypothesis. In general these design parameters are chosen so that the Type I error rate is controlled at a significance level α, and the power at a specified alternative value θ_1 is maintained at a level of $1 - \beta$. Note that the fixed size test that rejects H_0 if $|W(t)| > \sqrt{t}\Phi^{-1}(1-\alpha/2)$ has significance level α for each fixed t, and the information needed to achieve the power is

$$t = \left[\frac{\Phi^{-1}(1-\alpha/2)+\Phi^{-1}(1-\beta)}{\theta_1}\right]^2. \tag{6-3}$$

For a group sequential test, the null hypothesis may be rejected at any of the K interim analyses. Therefore, the Type I error constraint gives

$$\sum_{k=1}^{K} P_0(|W(t_j)| \le c_j\sqrt{t_j}, j \le k-1, |W(t_k)| > c_k\sqrt{t_k}) = \alpha, \tag{6-4}$$

where P_θ represents the probability computed when the drift parameter is θ. The power constraint yields

$$\sum_{k=1}^{K} P_{\theta_1}(|W(t_j)| \le c_j\sqrt{t_j}, j \le k-1, |W(t_k)| > c_k\sqrt{t_k}) = 1-\beta. \tag{6-5}$$

Due to repeated testing of the null hypothesis, the Type I error of a group sequential test can be substantially inflated if we set each c_k to be $\Phi^{-1}(1 - \alpha/2)$, the critical value used for a fixed sample size test. For example, with $\alpha = 0.05$, the Type I error probabilities for $2 \le K \le 10$ are 0.08, 0.11, 0.13, 0.14, 0.15, 0.17, 0.18, 0.19, and 0.20, respectively, if we set $c_k = 1.96$ for each k. The Type I error can approach 1 if K is large.

A number of group sequential methods have been proposed in the clinical trial literature to control Type I errors. The procedure by Pocock (1977) considers equally spaced tests, that is, $t_k = (k/K)t_K$, and defines the stopping boundary $c_k = C_P(K, \alpha)$. The procedure proposed in O'Brien and Fleming (1979) is also equally spaced, with stopping boundaries given by $c_k = C_B(K,\alpha)\sqrt{K/k}$. Here C_P and C_B are constants that depend only on the significance level α and the number K of interim analyses and can be determined by the Type I error constraint Equation (6-4). The total information t_K for each procedure is computed from the power constraint Equation (6-5) and is often converted to produce the sample sizes needed. The O'Brien and Fleming boundaries are more commonly used in monitoring clinical trials, since they tend to be more conservative in the sense that early stopping of a test is less likely. Moreover, the critical values and sample sizes at the last analysis are much closer to those for a fixed size test.

Wang and Tsiatis (1987) generalized the above two procedures by considering $c_k = C_{WT}(K, \alpha, \Delta)(k/K)^{\Delta-1/2}$, where Δ defines the shape of the boundary and C_{WT} is a constant for given K, α, and Δ. Thus setting $\Delta = 1/2$ yields Pocock's (1977) boundary and $\Delta = 0$ gives the O'Brien and Fleming (1979) boundary. The shape parameter Δ allows practitioners to design a group sequential test that can be more conservative than Pocock's but less conservative than O'Brien and Fleming's. For various K, α, and Δ, the values of the constant C_{WT} are well tabulated in Jennison and Turnbull (2000), who also provided comparisons among different tests in terms of maximum sample sizes and expected sample sizes for certain alternatives.

In practice, it may be unrealistic to have equally spaced interim analyses since the Fisher information must be estimated from the data. The error spending approach of Lan and DeMets (1983) allows unequally spaced information time and does not require the number K of interim analyses be fixed. However, the maximum information t_K must be fixed to use such an approach. Lan and DeMets define an error spending function $e(t)$ as a function on [0, 1] such that $e(t)$ is strictly increasing in t with $e(0) = 0$ and $e(1) = \alpha$, the significance level of the test. With this error spending function, the first interim analysis can be conducted at any $t_1 < t_K$ with boundary value c_1 and Type I error no larger than $e(t_1/t_K)$, that is,

$$P_0(|W(t_1)| > c_1\sqrt{t_1}) = 2\{1 - \Phi(c_1)\} = e(t_1/t_K),$$

yielding

$$c_1 = \Phi^{-1}\left\{1 - \frac{1}{2}e(t_1/t_K)\right\}.$$

If $|W(t_1)| > c_1\sqrt{t_1}$, the test stops and H_0 is rejected. Otherwise, the test continues to the second analysis at $t_1 < t_2 \le t_K$, with boundary value c_2 and cumulative Type I error no larger than $e(t_2/t_K)$, that is, $P_0(|W(t_1)| > c_1\sqrt{(t_1)} + P_0(|W(t_1)| \le c_1\sqrt{t_1}, |W(t_2)| > c_2\sqrt{(t_2)} = e(t_2/t_K)$, or equivalently $P_0(|W(t_1)| \le c_1\sqrt{t_1}, |W(t_2)| > c_2\sqrt{(t_2)} = e(t_2/t_K) - e(t_1/t_K)$, yielding a c_2 value that may only be computed numerically. If the test continues to the kth stage at t_k ($t_1 < \ldots < t_k < t_K$), the boundary value c_k can be numerically calculated from $P_0(|W(t_j)| \le c_j\sqrt{t_j}, j \le k-1, |W(t_k)| > c_k\sqrt{(t_k)} = e(t_k/t_K) - e(t_{k-1}/t_K)$, which involves calculation of multiple integrations.

Popular error spending functions include

$$e(t) = \begin{cases} \alpha(1-e^{-\gamma t})/(1-e^{-\gamma}), & \text{if } \gamma \neq 0, \\ \alpha t, & \text{if } \gamma = 0, \end{cases}$$

by Hwang et al. (1990), and $e(t) = \min\{\alpha t^{\rho}, \alpha\}$ for some positive value $\rho > 0$, by Kim and DeMets (1987). A list of common error spending functions can be found in Jennison and Turnbull (2000).

As an illustration, let us consider a group sequential test (two-sided) with 10 interim analyses and significance level $\alpha = 0.05$. Figure 6.1 plots the upper boundary for $W(t)$ versus t derived from the methods of Pocock, O'Brien and Fleming, and Wang and Tsiatis with $\Delta = 0.1$, and Hwang et al. with $\gamma = 0$. For better illustration, the maximum information t_K is rescaled as 1. From Jennison and Turnbull (2000), the constants are $C_P = 2.56$, $C_B = 2.09$, and $C_{WT} = 2.12$. The boundary values of Hwang et al. are 2.80, 2.74, 2.67, 2.62, 2.56, 2.51, 2.47, 2.42, 2.39, and 2.35 for the standardized test statistics $(W(t)/\sqrt{t})$, determined by using the free software downloaded from http://www.biostat.wisc.edu/software/index.htm developed by a biostatistics group at the University of Wisconsin. This gives the boundary values for $W(t)$ as 0.89, 1.23, 1.46, 1.66, 1.81, 1.94, 2.07, 2.16, 2.27, and 2.35.

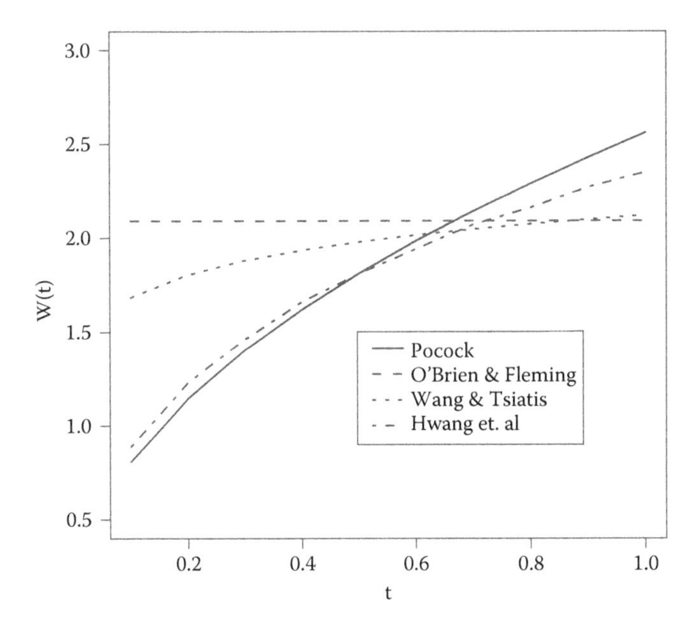

FIGURE 6.1
Stopping boundaries of various types.

6.3 Sequential Evaluation of Single ROC Curve

In a diagnostic accuracy study to evaluate a single test, the question of interest is typically whether the diagnostic test under investigation is useful for distinguishing diseased subjects from healthy subjects. Suppose that the diagnostic test yields continuous test outcomes and its diagnostic accuracy is measured by its AUC. Then the null hypothesis can be set to be H_0: $\theta = AUC - 0.5 = 0$, that is, the diagnostic test performs no better than a random decision. An AUC differing from half indicates that a test has higher accuracy than random assignment of disease status. A group sequential testing procedure will be based on test outcomes $X_1, X_2, \ldots$ from healthy subjects and $Y_1, Y_2, \ldots$ from diseased subjects.

6.3.1 Binormal Model

The binormal model assumes that test outcomes, possibly after certain transformations (e.g., logarithms), from healthy and diseased populations are normally distributed with $X \sim N(\mu_X, \sigma_X^2)$, $Y \sim N(\mu_Y, \sigma_Y^2)$. The ROC curve and its AUC under this model are given by

$$\mathrm{ROC}(FPF) = \Phi(a + b\,\Phi^{-1}(FPF)), \quad \mathrm{AUC} = \Phi\left(\frac{a}{\sqrt{1+b^2}}\right),$$

respectively, where

$$a = \frac{\mu_Y - \mu_X}{\sigma_Y}, \quad b = \frac{\sigma_X}{\sigma_Y}.$$

See, e.g., Pepe (2003). Define

$$\hat{\mu}_Y = \frac{1}{n^1}\sum_{j=1}^{n^1} Y_i, \quad \hat{\sigma}_Y^2 = \frac{1}{n^1}\sum_{j=1}^{n^1}(Y_i - \hat{\mu}_Y)^2,$$

and

$$\hat{\mu}_X = \frac{1}{n^0}\sum_{i=1}^{n^0} X_i, \quad \hat{\sigma}_X^2 = \frac{1}{n^0}\sum_{i=1}^{n^0}(X_i - \hat{\mu}_X)^2,$$

where the maximum likelihood estimate (MLE) of the corresponding parameters n^0 and n^1 are, respectively, the numbers of healthy and diseased subjects. The MLE of the AUC is thus given by

$$\widehat{\text{AUC}} = \Phi\left(\frac{\hat{a}}{\sqrt{1+\hat{b}^2}}\right), \tag{6-6}$$

where

$$\hat{a} = \frac{\hat{\mu}_Y - \hat{\mu}_X}{\hat{\sigma}_Y}, \quad b = \frac{\hat{\sigma}_X}{\hat{\sigma}_Y},$$

are the MLEs of the binormal parameters.

The asymptotic variance of $\widehat{\text{AUC}}$ can be derived using the so-called *delta method* (Rao, 1973) based on Taylor's expansion; see Lehmann (1999). Obuchowski and McClish (1997), Mazumdar and Liu (2003), and Liu and Schisterman (2003) all use this method to obtain an expression for the variance. For example, an expression derived by Liu and Schisterman (2003) takes the form (after minor modification of their original expression):

$$V(\widehat{\text{AUC}}) = \frac{1}{1+b^2}\phi^2\left(\frac{a}{\sqrt{1+b^2}}\right)\left(\frac{b^2}{n^0}+\frac{1}{n^1}\right)\left[1+\frac{a^2}{2(1+b^2)}\right],$$

which reduces to a simpler expression

$$V(\widehat{\text{AUC}}) = \frac{1}{n^1}\phi^2\left(\frac{a}{\sqrt{1+b^2}}\right)\left[1+\frac{a^2}{2(1+b^2)}\right],$$

when $n^0 = n^1$.

Therefore, an estimate of the variance of the estimated AUC can be conveniently obtained by replacing the parameters in the variance expression with their MLEs. This gives

$$\hat{V}(\widehat{\text{AUC}}) = \frac{1}{1+\hat{b}^2}\phi^2\left(\frac{\hat{a}}{\sqrt{1+\hat{b}^2}}\right)\left(\frac{\hat{b}^2}{n^0}+\frac{1}{n^1}\right)\left[1+\frac{\hat{a}^2}{2(1+\hat{b}^2)}\right]. \tag{6-7}$$

With these developments, a group sequential test for H_0: AUC = 0.5 with two-sided alternative H_1: AUC ≠ 0.5 can now be straightforwardly carried out by defining

$$t = \frac{1}{\hat{V}(\widehat{\text{AUC}})}, \quad \text{and } W(t) = \frac{\widehat{\text{AUC}} - 0.5}{\hat{V}(\widehat{\text{AUC}})}, \tag{6-8}$$

which resembles a Brownian motion with drift θ = AUC – 0.5. The group sequential test stops and rejects H_0 if $|W(t_k)| > c_k\sqrt{t_k}$ at some stage k.

Example 6.1. We describe in some detail a simple group sequential procedure of two interim analyses with significance level $\alpha = 0.05$ using the

O'Brien and Fleming boundary. Suppose we plan to conduct interim analyses after every 50 test outcomes from healthy samples and 50 outcomes from diseased samples. If the sampling continues to the second analysis, we will have a total number of 100 healthy outcomes and 100 diseased outcomes.

The constant $C_B(2, 0.05)$ is 1.977, as tabulated in Table 2.3 of Jennison and Turnbull (2000). Thus, at the first analysis, we use observations $\{X_1, \ldots, X_{50}; Y_1, \ldots, Y_{50}\}$ to calculate t_1 and $W(t_1)$ according to Equation (6-8). If

$$\frac{|W(t_1)|}{\sqrt{t_1}} > \sqrt{2}C_B = 2.796,$$

we stop the test and reject H_0. If $|W(t_1)|/\sqrt{t_1} \le 2.796$, we continue the test and collect healthy outcomes, $\{X_{51}, \ldots, X_{100}\}$, and diseased outcomes $\{Y_{51}, \ldots, Y_{100}\}$. For the second analysis, we use all observations $\{X_1, \ldots, X_{100}; Y_1, \ldots, Y_{100}\}$ to calculate t_2 and $W(t_2)$, again according to Equation (6-8). At this stage, H_0 is rejected if

$$\frac{|W(t_2)|}{\sqrt{t_2}} > C_B = 1.977.$$

Otherwise, H_0 will not be rejected. Regardless of the decision about rejection of H_0, no more test outcomes will be collected after the second stage. Note that the critical value C_B is only slightly larger than 1.96, the critical value for the fixed size test.

6.3.2 Nonparametric Model

Use of the binormal model may result in a loss of efficiency when test outcomes depart from the assumed normalities. If we are uncertain about the distributional assumptions, we can use nonparametric testing which is robust against the distributional assumptions. For continuous outcomes, we can show (see Bamber, 1975; Pepe, 2003) that $AUC = P(Y > X)$, with an addition of $P(Y = X)/2$ for ties. Thus with n^0 healthy and n^1 diseased test outcomes, the empirical estimator of the AUC is given by

$$\widehat{AUC} = \frac{1}{n^0 n^1} \sum_{i=1}^{n^0} \sum_{j=1}^{n^1} I(Y_j > X_i), \tag{6-9}$$

where $I(y > x) = 1$ if $y > x$ and 0 if otherwise.

This empirical estimator is always unbiased for AUC regardless of sample sizes and distributions of the test outcomes. It is a U-statistic best known as the Wilcoxon two-sample statistic (Lehmann, 1999) and is widely used in two-sample comparisons as an alternative to the two-sample t-test. The empirical estimator, like any U-statistic, is asymptotically normally distributed. Its mean is the AUC and its (asymptotic) variance $V(\widehat{AUC})$ may be obtained via tedious but straightforward algebraic manipulations. Here we present one expression from Lehmann (1999). Define

$$\sigma_{10}^2 = P(X_1 < \text{both } Y_1 \text{ and } Y_2) - AUC^2, \sigma_{01}^2 = P(Y_1 > \text{both } X_1 \text{ and } X_2) - AUC^2,$$

the probability that a healthy (diseased) outcome is smaller (larger) than two independent diseased (healthy) outcomes, minus the squared AUC. Then

$$V(\widehat{AUC}) \approx \frac{\sigma_{10}^2}{n^0} + \frac{\sigma_{01}^2}{n^1}.$$

The two parameters σ_{10}^2 and σ_{01}^2 can be estimated empirically by

$$\hat{\sigma}_{10}^2 = \frac{2}{n^0 n^1 (n^1 - 1)} \sum_{i=1}^{n^0} \sum_{1 \le j_1 < j_2 \le n^1} I(X_i < \min(Y_{j_1}, Y_{j_2})) - \widehat{AUC}^2, \quad \text{and}$$

$$\hat{\sigma}_{01}^2 = \frac{2}{n^1 n^0 (n^0 - 1)} \sum_{j=1}^{n^1} \sum_{1 \le i_1 < i_2 \le n^0} I(Y_j > \max(X_{i_1}, X_{i_2})) - \widehat{AUC}^2.$$

The empirical estimator of $V(\widehat{AUC})$ is then given by

$$\hat{V}(\widehat{AUC}) = \frac{\hat{\sigma}_{10}^2}{n^0} + \frac{\hat{\sigma}_{01}^2}{n^1}. \tag{6-10}$$

It is well known that *U*-statistics such as the Wilcoxon two-sample may be asymptotically expressed as sums of independent variables. Thus if we define

$$t = \frac{1}{\hat{V}(\widehat{AUC})}, \quad W(t) = \frac{\widehat{AUC} - 0.5}{\hat{V}(\widehat{AUC})}, \tag{6-11}$$

$W(t)$ resembles a Brownian motion with AUC – 0.5 as its drift parameter θ. Based on t and $W(t)$, a group sequential testing procedure for H_0: $AUC = 0.5$ can be conducted similar to the binormal model case. At each stage, t and $W(t)$ are calculated using all the test outcomes available at this stage, and the decision to stop and reject H_0 is made according to the error spending function chosen for the study.

Example 6.2. Consider the two-stage group sequential test in Example 6.1 using the same stopping boundaries. However, this time the nonparametric estimation is used. At the first interim analysis we compute

$$\widehat{AUC} = \frac{1}{50 \times 50} \sum_{i=1}^{50} \sum_{j=1}^{50} I(Y_j > X_i),$$

$$\hat{\sigma}_{10}^2 = \frac{1}{25 \times 50 \times 49} \sum_{i=1}^{50} \sum_{1 \le j_1 < j_2 \le 50} I(X_i < \min(Y_{j_1}, Y_{j_2})) - \widehat{\mathrm{AUC}}^2,$$

$$\hat{\sigma}_{01}^2 = \frac{1}{25 \times 50 \times 49} \sum_{j=1}^{50} \sum_{1 \le i_1 < i_2 \le 50} I(Y_j > \max(X_{i_1}, X_{i_2})) - \widehat{\mathrm{AUC}}^2.$$

Using these estimates, we can construct the first-stage Brownian motion approximations t_1 and $W(t_1)$ using Equations (6-10) and (6-11). If $|W(t_1)|/\sqrt{t_1} > 2.796$, we stop and reject H_0. Otherwise, we observe 50 more healthy outcomes $\{X_{51}, \ldots, X_{100}\}$ and 50 more diseased outcomes $\{Y_{51}, \ldots, Y_{100}\}$. We update the estimates for AUC, σ_{10}^2 and σ_{01}^2 based on all observations $\{X_1, \ldots, X_{100}; Y_1, \ldots, Y_{100}\}$, and then construct the second-stage Brownian motion approximations t_2 and $W(t_2)$, again using Equations (6-10) and (6-11). A decision to reject H_0 is made at this stage if $|W(t_2)|/\sqrt{t_2} > 1.977$.

6.4 Sequential Comparison of Two ROC Curves

It is common in comparative diagnostic accuracy studies to determine whether a newly developed diagnostic test is more accurate than a standard diagnostic test in identifying diseased subjects. When the two diagnostic tests under investigation yield continuous outcomes, their diagnostic accuracy is usually measured by the AUC. The null hypothesis is set as H_0: $\theta = 0$, where θ is the difference between the AUCs.

Consider a group sequential test with K interim analyses. We choose an error spending function $e(t)$ that yields stopping boundary values c_k. Suppose the kth analysis, $k = 1, \ldots, K$, is conducted with n_k^0 healthy outcomes denoted by $X_{l1}, \ldots, X_{ln_k^0}$ and n_k^1 diseased outcomes denoted by $Y_{l1}, \ldots, Y_{ln_k^1}$ from the lth ($l = 1$ if standard and 2 if new) diagnostic test. Using data accumulated at this stage we compute an estimate of the AUC, $\widehat{\mathrm{AUC}}_l$, and its estimated variances $\hat{V}_l(\widehat{\mathrm{AUC}}_l)$, for the lth diagnostic test. These estimates can be derived using a parametric or nonparametric method as described in Section 6.3 concerning a single ROC curve. The diagnostic accuracy difference θ can then be estimated at the kth stage by $\hat{\theta} = \widehat{\text{AUC}}_2 - \widehat{\text{AUC}}_1$, with its variance given by

$$V(\hat{\theta}) = V(\widehat{\text{AUC}_1}) + V(\widehat{\text{AUC}_2}) - 2\text{COV}\left(\widehat{\text{AUC}_1}, \widehat{\text{AUC}_2}\right).$$

Now it suffices to obtain a consistent estimate of $V(\hat{\theta})$, say $\hat{V}(\hat{\theta})$, so that

$$t = \frac{1}{\hat{V}(\hat{\theta})}, \quad W(t) = \frac{\hat{\theta}}{\hat{V}(\hat{\theta})}, \tag{6-12}$$

which in general resembles a Brownian motion. The null hypothesis H_0: $\theta = 0$ is thus rejected if $|W(t_k)|/\sqrt{t_k} > c_k$.

The covariance between the two estimated AUCs depends on the model used to characterize the test outcomes and the study designs that yield these outcomes. If a study is designed such that the two diagnostic tests are applied to unrelated subjects, the outcomes are independent and so are the two ROC curves. In this case the covariance is 0 and the variance of θ is simply the sum of the variances of the estimated AUCs.

When the two diagnostic tests are applied to the same subjects, as in most diagnostic accuracy studies, the outcomes from the two tests applying to the same subject, X_{1i} and X_{2i}, or Y_{1j} and Y_{2j}, are usually not independent. This results in correlated ROC curves and subsequent AUCs. The covariance of the two correlated AUCs depends on the joint distributions of X_{1i} and X_{2i} and of Y_{1j} and Y_{2j}. The next sections focus on the correlated cases.

6.4.1 Binormal Model

Mazumdar and Liu (2003) considered a group sequential comparison of two AUCs under a general binormal model, assuming that

$$\begin{pmatrix} X_{1i} \\ X_{2i} \end{pmatrix} \sim N\left(\begin{pmatrix} \mu_{1X} \\ \mu_{2X} \end{pmatrix}, \begin{pmatrix} \sigma_{1X}^2 & \rho_X\sigma_{1X}\sigma_{2X} \\ \rho_X\sigma_{1X}\sigma_{2X} & \sigma_{2X}^2 \end{pmatrix}\right),$$

and

$$\begin{pmatrix} Y_{1j} \\ Y_{2j} \end{pmatrix} \sim N\left(\begin{pmatrix} \mu_{1Y} \\ \mu_{2Y} \end{pmatrix}, \begin{pmatrix} \sigma_{1Y}^2 & \rho_Y\sigma_{1Y}\sigma_{2Y} \\ \rho_Y\sigma_Y\sigma_{2Y} & \sigma_{2Y}^2 \end{pmatrix}\right).$$

Under the above model, $\widehat{\text{AUC}_l}$ and its estimated variances $\hat{V}_l(\widehat{\text{AUC}_l})$ are given by Equations (6-6) and (6-7), respectively, for the lth diagnostic test. The covariance term again can be derived using the delta method. We have

$$\mathrm{COV}\left(\widehat{\mathrm{AUC}_1}, \widehat{\mathrm{AUC}_2}\right) = \left(\frac{\rho_X \sigma_{1X} \sigma_{2X}}{n^1} + \frac{\rho_Y \sigma_{1Y} \sigma_{2Y}}{n^0}\right) \times$$

$$\frac{\phi(\Phi^{-1}(\mathrm{AUC}_1))\phi(\Phi^{-1}(\mathrm{AUC}_2))}{\sqrt{(\sigma_{1X}^2 + \sigma_{1Y}^2)(\sigma_{2X}^2 + \sigma_{2X}^2)}} \left(1 + \frac{\Phi^{-1}(\mathrm{AUC}_1)\Phi^{-1}(\mathrm{AUC}_2)}{\sqrt{(\sigma_{1X}^2 + \sigma_{1Y}^2)(\sigma_{2X}^2 + \sigma_{2Y}^2)}}\right). \tag{6-13}$$

At the kth interim analysis, the two correlation coefficients ρ_X and ρ_Y are estimated, as usual, by

$$\hat{\rho}_X = \frac{\sum_{i=1}^{n_k^0} (X_{1i} - \hat{\mu}_{1X})(X_{2i} - \hat{\mu}_{2X})/n_k^0}{\hat{\sigma}_{1X}\hat{\sigma}_{2X}},$$

and

$$\hat{\rho}_Y = \frac{\sum_{i=1}^{n_k^1} (Y_{1i} - \hat{\mu}_{1Y})(X_{2i} - \hat{\mu}_{2Y})/n_k^1}{\hat{\sigma}_{1Y}\hat{\sigma}_{2Y}},$$

respectively, where the $\hat{\mu}$ and $\hat{\sigma}$ values are the MLEs of the corresponding parameters. We can then obtain an estimate $\widehat{\mathrm{COV}\left(\mathrm{AUC}_1, \mathrm{AUC}_2\right)}$ of the covariance term by replacing the unknown parameters in Equation (6-13) with their estimates. Using this covariance estimate, we can construct the Brownian statistics t and $W(t)$ in Equation (6-12), conduct the kth analysis, and reject H_0: $\theta = 0$ if $|W(t_k)|/\sqrt{t_k} > c_k$.

Obuchowski and McClish (1997) and Liu and Schisterman (2003) gave alternative asymptotic expressions for the covariance term that may also be used to construct the Brownian statistics.

6.4.2 Nonparametric Model

Nonparametric group sequential procedures for testing the equality of two AUCs were developed by Liu et al. (2008) and Zhou et al. (2008). At the kth stage, the AUC of the lth diagnostic test $\mathrm{AUC}_l = P(Y_{l1} > X_{l1})$ is estimated using the Wilcoxon two-sample statistic, Equation (6-9)

$$\widehat{AUC_l} = \frac{1}{n_k^0 n_k^1} \sum_{i=1}^{n_k^0} \sum_{j=1}^{n_k^1} I(Y_{lj} > X_{li}),$$

with an estimate of its variance $V(\widehat{AUC_l})$ given by Equation (6-10).

Liu et al. (2008) derived the covariance $\mathrm{COV}(\widehat{AUC_1}, \widehat{AUC_2})$ by expressing $\widehat{AUC_l}$ as the sum of independent variables. Define

$$\psi_{10} = P(Y_{11} > X_{11}, Y_{21} > X_{22}) - \text{AUC}_1\text{AUC}_2,$$

and

$$\psi_{01} = P(Y_{11} > X_{11}, Y_{22} > X_{21}) - \text{AUC}_1\text{AUC}_2.$$

Then

$$\text{COV}(\widehat{AUC}_1, \widehat{AUC}_2) = \frac{1}{n_k^0}\psi_{01} + \frac{1}{n_k^1}\psi_{10}.$$

Note that ψ_{10} and ψ_{01} can be estimated empirically by

$$\hat{\psi}_{10} = \frac{2}{n_k^1 n_k^0 (n_k^0 - 1)} \sum_{j=1}^{n_k^1} \sum_{1 \le i_1 < i_2 \le n_k^0} I(Y_{1j} > X_{1i_1}, Y_{2j} > X_{2i_2}) - \widehat{\text{AUC}}_1\widehat{\text{AUC}}_2,$$

and

$$\hat{\psi}_{01} = \frac{2}{n_k^1 n_k^0 (n_k^1 - 1)} \sum_{i=1}^{n_k^0} \sum_{1 \le j_1 < j_2 \le n_k^1} I(Y_{1j_1} > X_{1i}, Y_{2j_2} > X_{2i}) - \widehat{\text{AUC}}_1\widehat{\text{AUC}}_2.$$

This yields an estimate of the covariance as

$$\widehat{\text{COV}}(\widehat{AUC}_1, \widehat{AUC}_2) = \frac{1}{n_k^0}\hat{\psi}_{01} + \frac{1}{n_k^1}\hat{\psi}_{10}. \tag{6-14}$$

With these estimates of the AUC, the variances and covariance, the nonparametric statistics

$$t = \frac{1}{\hat{V}(\hat{\theta})}, \qquad W(t) = \frac{\hat{\theta}}{\hat{V}(\hat{\theta})},$$

can be obtained. Because $\hat{\theta}$ is asymptotically equivalent to sums of independent variables, the two statistics behave like a Brownian motion with drift θ, enabling the implementation of group sequential testing based on Brownian motion theory. The null hypothesis H_0: $\theta = 0$ is thus rejected if $|W(t_k)|/\sqrt{t_k} > c_k$.

Asymptotically equivalent variance and covariance expressions exist in the literature; see Hanley and McNeil (1982) and DeLong et al. (1988). These expressions can also be used in constructing Brownian statistics to implement a group sequential testing procedure; see Tang et al. (2008).

Wieand et al. (1989) proposed a general measure for comparison of two ROC curves. Denote by S_{lX} and S_{lY}, respectively, the (marginal) survival function of a healthy outcome X_{l1} and a diseased outcome Y_{l1}. The ROC curve is given by $(u_1\ S_{iY}(S_{iX}(u)))$ with $0 \le u \le 1$. Instead of evaluating the area under the whole ROC curve, Wieand et al. suggested evaluating a weighted area $\mathrm{wAUC}_l = \int_0^1 S_{lY}(S_{lX}^{-1}(u))dR(u)$, where $R(u)$ is some probability measure on [0,1]. This general index includes AUC if $R(u) = u$, partial area pAUC on $[u_1, u_2]$ if $R(u) = uI(u_1 \le u \le u_2)$, and sensitivity at a given level of FPF if $R(u)$ is a degenerated density function. The two tests are then compared via the difference between wAUCs:

$$\theta = \mathrm{wAUC}_2 - \mathrm{wAUC}_1 = \int_0^1 [S_{2Y}(S_{2X}^{-1}(u)) - S_{1Y}(S_{1X}^{-1}(u))]dR(u),$$

which can be estimated conveniently by replacing the survival functions by their empirical counterparts:

$$\hat{\theta} = \int_0^1 [\hat{S}_{2Y}(\hat{S}_{2X}^{-1}(u)) - \hat{S}_{1Y}(\hat{S}_{1X}^{-1}(u))]dR(u).$$

Wieand et al. (1989) showed that $\hat{\theta}$ is asymptotically equal to the sum of independent variables, and obtained an asymptotic variance of $\hat{\theta}$. Let $\hat{V}(\hat{\theta})$ be the empirical estimate of variance. Then, as argued by Tang et al. (2008), the two statistics $t = 1/\hat{V}(\hat{\theta})$, $W(t) = \hat{\theta}/\hat{V}(\hat{\theta})$, resemble a Brownian motion and a group sequential procedure can be implemented using these statistics.

6.5 Sequential Evaluation of Binary Outcomes

Diagnostic tests often yield binary outcomes such as "testing positive" and "testing negative." Even when the results are measured on a continuous scale, they are often dichotomized using some cut point to generate binary outcomes. The diagnostic accuracy of a binary test is usually evaluated using its sensitivity, specificity, or a proper function of the two indices such as their sum or weighted sum. Let $X_1, \ldots, X_{n^0}$ be the outcomes of a diagnostic test of n^0 healthy subjects and $Y_1, \ldots, Y_{n^1}$ be the outcomes from n^1 diseased subjects, taking value 1 if the test results are positive and 0 if otherwise. The sensitivity (Se) and specificity (Sp) are estimated empirically by

$$\widehat{\mathrm{Se}} = \frac{1}{n^1}\sum_{j=1}^{n^1} Y_j, \quad \widehat{\mathrm{Sp}} = \frac{1}{n^0}\sum_{i=1}^{n^0}(1 - X_i). \tag{6-15}$$

Note that $n^1\widehat{\mathrm{Se}}$ and $n^0\widehat{\mathrm{Sp}}$ both follow binomial distributions. Exact calculations are possible but may be complicated and extensive. Note also that $\widehat{\mathrm{Se}}$

and $\widehat{\text{Sp}}$ are both sums of independent variables and thus functions (with continuous second derivatives) of $\widehat{\text{Se}}$ and $\widehat{\text{Sp}}$. This makes large sample approximation via Brownian motion also feasible.

6.5.1 Evaluating Accuracy of Diagnostic Tests

An ideal diagnostic test should exhibit high levels of sensitivity and specificity. In a study that investigates the diagnostic accuracy of newly developed tests, the case control sampling method is usually used to determine whether one or more diagnostic tests meet minimally acceptable levels for sensitivity and specificity. A diagnostic test that meets the minimal criteria and appears promising for further development may undergo evaluation in larger case control studies, possibly involving comparison with standard diagnostic tests.

Conversely, if early evidence fails to show promising accuracy results for a diagnostic test, the test should not be evaluated further. By discontinuing unpromising diagnostic tests early, resources can be reallocated to evaluate more promising tests. This strategy is similar to a Phase II cancer clinical trial in which patient responses to a therapeutic drug are evaluated sequentially. A drug would be excluded from future investigation if response rates were low at an early stage; see Gehan (1961), Fleming (1982), and Simon (1989).

Consider a diagnostic test that will be declared unpromising if its sensitivity is not above a threshold Se_0 or its specificity is not above a threshold Sp_0. We can set the null hypothesis to:

$$H_0 : \text{Se} \le \text{Se}_0 \text{ or } \text{Sp} \le \text{Sp}_0, \tag{6-16}$$

with the alternative

$$H_1 : \text{Se} > \text{Se}_0 \text{ and } \text{Sp} > \text{Sp}_0. \tag{6-17}$$

The Se_0 and Sp_0 threshold values are prespecified minimally acceptable values of sensitivity and specificity—usually decided based on data from previous studies. If the null hypothesis is rejected, the conclusion is that the test meets the minimal criteria and a larger scale case control study may be recommended; otherwise the test will be excluded from further evaluations.

For a fixed sample size testing procedure, we reject the null hypothesis if $\widehat{\text{Se}} > c_X$ and $\widehat{\text{Sp}} > c_Y$, where the two critical values satisfy error requirements. Let

$$\text{Bin}(c,n,p) = \sum_{i=0}^{c} \binom{n}{i} p^i (1-p)^{n-i}$$

stand for the cumulative binomial function. Then the power (Pw) of the test as a function of Se and Sp is given by

$$\begin{aligned}\text{Pw}(\text{Se},\text{Sp}) &= P\left(\widehat{\text{Se}} > c_X, \widehat{\text{Sp}} > c_Y\right) = P\left(\widehat{\text{Se}} > c_X\right)P\left(\widehat{\text{Sp}} > c_Y\right) \\ &= (1-\text{Bin}(n^0 c_X, n^0, \text{Se}))(1-\text{Bin}(n^1 c_Y, n^1, \text{Sp})).\end{aligned} \tag{6-18}$$

We choose c_X and c_Y such that $\sup_{\Theta_0}\text{Pw}(\text{Se},\text{Sp}) = \alpha$, where Θ_0 represents the values of Se and Sp under the null hypothesis. This fixed sample size procedure can be extended to a *K*-stage group sequential procedure as follows. Suppose there are n_k^1 diseased and n_k^0 healthy test outcomes available to conduct a *k*th interim analysis that yields $\widehat{\text{Se}}_k$ and $\widehat{\text{Sp}}_k$, the empirical estimates of sensitivity and specificity. We stop and reject the null hypothesis if $\widehat{\text{Se}}_k > c_{kX}$ and $\widehat{\text{Sp}}_k > c_{kY}$ where c_{kX} and c_{kY} are the critical values at the *k*th analysis. The power *Pw*(Se, Sp) of this sequential procedure at Se and Sp is given by

$$\sum_{k=1}^{K} P_{\text{Se},\text{Sp}}\left(\widehat{\text{Se}}_i \le c_{iX} \text{ or } \widehat{\text{Sp}}_i \le c_{iY}, i \le k-1, \widehat{\text{Se}}_k > c_{kX} \text{ and } \widehat{\text{Sp}}_k > c_{kY}\right). \tag{6-19}$$

The critical values c_{kX} and c_{kY} can be derived numerically using binomial distributions so that the power of the test will not exceed α for (Se, Sp) ∈ Θ_0, that is, $\sup_{\Theta_0}\beta(\text{Se},\text{Sp}) = \alpha$.

Shu et al. (2007) suggested using an error spending function to determine the critical values. Suppose we fix the total number of diseased and healthy outcomes, n_K^1 and n_K^0, and write $t_k = N_k/N_K$, with *N* indicating total sample size of both diseased and healthy subjects. With an error spending function *e*(*t*), the first stage critical values c_{1X} and c_{1Y} are computed from $\sup_{\Theta_0} P\left(\widehat{\text{Se}}_1 > c_{1X}, \widehat{\text{Sp}}_1 > c_{1Y}\right) = e(t_1)$. After c_{iX} and c_{iY} are determined for $1 \le i \le k-1$, the *k*th stage critical values c_{kX} and c_{kY} are then computed from

$$\sup_{\Theta_0} P\left(\widehat{\text{Se}}_i \le c_{iX} \text{ or } \widehat{\text{Sp}}_i \le c_{iY}, i \le k-1, \widehat{\text{Se}}_k > c_{kX} \text{ and } \widehat{\text{Sp}}_k > c_{kY}\right) = e(t_k) - \sum_{i=1}^{k-1} e(t_i).$$

These calculations are based on binomial distributions rather than large sample approximations and are thus "exact." For a two-stage ($K = 2$) procedure, Shu et al. (2007) presented optimal designs that minimize the expected total sample sizes at certain values of sensitivity and specificity. In general, exact calculations of these optimal designs involve global search for the group sizes n_k^1 and n_k^0 and critical values c_{kX} and c_{kY} ($1 \le k \le K$).

6.5.2 Comparison of Two Diagnostic Tests

In a comparative accuracy study with two diagnostic tests in which the outcomes of each test $l = 1, 2$ are continuous, comparison of the accuracy usually involves testing the null hypothesis that the AUC or pAUC values of the two ROC curves are equal, as discussed in Section 6.4. When the two diagnostic tests under comparison yield binary outcomes, the null hypothesis can be set to be that the two tests have equal sensitivities and specificities, that is,

$$H_0\colon \Delta_Y = \mathrm{Se}_2 - \mathrm{Se}_1 = 0, \quad \Delta_X = \mathrm{Sp}_2 - \mathrm{Sp}_1 = 0. \tag{6-20}$$

Suppose that the two diagnostic tests involve the same subjects. We write $X_{l1}, \ldots, X_{ln^0}$ as the test outcomes from n^0 healthy subjects and $Y_{l1}, \ldots, Y_{ln^1}$ as the test outcomes from n^1 diseased subjects, for diagnostic test l. According to this design structure, the n^0 pairs $(X_{11}, X_{21}), \ldots, (X_{1n^0}, X_{2n^0})$ are i.i.d. random vectors, each consisting of two correlated binary outcomes. The n^1 pairs, $(Y_{11}, Y_{21}), \ldots, (X_{1n^1}, X_{2n^1})$, are also i.i.d. with correlated binary variables in each pair. The sensitivity and specificity of each test can be estimated by

$$\widehat{\mathrm{Se}}_l = \frac{1}{n^1}\sum_{j=1}^{n^1} Y_{lj}, \quad \widehat{\mathrm{Sp}}_l = \frac{1}{n^0}\sum_{i=1}^{n^0}(1 - X_{li}), \; l = 1, 2. \tag{6-21}$$

A fixed size procedure with sizes n^0 and n^1 rejects H_0 if $|\hat{\Delta}_Y| > c_Y$ or $|\hat{\Delta}_X| > c_X$, where

$$\hat{\Delta}_Y = \widehat{\mathrm{Se}}_2 - \widehat{\mathrm{Se}}_1, \hat{\Delta}_X = \widehat{\mathrm{Sp}}_2 - \widehat{\mathrm{Sp}}_1. \tag{6-22}$$

The healthy outcomes are assumed to be independent of the diseased outcomes. Given a significance level α, the Type I error constraint yields

$$\begin{aligned}
\alpha &= P_{H_0}\left(|\hat{\Delta}_Y| > c_Y \text{ or } |\hat{\Delta}_X| > c_X\right) \\
&= P_{H_0}\left(|\hat{\Delta}_Y| > c_Y\right) + P_{H_0}\left(|\hat{\Delta}_X| > c_X\right) \\
&\quad - P_{H_0}\left(|\hat{\Delta}_Y| > c_Y \text{ and } |\hat{\Delta}_X| > c_X\right) \\
&= \alpha_Y + \alpha_X - \alpha_Y\alpha_X,
\end{aligned} \tag{6-23}$$

where $\alpha_Y = P_{H_0}\left(|\hat{\Delta}_Y| > c_Y\right)$ is the Type I error probability of the test that rejects the null hypothesis $H_{0Y}\colon \Delta_Y = 0$ if $|\hat{\Delta}_Y| > c_Y$, and $\alpha_X = P_{H_0}\left(|\hat{\Delta}_X| > c_X\right)$ is the Type I error probability of the test that rejects the null hypothesis H_{0X}: $\Delta_X = 0$ if $|\hat{\Delta}_X| > c_X$.

By fixing α_X and α_Y, we can test H_0 for H_{0X} and H_{0Y} separately, using the Bonferroni procedure; see Chapter 15 of Jennison and Turnbull (2000). Because the $\widehat{\Delta}_X$ and $\widehat{\Delta}_Y$ statistics are independent, we can provide exact control of the Type I error rate. We can allocate different significance levels ($\alpha_X \neq\approx \alpha_Y$) to emphasize the importance of sensitivity over specificity ($\alpha_Y < \alpha_X$), or specificity over sensitivity ($\alpha_X < \alpha_Y$). Otherwise, we can set $\alpha_X = \alpha_Y$ in which case we have $\alpha_Y = \alpha_X = 1 - \sqrt{1-\alpha}$.

With a specified α_Y significance level, a K-stage group sequential procedure for testing H_{0Y} can then be implemented. The maximum sample sizes n_K^1 and n_K^0 must be fixed prior to the test. Suppose an error spending function $e(t)$, $0 \le t \le 1$, is used for the interim analysis. At the kth stage with n_K^0 healthy outcomes and n_K^1 diseased outcomes, the null hypothesis H_{0Y} is rejected if $|\Delta_{kY}| > c_{kY}$. The Type I error constraint requires that

$$\alpha_Y = \sum_{k=1}^{K} P_{\Delta_X=\Delta_Y=0}\left(|\widehat{\Delta}_{iY}| \le c_{iY}, i \le k-1, |\widehat{\Delta}_{kY}| \le c_{kY}\right). \tag{6-24}$$

With relatively large sample sizes, the c_{kY} critical values can be obtained via Brownian motion approximations. Note that $\widehat{\Delta}_Y$ is sum of i.i.d. random variables:

$$\widehat{\Delta}_Y = \frac{1}{n^1}\sum_{j=1}^{n^1}(Y_{1j} - Y_{2j}).$$

Its variance is given by

$$V\left(\widehat{\Delta}_Y\right) = \frac{1}{n^1}V(Y_{11} - Y_{21})$$

$$= \frac{1}{n^1}(V(Y_{11}) + V(Y_{21}) - 2COV(Y_{11}, Y_{21}))]$$

$$= \frac{1}{n^1}\{Se_1(1-Se_1) + Se_2(1-Se_2) - 2(E(Y_{11}Y_{21}) - Se_1Se_2)\}. \tag{6-25}$$

The empirical estimate $\widehat{V}\left(\widehat{\Delta}_Y\right)$ of the variance is obtained by replacing Se_1 and Se_2 by $\widehat{Se}_1$ and $\widehat{Se}_2$, respectively, and $E(Y_{11}Y_{21})$ by

$$\hat{E}(Y_{11}Y_{21}) = \frac{1}{n^1}\sum_{i=1}^{n^1}Y_{1i}Y_{2i} = \frac{1}{n^1}\sum_{i=1}^{n^1}I(Y_{1i} = Y_{2i} = 1).$$

Thus, the Brownian motion can be constructed by defining

$$t = \frac{1}{\widehat{V}\left(\widehat{\Delta}_Y\right)}, \quad W(t) = \frac{\widehat{\Delta}_Y}{\widehat{V}\left(\widehat{\Delta}_Y\right)}.$$

The null hypothesis is rejected at the kth stage if $|W(t_k)|/\sqrt{t_k} > c_k$, or $|W(t_k)| > \sqrt{t_k}c_k$. This gives $c_{kY} = \sqrt{t_k}c_k = \sqrt{\widehat{V}(\widehat{\Delta}_Y)}c_k$. A sequential procedure for testing H_{0X} can be carried out in a similar manner.

6.6 Sample Size Estimation

A sample size required for a comparative diagnostic accuracy study usually consists of a number of diseased and healthy subjects. The sample size must be relatively large for a study to have sufficient power to detect a meaningful difference in the accuracies of two diagnostic tests under investigation. Many factors affect the calculation of sample size including the significance level α, power $1 - \beta$ at certain alternative values of the accuracy difference, nuisance parameters, and test procedure (test statistics and decision to reject a null hypothesis of no difference in diagnostic accuracy). For fixed sample size tests, Obuchowski (1994, 1997, 1998) and Obuchowski and McClish (1997) described procedures to compute sample sizes based on the binormal model or the Wilcoxon statistics. These and other methods are elaborated in Pepe (2000).

When a group sequential testing procedure is used, the sample size is defined as the number of subjects at the final analysis. This sample size is in general larger than that required by a fixed sample size procedure due to repeated significance tests. To this end, let n_F^0 and n_F^1 be the number of healthy and diseased subjects, respectively, for a fixed size testing procedure, and n_S^0 and n_S^1 be the values for a group sequential procedure. Write $n_F = n_F^0 + n_F^1$ and $n_S = n_S^0 + n_S^1$, and define $\Upsilon = n_S/n_F$, the ratio of sample sizes. Then, if it is more convenient to compute fixed size n_F and size ratio ¡, the sequential size n_S is the product of these two.

For a given error spending function $e(t)$ with specified numbers of interim analyses K and analysis times t_k, $1 \le k \le K$, the size ratio Υ depends only on the error constraints α and β; see Liu et al. (2000). For several popular group sequential procedures, including those of Pocock (1977), O'Brien and Fleming (1979), and Wang and Tsiatis (1987), the Υ values are well tabulated in Jennison and Turnbull (2000). The sequential sample sizes can then be derived from n_F and Υ.

As an example, consider a fixed size procedure testing the null hypothesis that two diagnostic tests have equal AUCs. Suppose that a nonparametric test based on the Wilcoxon two-sample statistics is used and the fixed size procedure requires $n_F^0 = 100$ healthy and $n_F^1 = 150$ diseased subjects, with level of significance $\alpha = 0.05$ and power $1 - \beta = 0.9$ when $AUC_2 - AUC_1 = 0.15$. Suppose instead that a group sequential procedure is carried out using Pocock's boundary with five interim analyses. From Table 2.2 of Jennison and Turnbull (2000), we find $\Upsilon = 1.23$. Hence the sequential sample sizes are given, respectively, by

$$n_S^0 = n_F^0 \times \Upsilon = 100 \times 1.23 = 123;\ n_S^1 = n_F^1 \times \Upsilon = 150 \times 1.23 = 185.$$

6.7 Remarks and Further Reading

6.7.1 Inference upon Termination

After a sequential procedure is terminated in the course of evaluation of a diagnostic test or comparison of two diagnostic tests, a decision is made whether the diagnostic test deserves further examination or whether one diagnostic test has greater diagnostic accuracy than the other. In addition to such terminal decisions, investigators may also be interested in other inferential issues such as construction of a point or interval estimate of the sensitivity, specificity, AUC or pAUC of a test, the difference in these indices between two diagnostic tests, or the calculation of a p-value as strength of evidence against the null hypothesis. In general, inferential methods developed in the clinical trial literature can be applied or straightforwardly extended to solve these issues.

Inference on the accuracy difference parameter θ is based on the statistic $(t, W(t))$ upon stopping. The functional forms of the maximum likelihood estimates are not affected by a sequential procedure, but their distributions are because the terminal sample size (number of diseased and healthy subjects) is a random variable. Consequently, the maximum likelihood estimates are biased and possess inflated variances. Two common approaches were proposed in the literature. One is Whitehead's (1986a, 1986b) bias adjusted estimator aimed at reducing the bias of the maximum likelihood estimate. The other is Emerson and Fleming's (1990) unbiased estimator obtained from the Rao–Blackwell theorem. Numerical results demonstrated that the bias adjusted estimator usually has a smaller mean squared error than the unbiased estimator. See also Liu and Hall (2000, 2001), Whitehead (1997), Jennison and Turnbull (2000), and Proschan et al. (2006), among others.

P-values and confidence intervals concerning θ can be constructed by ordering the two-dimensional sample space of $(t, W(t))$ that tells which observation is more extreme. A few popular orderings have been proposed by Siegmund (1978), Fairbanks and Madsen (1982), Tsiatis et al. (1984), Chang (1989), and Emerson and Fleming (1990). For a specific ordering, we can compute the probability, as a function $p(\theta)$ of θ, that $(t,W(t))$ is more extreme than the observed one. Then the p-value is given by $p(0)$, and the $1 - \alpha$ confidence limits are obtained by setting $p(\theta)$ to be $\alpha/2$ and $1 - \alpha/2$, respectively. For more details, see Jennison and Turnbull (2000) and Proschan et al. (2006).

6.7.2 Sample Size Re-Estimation

Calculation of sample size for a comparative diagnostic accuracy study usually involves a number of nuisance parameters that must be specified; the required power of a study is achieved through these specified values. If the true values of these parameters are different from the specified values, a study may be substantially under-powered. To ensure adequate power, we can derive estimates of the nuisance parameters using data available during the mid-course of the study and re-estimate the sample size based on the updated parameter estimates. As a function of the mid-course data, the re-estimated sample size is a random variable. Such an adaptive approach as demonstrated by Wu et al. (2008) and Tang and Liu (2010) is very effective in maintaining the power of a study regardless of the parameter values.

6.7.3 Computing Software

The implementation of a group sequential test requires computation of boundary values and error probabilities involving multiple integrations arising from the joint distribution of Brownian sequences. A number of commercial and free software programs can perform these calculations. Wassmer and Vandemeulebroecke (2006) provide a brief overview. Popular software includes EaSt developed by Cytel Software Corporation (http://www.cytel.com/Products/East/), PEST developed by the Medical and Pharmaceutical Statistics research group led by Whitehead (http://www.maths.lancs.ac.uk/department/research/statistics/mps/pest), Modules SEQ, SEQSCALE, and SEQSHIFT in SAS Version 9.2 developed by the SAS Institute (http://www.sas.com), and an S-PLUS module S+SeqTrial developed by Insightful Corporation (http://www.insightful.com/products/seqtrial). Two free sources of FORTRAN codes are Jennison's homepage at http://www.bath.ac.uk/~mascj/book/programs/general and http://www.biostat.wisc.edu/software/index.htm developed by a biostatistics group at the University of Wisconsin.

References

Bamber, D. 1975. The area above the ordinal dominance graph and the area below the receiver operating characteristics graph. *Journal of Mathematical Psychology* 12: 387–415.

Chang, M.N. 1989. Confidence intervals for a normal mean following a group sequential test. *Biometrics* 45: 247–254.

DeLong, E.R., DeLong, D.M., and Clarke-Pearson, D.L. 1988. Comparing the areas under two or more correlated receiver operating characteristic curves: a nonparametric approach. *Biometrics* 44: 837–845.

Emerson, S.S. and Fleming, T.R. 1990. Parameter estimation following sequential hypothesis testing. *Biometrika* 77: 875–892.

Fairbanks, K. and Madsen, R. 1982. P values for tests using a repeated significance design. *Biometrika* 69: 69–74.

Fleming, T.R. 1982. One-sample multiple testing procedure for phase II clinical trials. *Biometrics* 38: 143–151.

Gehan, E.A. 1961. The determination of the number of patients required in a preliminary and a follow-up trial of a new chemotherapeutic agent. *Journal of Chronic Diseases* 13: 346–353.

Hanley, J.A. and McNeil, B.J. 1982. The meaning and use of the area under a receiver operating characteristic (ROC) curve. *Radiology* 143: 29–36.

Hwang, I.K., Shih, W.J., and DeCani, J. 1990. Group sequential designs using a family of type I error probability spending functions. *Statistics in Medicine* 9: 1439–1445.

Jennison, C. and Turnbull, B.W. 2000. *Group Sequential Methods with Applications to Clinical Trials*. New York: Chapman & Hall.

Kim, K. and DeMets, D.L. 1987. Design and analysis of group sequential tests based on the type I error spending rate function. *Biometrika* 74: 149–154.

Lan, K.K.G. and DeMets, D.L. 1983. Discrete sequential boundaries for clinical trials. *Biometrika* 70: 659–663.

Lehmann, E.L. 1999. *Elements of Large-Sample Theory*. New York: Springer.

Liu, A. and Hall, W.J. 1999. Unbiased estimation following a group sequential test. *Biometrika* 86: 71–78.

Liu, A. and Hall, W.J. 2001. Unbiased estimation of secondary parameters following a sequential test. *Biometrika* 88: 895–900.

Liu, A. and Schisterman, E.F. 2003. Comparison of diagnostic accuracy of biomarkers with pooled assessments. *Biometrical Journal* 45: 631–644.

Liu, A. Boyett, J., and Xiong, X.P. 2000. Sample size calculation for planning group sequential longitudinal trials. *Statistics in Medicine* 19: 205–220.

Liu, A., Wu, C.Q. and Schisterman, E.F. 2008. Nonparametric sequential evaluation of diagnostic biomarkers. *Statistics in Medicine* 27: 1667–1678.

Mazumdar, M. 2004. Group sequential design for comparative diagnostic accuracy studies: implications and guidelines for practitioners. *Medical Decision Making* 24: 525–533.

Mazumdar, M. and Liu, A. 2003. Group sequential design for comparative diagnostic accuracy studies. *Statistics in Medicine* 22: 727–739.

Obuchowski, N.A. 1994. Computing sample size for receiver operating characteristic studies. *Investigative Radiology* 29: 238–243.

Obuchowski, N.A. 1997. Nonparametric analysis of clustered ROC curve data. *Biometrics* 53: 567–578.

Obuchowski, N.A. 1998. Sample size considerations in studies of test accuracy. *Statistical Methods in Medical Research* 7: 371–392.

Obuchowski, N.A. and McClish, D.K. 1997. Sample size determination for diagnostic accuracy studies involving binormal ROC curve indices. *Statistics in Medicine* 16: 1529–1542.

O'Brien, P.C. and Fleming, T.R. 1979. A multiple testing procedure for clinical trials. *Biometrics* 35: 549–556.

Pepe, M.S. 2003. *The Statistical Evaluation of Medical Tests for Classification and Prediction*. Oxford: University Press.

Pocock, S.J. 1977. Group sequential methods in the design and analysis of clinical trials. *Biometrika* 64: 191–199.

Proschan, M.A., Lan, K.K.G., and Wittes, J.T. 2006. *Statistical Monitoring of Clinical Trials: A Unified Approach*. New York: Springer.

Rao, C.R. 1973. *Linear Statistical Inference and Its Applications*, 2nd ed. New York: Wiley.

Rosner, G.L. and Tsiatis, A.A. 1988. Exact confidence intervals following a group sequential trial: A comparison of methods. *Biometrika* 75: 723–729.

Siegmund, D. 1978. Estimation following sequential tests. *Biometrika* 65: 295–297.

Shu, Y., Liu, A., and Li, Z.H. 2007. Sequential evaluation of a medical diagnostic test with binary outcomes. *Statistics in Medicine* 26: 4416–4427.

Simon, R. 1989. Optimal two-stage designs for phase II clinical trials. *Controlled Clinical Trials* 10: 1–10.

Tang, L. and Liu, A. 2010. Sample size recalculation in sequential diagnostic trials. *Biostatistics* 11: 151–163.

Tang, L., Emerson, S.S., and Zhou, X.H. 2008. Nonparametric and semiparametric group sequential methods for comparing accuracy of diagnostic tests. *Biometrics* 64: 1137–1145.

Wald, A. 1945. Sequential tests of statistical hypotheses. *Annals of Mathematical Statistics* 16: 117–186.

Wang, S.K. and Tsiatis, A.A. 1987. Approximately optimal one-parameter boundaries for group sequential trials. *Biometrics* 43: 193–199.

Wassmer, G. and Vandemeulebroecke, M. 2006. A brief review on software developments for group sequential and adaptive designs. *Biometrical Journal* 48: 732–737.

Wieand, S., Gail, M.H., James, B.R. et al. 1989. A family of nonparametric statistics for comparing diagnostic markers with paired or unpaired data. *Biometrika* 75: 585–592.

Whitehead, J. 1986a. On the bias of maximum likelihood estimation following a sequential test. *Biometrika* 73: 573–581.

Whitehead, J. 1986b. Supplementary analysis at the conclusion of a sequential clinical trial. *Biometrics* 42: 461–471.

Whitehead, J. 1997. *The Design and Analysis of Sequential Clinical Trials*, 2nd ed. Chichester: Wiley.

Whitehead, J. 1999. A unified theory for sequential clinical trials. *Statistics in Medicine* 18: 2271–2286.

Wu, C., Liu, A., and Yu, K.F. 2008. An adaptive approach to designing comparative diagnostic accuracy studies. *Journal of Biopharmaceutical Statistics* 18: 116–125.

Zhou, X.H., Li, S., and Gatsonis, C. 2008. Wilcoxon based group sequential designs for comparison of areas of two correlated ROC curves. *Statistics in Medicine* 27: 213–223.

7

Multireader ROC Analysis

7.1 Introduction

In a clinical environment, trained human observers are often necessary components of a diagnostic system (e.g., interpretation of cardiograms or the assessment of mammograms). Because of the incorporation of human observers (readers), the accuracy of a system may reflect personal characteristics of the human observers such as experience, physiological abilities, and personal preferences. Unfortunately. Even within a well defined group, the characteristics of trained observers differ substantially (e.g., Beam, 1998; Gur et al., 2007). When assessing system accuracy, it is often appropriate to consider a target "population of readers" as a part of the conceptual framework. In other words, one visualizes the results of the evaluation of a diagnostic system not in terms of the readers who happen to have participated in the study but in the context of the target population of radiologists likely to use the technology. The selection of radiologists and design of multireader studies are described in several books (Swets and Pickett, 1982; Zhou et al., 2002).

Since readers' characteristics can affect the apparent diagnostic accuracy of a technology or the relative accuracies of two systems, it has become standard to use multiple readers in studies of diagnostic systems. Although a larger number of readers should increase efficiency of the comparison, large multireader studies are associated with substantial costs. Many studies utilize 5 to 10 radiologists, and studies with large numbers of radiologists (Beam 2005) are exceptions.

Because of a likely increase of variability when diagnostic results are obtained from different samples of subjects (often termed "cases"), the most common design for multireader studies is a fully crossed (or completely paired) design in which each subject is assessed by every radiologist under every modality investigated. However, this practice may not be feasible or cost-effective in some cases due to clinical or resource-related issues (Obuchowski, 1995; 2009).

The nature of multireader studies generates multiple challenges for obtaining reliable and practically relevant conclusions. The natural differences in performances and behaviors of human observers exerted a significant impact on the current structure of the multireader ROC analysis, affecting the choice of performance measure, methods for estimation of variability, and strategies for study design. Many of the methods for multireader studies were developed in radiology and related areas and are applicable to a variety of ROC summary indices. Several major techniques for multireader analysis are covered in detail in several books and papers (Zhou et al., 2002, Hillis, 2009). This chapter describes the general statistical methodology for analysis of multireader studies while focusing on the aspects that are under-emphasized or not covered in existing books. We focus on the most commonly used fully-crossed design and empirical AUC, but many of the procedures covered can be used with other summary indices and adjusted for other types of designs. Consideration of the empirical AUCs under fully-crossed designs permits closed-form solutions for many approaches for evaluating a single modality or comparing two diagnostic modalities, thereby helping reveal important relationships and similarities of different methods.

7.2 Overall ROC Curve and Its AUC

The cornerstone of ROC analysis is the ROC curve and most standard indices are derived from this curve. Thus, it is most instructive to consider the overall summary indices from the perspective of the ROC curve. For each observer, the ROC curve can be constructed using standard methods (Chapters 1, 3, 4). However, the definition of the overall ROC curve is not trivial and can be considered a two-stage process: (1) define which points on the observer-specific ROC curves should be combined; (2) define how to combine corresponding points.

For example, a pooled approach in which the observations from all readers are put together combines the points that correspond to the same rating threshold. Combining of points is done by a weighted-average (weights reflect the relative number of cases interpreted by each reader). The overall *TPF* at threshold ξ is a weighted average of the reader-specific *TPF*s at the same threshold, $TPF^{pooled}(\xi) = \int TPF_r(\xi)dG(r)$, where *G(r)* describes the distribution of cases among readers. The overall *FPF* has a similar expression. This approach was, for example, used in Lee and Rosner (2001). The area under the pooled empirical ROC curve can be expressed as follows:

$$A^{pooled} = \frac{\sum_{r=1}^{n^R}\sum_{s=1}^{n^R}\sum_{i=1}^{n^0}\sum_{j=1}^{n^1}\psi(x_{ir}, y_{js})}{n^0 n^1 (n^R)^2} \quad where \quad \psi(x_i, y_j) = \begin{cases} 0 & x_i > y_j \\ 0.5 & x_i = y_j \\ 1 & x_i < y_j \end{cases} \tag{7-1}$$

where x_{ir} denotes the rating assigned by the rth reader ($r = 1,\ldots, n^R$) for the ith normal subject ($I = 1,\ldots, n^0_r$), and y_{js} denotes the rating assigned by the sth reader ($s = 1,\ldots, n^R$) for the jth abnormal subject ($I = 1,\ldots, n^1_r$). In other words, the implied index is the discrimination probability among the observations from the mixture distribution of ratings for normal and abnormal subjects, i.e., $E(A^{pooled}) = P(X_R < Y_S) + \frac{1}{2}P(X_R = Y_S)$.

A more conventional approach is the vertical averaging method combining the points that correspond to the same level of *FPF*, let's say fpf_0. The combining is done by simple averaging. The overall *TPF* at a given fpf_0 is a simple average of the reader-specific *TPFs* at the reader-specific thresholds that result in fpf_0, i.e., $TPF^{average}\big|_{fpf_0} = \int TPF_r\left(FPF_r^{-1}(fpf_0)\right)dr$. Naturally, the area under the average empirical ROC curve is the traditional average AUC, i.e.,

$$A^{average} = \overline{A_\bullet} = \frac{\sum_{r=1}^{n^R}\sum_{i=1}^{n^0}\sum_{j=1}^{n^1}\psi(x_{ir}, y_{jr})}{n^R n^0 n^1} \tag{7-2}$$

In other words, the implied index is the average discrimination probability among ratings for normal and abnormal subjects assigned by the same reader, i.e. $E(A^{average}) = E\{P(X_R < Y_R \mid R) + \frac{1}{2}P(X_R = Y_R \mid R)\}$. A hybrid of "pooled" and "average" types of analysis can be constructed but the practice is not common in multireader ROC analysis.

The choice of approaches to calibrating and combining points for the overall ROC curve should be driven by the nature of the problem and the specific questions of interest. For example, the pooled approach may be suitable for a well defined rating scale that is directly related to clinical actions (e.g., BIRADS in radiology). At the same time, pooling is usually considered inappropriate for experimental scales (e.g., 0 to 100) that are not routinely utilized in clinical practice, since the interpretation of these scales may differ substantially across readers.

The vertical calibration may be interpreted as implying that different readers may be prompted simultaneously to operate at the same level of *FPF*—that also may or may not be appropriate, depending on the specific diagnostic task. The weighted-average combination of *TPF* and *FPF* represents a population-averaged type of summary and is naturally appropriate where the interest lies in the performance of a group of radiologists. The simple average of *TPF* and *FPF* represents the performance of a single reader, which is useful whenever an interpretation in terms of a single, although abstract, reader is appropriate.

7.3 Statistical Analysis of Cross-Correlated Multireader Data

Under a fully-crossed (completely paired) multireader study design, every case is evaluated by every reader under every diagnostic modality investigated. The corresponding cross-correlated data obtained from a study with n^R readers, n^M modalities, and n^0 normal and n^1 abnormal cases can be presented as follows:

$$\left\{x_{ir}^{m}\right\}_{i=1,\, r=1,\, m=1}^{n^0,\, n^R,\, n^M} \quad \left\{y_{jr}^{m}\right\}_{j=1,\, r=1,\, m=1}^{n^1,\, n^R,\, n^M}, \tag{7-3}$$

where $x_{ir}^{\ m}$ denotes the rating assigned by the rth reader for the ith normal subject under modality m, and $y_j^{\ m}$ denotes the rating assigned by the rth reader for the jth abnormal subject under modality m. The data in tabular format may be presented as follows:

	X_1			...	X_{n^0}			Y_1			...	Y_{n^1}		
	mod^1	...	mod$^{n^M}$	...	mod^1	...	mod$^{n^M}$	mod^1	...	mod$^{n^M}$	...	mod^1	...	mod$^{n^M}$
reader$_1$	x_{11}^1		x_{11}^2		$x_{n^0 1}^1$		$x_{n^0 1}^2$	y_{11}^1		y_{11}^2		$y_{n^1 1}^1$		$y_{n^1 1}^2$
reader$_2$	x_{12}^1	...	x_{12}^2	...	$x_{n^0 2}^1$	...	$x_{n^0 2}^2$	y_{12}^1	...	y_{12}^2	...	$y_{n^1 2}^1$	...	$y_{n^1 2}^2$
...	$\vdots$		$\vdots$		$\vdots$		$\vdots$							
reader$_{n^R}$	$x_{1n^R}^1$		$x_{1n^R}^2$		$x_{n^0 n^R}^1$		$x_{n^0 n^R}^2$	$y_{1n^R}^1$		$y_{1n^R}^2$		$y_{n^1 n^R}^1$		$y_{n^1 n^R}^2$

Note that the observations in the same row or column block corresponding to the same subject are correlated. This cross-correlated structure presents one of the primary challenges in multireader analysis.

An important distinction in the design and analysis of multireader studies is whether readers are treated as fixed or random. If the desire is to make inferences only about a group of readers who rated images in the study, treating readers as a fixed component is acceptable. However, if the desire is to generalize to a population of readers, readers should be selected in a representative manner and treated as random to reflect uncertainty related to the incomplete sampling. In general, treating readers as a random factor when designing a study tends to result in wider confidence intervals and thus requires a greater number of readings due to the formal incorporation of reader variability.

Some of the methods discussed in this chapter permit fixed reader inferences only, while others permit inferences for either fixed or random reader inference that may be combined with different treatments of the factors (Hillis et al., 2008). Many procedures have been developed for simple comparisons of several diagnostic modalities. They are usually nonparametric or employ only mild assumptions about a data structure, but they do not permit easy incorporation of covariates. Model-based methods permit a natural framework for incorporating covariates, but require more restrictive assumptions.

Finally, while some of the methods apply to a specific ROC index (AUCs or other parameter of ROC curves), some of the methods are applicable to any type of index.

7.3.1 Covariate-Free Approaches

7.3.1.1 Methods for Fixed Reader Inferences

Early analyses of multireader ROC studies often entailed a separate analysis for each reader or application of a paired t-test to test the hypothesis that the average over all readers was equal for two modalities (Swets and Pickett, 1982). However, since the study design often included a group of readers rating the same set of images under two modalities, correlations were induced by both multiple readings of the same case and by multiple readings by the same reader. A paired t-test fails to address correlations resulting when readers rate the same cases, leading to an invalid Type I error rate (Obuchowski and Rockette, 1995). However, some of the approaches developed for comparison of the modalities under the paired design can be easily extended to analyses of multireader data.

DeLong et al. (1988) proposed a nonparametric test for comparison of nonparametric AUCs under a paired design. Since the test has a general multivariate formulation, it is suitable to estimate the accuracy of a single modality and to compare modalities under the multireader design. The multireader application of this test was noted by Song (1997) in her paper on various techniques for analyzing correlated AUCs. In particular, she noted that DeLong's procedure permits a simple comparison of two diagnostic modalities using the average AUC (area under the vertically averaged ROC curve). Technically the procedure is a particular case of a general hypothesis testing procedure described in DeLong et al. (1988), in which a specific contrast results in a difference of average areas, i.e.,

$$\left(\frac{1}{n^R}, \quad \cdots \quad \frac{1}{n^R}, \quad -\frac{1}{n^R}, \quad \cdots \quad -\frac{1}{n^R}\right) \times \begin{pmatrix} A_1^1 \\ \vdots \\ A_{n^R}^1 \\ A_1^2 \\ \vdots \\ A_{n^R}^2 \end{pmatrix} = \bar{A}_{\bullet}^1 - \bar{A}_{\bullet}^2 = \bar{D}_{\bullet}. \quad (7\text{-}4)$$

The general formula for variability of the above contrast can be found in papers of Song (1997) and DeLong et al. (1988). As noted by the latter authors, the proposed variance estimator is equivalent to a two-sample jack-knife variance (Arvesen, 1969). As types of U-statistics, the empirical AUC and the averaged difference under the paired design have a simple closed-form expression (Bandos et al., 2006):

$$V_{J2}\left(\bar{D}_{\bullet}\right)=\frac{\sum_{i=1}^{n^0}\left(\bar{w}_{i\bullet\bullet}-\bar{w}_{\bullet\bullet\bullet}\right)^2}{n^0(n^0-1)}+\frac{\sum_{j=1}^{n^1}\left(\bar{w}_{\bullet j\bullet}-\bar{w}_{\bullet\bullet\bullet}\right)^2}{n^1(n^1-1)} \text{ where } w_{ijr}=\psi\left(x_{ir}^1,y_{jr}^1\right)-\psi\left(x_{ir}^2,y_{jr}^2\right). \tag{7-5}$$

It is worth noting that the two-sample jack-knife variance (J2) above is different from the delete-two jack-knife variance used by Song (1989). The two-sample jack-knife generates a pseudovalue by eliminating one observation from normal subjects and one from abnormal; the delete-two jack-knife removes two observations regardless of their normal or abnormal status. Due to the completely paired design of the data, the difference in the average AUC and its variance estimator have the same structure as the AUC and its variance for a single reader. Indeed, $\bar{D}_{\bullet}=\sum_{i,j}w_{ij\bullet}/n^0n^1$ and both the point estimator and its variability for a single AUC may be obtained by using ψ_{ij} instead of $w_{ij\bullet}$. A more general formulation of the procedure that may be useful for more complex hypotheses or testing designs other than fully-crossed is described in detail in Zhou et al. (2003).

A similar nonparametric technique was developed for multireader analysis by Lee and Rosner (2001). This technique uses differences in areas under the pooled ROC curves rather than the difference between areas under the combined ROC curves obtained by averaging the TPFs of individual readers at a common FPF (vertical averaging). This summary statistic may be expressed in a form similar to the average difference but with indicators computed from all combinations of normal and abnormal ratings including those obtained from different readers:

$$D^{pooled}=\frac{\sum_{s=1}^{n^R}\sum_{r=1}^{n^R}\sum_{i=1}^{n^0}\sum_{j=1}^{n^1}w_{ijrs}}{\left(n^R\right)^2n^0n^1}=\frac{\sum_{i=1}^{n^0}\sum_{j=1}^{n^1}\bar{w}_{ij\bullet\bullet}}{n^0n^1} \text{ where } w_{ijrs}=\psi\left(x_{ir}^1,y_{js}^1\right)-\psi\left(x_{ir}^2,y_{js}^2\right). \tag{7-6}$$

Lee and Rosner (2001) developed the variance estimator of this summary index based on the approach of DeLong et al. Because of the structure similarities of average and pooled differences in Equations (7-1) and (7-2), this estimator can be obtained by replacing indicator $\bar{w}_{ij\bullet}$ with $\bar{w}_{ij\bullet\bullet}$ in Equation (7–5). It is important to note that using a certain variance estimator for a given statistic is not a matter of choice. Generally, the variance for the pooled estimator is appropriate only for the pooled difference—not for the average. However, in some cases, pooled and average differences estimate the same parameter (readers have the same distribution of scores). In such cases, the approaches based on the pooled difference are more efficient. However, in general, pooled and average summaries estimate different quantities, possibly leading to contradictory conclusions in comparisons of two diagnostic modalities.

An alternative approach for comparison of two averaged AUCs is a permutation test was developed by Bandos et al., 2006. The general permutation test in a multireader setting can be constructed by permuting the ratings that correspond to the same case and reader but are assigned under different diagnostic modalities. If the compared diagnostic modalities utilize different rating scales, the observations may be standardized frequently to the same scale by ranking them within each reader and modality (Venkatraman and Begg, 1996). By computing the selected test statistic for every permutation sample (obtained by permuting ratings between modalities), one obtains the permutation distribution of the test statistic. The permutation distribution can then be used as a reference to assess the frequency of obtaining the results that are more distant from zero than those initially observed. For example, for an analysis based on a nonparametric AUC computed from a sample consisting of n^0 normal and n^1 abnormal subjects, the two-sided p-value can be written as follows:

$$p = P_{\Omega}\left(\left|\bar{D}_{\bullet}^{*}\right| \geq \left|\bar{D}_{\bullet}^{0}\right| \right) = \frac{\#\left\{ \left|\bar{D}_{\bullet}^{*t}\right| \geq \left|\bar{D}_{\bullet}^{0}\right| \right\}}{2^{n^0+n^1}} \quad t = 1,\ldots,2^{n^0+n^1}, \tag{7-7}$$

where $2^{n^0+n^1}$ is the total number of all possible permutations, $\bar{D}_{\bullet}^{0}$ is the observed reader-averaged AUC difference, and $\bar{D}_{\bullet}^{*t}$ is the reader-averaged AUC difference computed from the tth permutation. As the sample size increases, the total number of permutations increases exponentially. Hence, it is common practice to implement an approximate permutation test on a large number of randomly selected permutations (known as the Monte Carlo or MC permutation test).

Technically the permutation test can be applied to any summary index. However, for the empirical AUC, a convenient closed-form approximation performs very well even for small sample sizes. This approximation is provided by a Wald-type test based on the exact variance of its permutation distribution (variance among $2^{n^0+n^1}$ permutation values) in the following form:

$$V_{\Omega}\left(\bar{D}_{\bullet}\right) = \frac{\sum_{i=1}^{n^0}\left(\bar{w}_{i\bullet\bullet}^{1\bullet}\right)^2}{\left(n^0\right)^2} + \frac{\sum_{j=1}^{n^1}\left(\bar{w}_{\bullet j\bullet}^{\bullet 1}\right)^2}{\left(n^1\right)^2} \quad \textit{where} \quad w_{ijr}^{pq} = w\left(x_{ir}^{p}, y_{jr}^{q}\right) = \psi\left(x_{ir}^{p}, y_{jr}^{p}\right) - \psi\left(x_{ir}^{3-p}, y_{jr}^{3-q}\right). \tag{7-8}$$

If the rating scales used under two modalities are the same or they can be standardized by ranking within the modalities, the permutation test (MC or asymptotic) is fractionally more powerful than the approach of DeLong and Song. Heuristically, this can be explained by the use of a larger number of comparisons both within and across the modalities. However, if the rating scales cannot be easily put into correspondence, the permutation test may reflect differences in rating scales between modalities, similar to the way Lee and Rosner's test captures the differences between rating scales of the readers.

Another specific characteristic of the permutation test is its null hypothesis and the corresponding interpretation of the results. Unlike standard tests for comparison of AUCs that have null hypotheses of equality of the AUCs, the permutation test has a null hypothesis of equality of the modality-specific ROC curves for each reader plus "exchangeability" of the original or transformed test result (note that exchangeability is not equivalence and perfect exchangeability does not imply perfect agreement). In this respect, the permutation test is similar to conventional tests for trends that test overall equality but are specifically sensitive to differences in a specific direction. This property, for example, may result in a rejection rate higher than nominal in cases where the true average AUCs are equal (crossing reader-specific curves with the same area). However, in practical scenarios, the elevation of the rejection rate is negligible.

7.3.1.2 Methods for Random Reader or Fixed Reader Inferences

One of the first analytical treatments of the multireader problem from the random reader perspective was proposed by Swets and Pickett (1982). They emphasized the uncertainty of estimated accuracy measures due to several sources of variability including incomplete sampling of cases, incomplete sampling of readers, and residual variance reflecting remaining sources of variability (e.g., variability of reader responses on repeated readings). As a result, the overall uncertainty of the multireader summary measure (for concreteness we use differences in AUCs) may be expressed as a combination of the variance components, i.e.,

$$V(D_{rc}) = \underbrace{V\{E(D_{cr} \mid c)\}}_{case-related\ component} + \underbrace{V\{E(D_{cr} \mid r)\}}_{reader-related\ component} + \underbrace{V\{D_{cr} - E(D_{cr} \mid r) - E(D_{cr} \mid c)\}}_{residual\ component}, \quad (7\text{–}9)$$

where D_{rc} represents the difference in area under the ROC curve corresponding to the rth reader and a set of cases c. Here we enumerate the set of cases for illustration purposes because the need for enumeration typically appears in resampling approaches. The decomposition in Equation (7–9) is applicable to any indices summarizing data from two independent factors (here readers and cases) and has the same structure as a standard ANOVA partitioning of variance. The only required assumption is independence of the random factors of readers and cases. The specific indices influence only the form of the components, not the general structure of the decomposition. This and more detailed decompositions for specific summary measures (Kupinski et al., 2005; Gallas et al., 2009) can be obtained by manipulating variances of conditional expectations and expectations of conditional variances.

The classification of variance components as related to reader, case, or residual follows directly from the nature of quantities over which the variability is taken (e.g., expectation conditional on r is a function of a random r only). Alternatively, these variance components may be classified based on their dependence on the numbers of readers and cases. The reader variance component decreases with an increasing number of readers but not with the number of cases. In contrast, the case-related variance component decreases with the number of cases but not with the number of readers. The residual component may be set arbitrarily close to zero by increasing either of these numbers, i.e., by the product of the number of cases and readers. Using these properties, the variance of a summary measure estimated from a multireader study with n^R readers and $n^0 + n^1$ cases can be written in terms of more basic variance components, for example:

$$V(\bar{D}_{\bullet}) = \frac{1}{n^0 + n^1}\gamma_C + \frac{1}{n^R}\gamma_R + \frac{1}{n^R(n^0 + n^1)}\gamma_{RC}, \tag{7-10}$$

where, with increasing sample size, the variance components γ approach certain constants. The fully-crossed multireader design detailed in this chapter permits consideration of the same structure of variance decomposition for both individual indices and their differences. However, it is important to note that the interpretation of the variance components differs. For example, the reader-related variance component γ_r in Equation (7-10) is actually a reader-by-modality variance component in the decomposition of a single index.

We will call the decomposition in Equation (7-10) "Swets and Pickett's" decomposition. Since many of the estimates of the conventional summary indices are asymptotically normal, knowledge of the variance is frequently the primary factor enabling statistical inferences. If a consistent estimate of the variance is available, often an asymptotically appropriate statistical test can be based on comparison of $\bar{D}_{\bullet}/\sqrt{V(\bar{D}_{\bullet})}$ with the percentiles of a standard normal distribution. However, earlier works on random reader inferences in multireader settings (Swets and Pickett, 1982; Thompson and Zucchini, 1989) were too limited for practical application (Dorfman et al., 1992; Obuchowski and Rockette, 1995).

The first practical approach to analyzing fully-crossed multireader data was proposed by Dorfman, Berbaum and Metz (1992). This approach (frequently abbreviated DBM) capitalized on earlier developments but avoided the undesirable techniques of data splitting. The primary idea was to replicate the observed summary statistic using jack-knife pseudovalues and then apply a standard three-way ANOVA approach (the three factors are modalities, readers, and cases). Despite impressive empirical performance, this technique was criticized for the inadequate justification, including failure to account for the dependence of the jack-knife pseudovalues for finite sample sizes (Zhou et al., 2002; Song and Zhou, 2005). However, the approach was later shown to have a solid theoretical justification by Hillis et al. (2005). The theoretical justification of the DBM approach can be viewed as stemming from its relationship to another, originally theoretically grounded, method developed by Obuchowski and Rockette (1995); it is frequently called the OR method.

Obuchowski and Rockette proposed a method based on the two-way ANOVA model for correlated data (the two factors are modalities and readers). The procedure applies a method proposed by Pavur and Nath (1984) to correct the two-way ANOVA *F*-statistic for lack of independence between results obtained from the same reader. The correction adds a correlation term to the conventional denominator of the *F*-statistic. The implementation requires estimation of the variability of the test statistic due to cases and three types of correlation coefficients: between modalities for the same reader, between readers for the same modality, and between different modalities for different readers. When the nonparametric AUC is used as a summary statistic, it was originally proposed to estimate covariances using the approach of DeLong et al. (1988) for corresponding pairs of AUCs. However, the possibility of using other variance estimation approaches was also acknowledged.

The original OR method was based on using the actual accuracy indices in a two-way ANOVA setting, and developed in a more formal manner than the DBM method utilizing a somewhat heuristic approach based on three-way ANOVA on jack-knife pseudovalues. However, Hillis et al. (2005) show that the *F*-statistic for the two methods can be placed in the same general form. Differences occur because the methods use different accuracy measures (DBM uses a jack-knife-adjusted summary index), different methods of covariance estimation, or different degrees of freedom. Thus both DBM and OR approaches can be interpreted as particular realizations of the same general approach we will call DBM-OR.

The details of the implementation of the original methods and their subsequent improvement are well described in several papers (Dorfman et al., 1992; Hillis et al., 2005; Hillis, 2007; Hillis et al., 2008) and books (Zhou et al., 2002; Hillis, 2009). Here we focus on a specific but rather instructive and commonly encountered comparison of two diagnostic modalities based on the empirical area under the ROC curve in a fully-crossed method in which numbers of normal and abnormal cases are fixed by design. The details of the formulation are summarized in Appendix 7.A at the end of this chapter. For this scenario, the numerator of the *F*-statistic of a general DBM-OR approach can be shown as proportional to the squared difference in the empirical AUCs, i.e.,

$$MS(T) \propto (\bar{D}_\bullet)^2. \tag{7-11}$$

The coefficients of proportionality depend on the number of cases and readers and may differ for specific formulations of DBM-OR. However, when the F-statistics are formed, the coefficients of proportionality exert no effect since they appear in both numerator and denominator.

For the fixed reader inference, the denominator of the F-statistic in the DBM-OR approach can be shown to be proportional to the two variances of average difference in AUCs, i.e.,

$$MS(TC) \propto V_*(\bar{D}_\bullet), \tag{7-12}$$

where the subscript asterisk (*) designates a specific approach for variance estimation. For example, the original DBM method leads to a traditional one-sample jack-knife variance (J1), while the traditional OR methods lead to a two-sample (stratified) jack-knife variance (J2). For the empirical AUC or AUC difference under the paired design, these two and several other variances have closed-form formulations that reveal some of the interesting relationships (see Appendix 7.B). For example, it can be shown algebraically that the one-sample jack-knife variance estimator is always smaller than the two-sample jack-knife variance estimator (Appendix 7.B). This contributes to the conservative nature of the original DBM approach relative to the OR approach when both of them use the same reference distribution.

Thus, the DBM-OR test-statistic for fixed reader inferences based on the empirical AUC is the square of a Wald-type statistic with a corresponding jack-knife variance estimator, i.e.,

$$F_{fixed-readers} = \left(\frac{\bar{D}_\bullet}{\sqrt{V_*(\bar{D}_\bullet)}} \right)^2. \tag{7-13}$$

The test for random reader inferences has a somewhat more complex structure. First, it requires computation of the combination of the mean squares in the denominator of the F-statistic. In addition, the degrees of freedom have more complicated expressions. However, by following the steps outlined in Appendix 7.A, all required quantities for inferences based on empirical AUC can be computed in simple closed forms. The resulting F-statistic again is a ratio of the squared difference to its variance, where the variance can be expressed as follows:

$$V_{random-readers}(\bar{D}_\bullet) = \frac{\sum_{r=1}^{n^R} (D_r - \bar{D}_\bullet)^2}{n^R(n^R - 1)} + \frac{n^R}{n^R - 1} V_*(\bar{D}_\bullet) - \frac{1}{(n^R - 1)} \overline{V_*(D_r)}. \tag{7-14}$$

It is instructive to compare the overall variance (over both readers and cases), Equation (7-14), to the variance conditional on the readers, Equation (7-12). The increase in variance does not simply equal the additional variability among the reader-specific estimates of the differences (D_r). The increase is actually smaller (since the average variance tends to be greater than the variance of the average), which heuristically can be interpreted as the incorporation by the simple sample variance of both the variability of the readers and part of the residual variability.

In practice, the second term in the formulation for random reader variance in Equation (7-14) is usually greater than the absolute value of the third. As a result, the overall variance is greater than the sample variability of the reader-specific summary indices (first term). When this is not true, the overall variance becomes less than the first term. In this case, the original DBM approach and subsequent modifications (Hillis et al., 2008) suggested using only the mean square in the denominator of the F-statistic due to modality–reader interaction. In terms of Equation (7-14), it is equivalent to using the first term as an estimate of the random reader variance. In other words:

$$V^{c}_{random-readers}\left(\bar{D}_{\bullet}\right)=\max\left\{\frac{\sum_{r=1}^{n^R}\left(D_r-\bar{D}_{\bullet}\right)^2}{n^R\left(n^R-1\right)};\right.$$
$$\left.\frac{\sum_{r=1}^{n^R}\left(\hat{D}_r-\bar{D}_{\bullet}\right)^2}{n^R\left(n^R-1\right)}+\frac{n^R}{n^R-1}V_*\left(\bar{D}_{\bullet}\right)-\frac{1}{\left(n^R-1\right)}\overline{V_*\left(D_r\right)}\right\}. \tag{7-15}$$

As to the statistical properties of the test, this constraint for the variance corrects instances of inadmissible estimates of specific variance components, thereby resulting in a Type I error rate that is closer to the nominal value. Note that in cases of inadmissible estimates, the test statistic becomes the same as that of the naïve t-test. In general, the overall DBM-OR test statistic for random reader comparison of the average of empirical AUCs can also be written as a square of a Wald-type statistic, i.e.,

$$F_{random-readers}=\left(\frac{\bar{D}_{\bullet}}{\sqrt{V^{c}_{random-readers}\left(\bar{D}_{\bullet}\right)}}\right)^2. \tag{7-16}$$

To perform the statistical test, the computed value should be compared to the percentile of the F-distribution with the numerator degree of freedom of 1 and specific denominator degrees of freedom. Relatively recent developments of the overall DBM-OR approach (Hillis, 2007) suggested improved degrees of freedom, that when using empirical AUCs can be computed:

$$df_H = \left(n^R - 1\right)\left\{ V^c_{random-readers}\left(\bar{D}_\bullet\right) \Big/ \frac{\sum_{r=1}^{n^R}\left(D_r - \bar{D}_r\right)^2}{n^R\left(n^R-1\right)} \right\}^2. \quad (7\text{-}17)$$

Note that in specific cases when the variance estimator requires a constraint, the random reader variance becomes equivalent to the sample variance of the reader-specific summaries and the degrees of freedom reduce to $n^R - 1$. In such cases, the modified DBM-OR approach is exactly equivalent to the naïve t-test used earlier in developing multireader approaches. In addition to using the one- and two-sample jack-knife approaches employed correspondingly by original DBM and OR approaches, the general DBM-OR approach can be implemented using bootstrap and other variance estimation approaches.

The relationships of some of the variance statistics described in Appendix 7.B provide an idea about the relative performance of different variants of DBM-OR for fixed-effect inferences and may be used to gain insight into the relative differences for random effect inferences. In general, various approaches for variance estimation in cross-correlated multireader data have been developed. The next section discusses several approaches to estimation of variance components.

7.3.1.3 Variance Components Estimation

In multireader studies, the variance of the summary indices is affected by various sources of variability that are often reflected with the help of variance components. Understanding the components of a variance is instrumental in designing future studies and often helps develop improved estimation methods. Under the general DBM-OR approach, the three variance components of Equation (7-10), Swets and Pickett's decomposition, may be obtained using linear combinations of mean squares conventional for an ANOVA setting. When applied to the empirical AUC, these variance components have particularly instructive closed-form expressions:

$$\begin{aligned}
\gamma_C^{DBM} &\propto \left(n^0 + n^1\right) \times \left[\tfrac{n^R}{n^R-1} V_*\left(\bar{D}_\bullet\right) - \tfrac{1}{n^R-1}\overline{V_*\left(D_r\right)}\right], \\
\gamma_R^{DBM} &\propto n^R \times \left[\frac{\sum_{r=1}^{n^R}\left(D_r - \bar{D}_\bullet\right)^2}{n^R\left(n^R-1\right)} - \tfrac{1}{n^R-1}\left\{\overline{V_*\left(D_r\right)} - V_*\left(\bar{D}_\bullet\right)\right\}\right], \\
\gamma_{RC}^{DBM} &\propto n^R\left(n^0 + n^1\right) \times \left[\tfrac{1}{n^R-1}\left\{\overline{V_*\left(D_r\right)} - V_*\left(\bar{D}_\bullet\right)\right\}\right].
\end{aligned} \quad (7\text{-}18)$$

Despite the linear model representation conventionally used for presenting ANOVA-based methods, the decomposition to the variance components under this design does not require model-based assumptions. Rather, it can be viewed as grouping quantities according to their order of tendency to zero with increasing sample size.

One of the first systematic approaches to presenting the variance of a summary index under the fully-crossed multireader design was considered by Roe and Metz (1997). They presented a variance component model relating the overall variance to the sources of variability due to readers, cases, and their interactions with the modalities. The resulting decomposition of the variance was more detailed than the traditional Swets and Pickett's decomposition, but less detailed than methods proposed later (Gallas, 2006). However, Roe and Metz did not propose a practical approach for estimation of variance components.

The practical realization of the Roe and Metz decomposition of variance was proposed by Beiden, Wagner, and Campbell (2000)—frequently termed the BWC approach. The cornerstone was the consideration of bootstrap replicates of a summary index, where bootstrap replicates were generated by independently resampling cases and readers. However, instead of considering a single bootstrap space generated by case and reader resampling, they proposed to additionally consider resampling of cases for fixed readers. Using the variances estimated from different reader–modality combinations, they identified the necessary variance components using expressions of the various variances through the variance components. Using their approach, the three basic variance components of the Swets and Pickett's decomposition can be written:

$$
\begin{aligned}
\gamma_C^{BWC} &\propto \left(n^0+n^1\right)\times\left[\frac{n^R}{n^R-1}V_B\left(\bar{D}_\bullet\right)-\frac{1}{n^R-1}\overline{V_B\left(D_r\right)}\right],\\
\gamma_R^{BWC} &\propto n^R\times\left[\sum_{r=1}^{n^R}\left(D_r-\bar{D}_\bullet\right)^2\Big/\left(n^R\right)^2\right],\\
\gamma_{RC}^{BWC} &\propto n^R\left(n^0+n^1\right)\times\left[\frac{1}{n^R-1}\left\{\overline{V_B\left(D_r\right)}-V_B\left(\bar{D}_\bullet\right)\right\}\right].
\end{aligned}
\qquad (7\text{-}19)
$$

In a BWC formulation, the reader-related component is the sample variability of the reader-specific estimates or, equivalently, the bootstrap variance of the reader-averaged estimate given the original set of cases. For the difference in (or single) nonparametric AUC, the ideal bootstrap variance (V_B) can be obtained in closed form (Appendix 7.B), circumventing the sampling error resulting from using a traditional Monte Carlo (MC) bootstrap (Bandos et al., 2006). For other indices, the estimation can be conducted via the MC bootstrap originally used in the BWC approach based on drawing a large random sample (e.g., 3000) of cases and readers and estimating required sample variances. In many cases, the resulting BWC estimates of the three variance components approach the values from the DBM method (Beiden et al., 2000). However, under some scenarios, they may lead to a noticeable bias (Gallas et al., 2009).

Although the BWC approach uses bootstrap resampling and considers sources of variability due to readers and cases, it is different from a "pure" bootstrap in which both cases and readers are resampled. Some of the BWC variances are estimated by resampling cases for all pairs of readers that are constrained to be the same. This makes the corresponding quantities consistent with variances based on resampling readers *without*, rather than *with*, replacement. This deviation from the pure bootstrap approach leads to an actual improvement of properties of estimation, especially by reducing bias of the bootstrap estimate of the case-related variance component. Under a pure bootstrap approach where both cases and readers are resampled, the three variance components are simply rescaled bootstrap versions of the variances in Equation (7-9), i.e., (Bandos et al., 2007),

$$\begin{aligned}
\gamma_C^{Boot} &\propto (n^0+n^1)\times\left[V_B(\bar{D}_\bullet)\right],\\
\gamma_R^{Boot} &\propto n^R\times\left[\sum_{r=1}^{n^R}(D_r-\bar{D}_\bullet)^2\Big/(n^R)^2\right],\\
\gamma_{RC}^{Boot} &\propto n^R(n^0+n^1)\times\left[\frac{1}{n^R}\left\{\overline{V_B(D_r)}-V_B(\bar{D}_\bullet)\right\}\right].
\end{aligned} \tag{7-20}$$

Comparing expressions for the variance components under the DBM, BWC, and pure bootstrap approaches [Equations (7-18) through (7-20)] we notice that the BWC approach is a combination of the other two. Indeed, although BWC variance components can be expressed as linear combinations of the bootstrap variance operators, the structure of the combination of variance operators in case and residual-related variance components is the same as in the DBM approach (different from pure bootstrap). As noted earlier, this discrepancy arises from the use of an analog of resampling without replacement for estimation of some of the variances and leads to the reduction of bias in estimation. The use of the pure bootstrap estimate for the reader variance components leads to an increase of bias. Although the bias of the bootstrap approach is asymptotically negligible, it can be substantial in certain practical scenarios (Gallas et al., 2009).

The advantages of the BWC approach to variance component estimation agree with the general notions about bootstrap-based estimations in multifactor models. Davison and Hinckley (1997) argued in their book that for models depicting nested structures (e.g., cases within centers), resampling without replacement at the second stage leads to better-behaving estimators of the variance components. The BWC deviation from the pure bootstrap may be viewed as an application of the analogous principle to the multireader data. The completely paired multireader data has a fully-crossed (rather than nested) structure that offers a certain arbitrariness as to which effects to sample with and without replacement. However, for estimating variance components, it is possible to develop general guidelines to resolve this arbitrariness via an approach developed by Gallas et al. (2009) termed here HB. It exploits the fact that variance components can be represented as variances of the expectations (7-9) and suggests using the sampling with replacement for the outside operator. The resultant variance components have less bias than BWC components.

Although the approaches considered in this section are not limited to empirical AUCs, applications to other summary indices do not necessarily result in closed-form expressions for the variance components. Decompositions with more than three components are possible and frequently advantageous. For example, the variability due to cases can be further partitioned into separate sources of variability due to normal and abnormal cases, thus enabling more appropriate study design planning. For empirical AUCs, the variability under a single modality may be decomposed into the eight basic variance components, each of which can be estimated in an unbiased manner (Gallas, 2006).

All the discussed estimators of variance components are consistent under general conditions. The small sample performances of various estimators of the variance components of empirical AUCs are considered by Gallas et al. (2009). The DBM and HB estimates are similar to the unbiased ones in terms of both bias and mean square error. The pure bootstrap estimators have the smallest mean square error but may be substantially biased for smaller sample sizes. The BWC shares some of the deficiencies of the bootstrap for reader-related variance components but enjoys the advantages of HB approaches for other variance components. Assuming that relative properties hold in general. The less biased HB approach is theoretically more preferable. However, because of the overall proximity of the results, general awareness of the method, and the availability of well-tested software, the DBM approach may be the current method of choice.

7.3.2 Covariate Adjustment Approaches

Another general approach to analysis of multireader data consists of models incorporating general types of covariates. Most of these methods can reflect differences among readers as a level of a categorical covariate. The model-based approaches use the ratings or simple functions of the ratings (comparison indicators) that enter nonparametric estimators of the ROC curve or related indices as input to the model. In general, ROC-related models fall into three groups (Pepe, 1998): models for the test results, models for the ROC curves, and models for the summary indices. Many of the approaches discussed below are described in detail in recent books (Zhou et al., 2002; Pepe, 2003). Here we focus on aspects of using these models to analyze multireader data.

All ROC models assume a specific form in which covariates affect the quantity of interest. Some can be classified as generalized linear models that consider the effects of the linear combination of covariates on the mean transformed by the "link function." Others have specific non-linear forms. Models for test results are often termed "indirect" ROC or "distribution-based," since they estimate parameters of the distribution of the test results and use the parameters to infer the effects of the covariates on the ROC curve. In contrast, "direct" or "distribution-free" models for ROC curves usually exploit parametric assumptions regarding the ROC curve while leaving distribution of ratings incompletely specified (Pepe, 2003). Models for summary indices impose assumptions of the simple functions of the ratings (in contrast to the simple linear model of the summary index or its pseudovalues, as used in ANOVA-based approaches described above).

Typical multireader data have cross-correlated structures that complicate statistical modeling. Standard GEE methods (Liang and Zeger, 1986) used by many ROC models for multireader data are formulated for clustered data (correlated within but independent between clusters). However, although very versatile and robust, GEE methods do not offer an easy avenue for reflecting the increased variability due to incomplete sampling of readers or for directly specifying a cross-correlated structure (although some GEE-based approaches permit inferences with cross-correlated data; Song and Zhou, 2005). As a result, many model-based multireader approaches offer fixed-effect inferences only and assume the observations made by the same observer (on different cases) are independent once the fixed factor of the reader is included in the model.

7.3.2.1 Models for ROC Curves

One of the first model-based approaches for multireader analysis was developed by Toledano and Gatsonis (1996) for ordinal ratings data. Their model is based on the formulation of a binormal ROC model using ordinal regression previously proposed by Tosteson and Begg (1988) to analyze uncorrelated data. For cross-correlated multireader data, Toledano and Gatsonis (1996) used GEE to incorporate a correlation structure reflecting different types of dependencies between ratings of the same subjects obtained from the same reader and different modality; different readers and same modality; and different modalities and different readers.

The model and proposed robust variance estimator implicitly assume that, given the set of readers, the ratings assigned by the same reader to two different subjects are independent. Despite the availability of built-in procedures of a GEE approach for generalized linear models (e.g., PROC GENMOD SAS Version 9.2), implementation of the Toledano and Gatsonis model still requires custom software, due primarily to its deviation from a standard generalized linear formulation:

$$\Phi^{-1}\left\{P\left(T \le c \mid Z\right)\right\} = e^{-\beta^T Z_2} \times \xi_c - \alpha^T Z_1 \times e^{-\beta^T Z_2}$$
$$\Downarrow \tag{7-21}$$
$$ROC_Z\left(fpf\right) = \Phi\left(a\left(Z\right) + b\left(Z\right) \times \Phi^{-1}\left(fpf\right)\right),$$

where Z_1 and Z_2 are the two overlapping covariate vectors including an abnormality (gold standard) indicator. As the summary curve over all readers, Toledano and Gatsonis (1996) proposed the ROC curve obtained by using the average of the location (α) and scale (β) parameters corresponding to reader-specific curves. The proposed GEE approach enables only fixed reader inferences. For random reader inferences, Toledano (2003) later proposed adjustment of the model-based variability in the spirit of Swets and Pickett by adding a sample estimate of the reader-related variance. They found this approach conservative in simulation studies. One possible reason for this conservativeness is the upward bias of the sample variance of the reader-specific differences as an estimate of the reader-related variance component under the fully-crossed design (Section 7.3.1.3).

The analog of the model by Toledano and Gatsonis (1996) may be formulated for continuous data as well (Pepe, 1998). The assumption of such models is that the test results belong to the location-scale family based on a certain distribution with survival function S, i.e.,

$$\begin{array}{ll} T\,|_{D=0} = \mu_0\left(Z\right) + \sigma_0\left(Z\right)\varepsilon & \\ & \varepsilon, e \sim S \\ T\,|_{D=1} = \mu_1\left(Z\right) + \sigma_1\left(Z\right)e & \end{array}$$
$$\Downarrow \tag{7-22}$$
$$ROC\left(fpf\right) = S\left(\underbrace{-\frac{\mu_1\left(Z\right) - \mu_0\left(Z\right)}{\sigma_1\left(Z\right)}}_{a(Z)} + \underbrace{\frac{\sigma_0\left(Z\right)}{\sigma_1\left(Z\right)}}_{b(Z)} \times S^{-1}\left(fpf\right)\right).$$

Depending on whether S is assumed known or left unspecified, the model may be interpreted as parametric or semiparametric. For example, use of the standard normal distribution function ($S(\bullet) = \Phi(\bullet)$) results in the model for the binormal ROC curve.

For completely parametric indirect ROC models, the incorporation of random reader effects is straightforward. Such approaches model the test results for diseased and nondiseased subjects, then determine the ROC curve as the $S_{T|D=1}{}^0S^{-1}{}_{T|D=0}$ composition of the estimated survival functions. However, these distribution-based methods have several essential limitations (Zhou et al., 2002; Pepe, 2003). The limitations become even more severe for multireader problems in which the distributions of test results vary substantially among readers.

A more flexible and interpretable approach for continuous data is provided by distribution-free models of ROC curves (Pepe, 1997; Alonzo and Pepe, 2002; Pepe, 2003). These approaches typically specify a parametric form of the ROC curve while leaving the distribution of ratings incompletely specified. [The semiparametric analog of the technique was developed by Cai and Pepe (2002).] The model is grounded on a clever reformulation of the ROC curve as the average of appropriately defined binary indicators (for continuous data), i.e., $ROC(p) = E(U_{jp})$ where $U_{jp} = I\{S_0(Y_j) \leq p\}$ This formulation allows analysis of the ROC curve in a generalized linear modeling framework in which the probability of observing an indicator of 1 is related to the linear combination of covariates via the link function g, i.e.,

$$ROC_Z(fpf) = g[\alpha^T h(fpf) + \beta^T Z]. \quad (7\text{-}23)$$

As a specific case this approach includes the model for binormal ROC curves:

$$\begin{cases} g(\bullet) = \Phi(\bullet) \\ \alpha^T h(\bullet) = \alpha_0 + \alpha_1 \Phi^{-1}(\bullet) \end{cases} \Rightarrow ROC_Z(fpf) = \Phi[\alpha_0 + \alpha_1 \Phi^{-1}(fpf) + \beta^T Z]. \quad (7\text{-}24)$$

To analyze multireader data via the ROC-GLM approach, the readers can be included as fixed factors. The estimation of this ROC-GLM model is achieved using an estimating equation, and statistical testing is proposed to be based on the robust estimator of the variance accounting for the correlation due to the same subjects (Pepe, 2003).

7.3.2.2 Models for Summary Indices

Another type of model-based approach useful for analyzing cross-correlated multireader data is the summary index model. This model type usually exploits the formulation of the summary index of interest as a mean of certain simple functions of observations. For example, the area under the ROC curve can be expressed as the mean of the ordering indicators for a pair of test results for diseased and nondiseased subjects, i.e.,

$$E(A) = E\left(\frac{\sum_{i=1}^{n^0}\sum_{j=1}^{n^1}\psi(x_i, y_j)}{n^0 n^1}\right) = E(\psi(x_i, y_j)) = E(\psi_{ij}). \quad (7\text{-}25)$$

Similarly the partial area can be expressed as the mean of the ordering indicators for test results that exceed a certain threshold. The regression models for the AUC and partial AUC (Dodd and Pepe 2003, 2004) can accommodate the cross-correlated multireader data using assumptions similar to those of the GEE models for ROC curves cited above. Specifically, the readers may be treated as levels of a categorical covariate; observations corresponding to the same reader and different cases are considered independent. These models use standard link functions (e.g., *logit*) for modeling the ordering indicators defined for continuous data, i.e., $g\{E(\psi_{ij})\} = \beta^T Z$.

Dodd and Pepe (2003) demonstrated that despite the cross-correlated nature of the ordering indicators (correlated due to sharing the same diseased or nondiseased subject), consistent estimates of the model's coefficients can be obtained by applying standard GEE. Song and Zhou (2005) further expanded the existing model for AUC (Dodd and Pepe 2003) by demonstrating consistency in the presence of an additional level of correlation structure due to readers and providing a robust variance estimator accounting for all types of correlation.

The substantial advantage of using the above-described models of summary indices is models' ability to handle the covariate information. However, this advantage comes at the cost of additional model-based assumptions and difficulty addressing random reader inferences. In contrast, the ANOVA-based approaches described in Section 7.3.1.2 cannot handle covariates but can easily address random reader inferences in covariate-free problems. In addition, for the simple and commonly encountered problems of covariate-free comparison of two diagnostic modalities under the fully-crossed design, the variance-decomposition methods are virtually assumption-free. Perhaps because of these properties, the ANOVA-based approaches are used most frequently.

7.3.2.3 Bayesian Approaches

Bayesian techniques (see Chapter 5) provide yet another class of approaches for analyzing multireader data. Most Bayesian approaches for multireader analysis impose a completely parametric model with a structure that can easily accommodate various covariates and random effects but inherit the rigidity of the assumed model. Although some Bayesian approaches to single reader ROC analyses use less rigid assumptions (Gu et al., 2008), their extensions to multireader analysis have not yet been developed. Similar to frequentist approaches, current Bayesian analyses of multireader data can handle indirect (distribution-based) ROC approaches for continuous and ordinal data as well, currently with direct analysis of ROC summary measures. However, Bayesian approaches for direct modeling of entire ROC curves are underdeveloped.

To analyze multireader ordinal data, Ishwaran and Gatsonis (2000) developed a hierarchical ROC model based on the latent variable approach. The model for the observed ordinal scores stems from the general form of the binormal ROC model for ordinal data (Tosteson and Begg, 1988; Toledano and Gatsonis, 1996). The proposed extensions permit modeling multiple correlations and sources of variability natural in multireader data and inclusion of the covariates at different levels of hierarchy. The essence of a simple model can be summarized as follows:

$$T^*_{irm} = \beta_0 d_i + \beta_1 z_{rm} + \left(\varepsilon_{irm} + \delta_{irm}\right) e^{\alpha_0 d_i + \alpha_1 u_{rm}} \text{ and } T_{irm} = \sum c_j I\left(\theta_{j-1} < T^*_{irm} < \theta_j\right), \quad (7\text{-}26)$$

where $\varepsilon_{irm} \sim N\left(0, R_i\right)$ and R_i is the correlation matrix for the results obtained for subject i; δ_{irm} follows a multinomial distribution over a fixed support set. The next two levels of hierarchy determine the prior distributions for the parameters of location (β), scale (α), and thresholds (θ). In contrast to a simpler model by Toledano and Gatsonis (1996), this approach models the correlations between assessments of the same subject (reflected by R_i) and can also incorporate the correlation and additional variability due to readers (with the help of δs and βs). This model can be further extended to permit different thresholds for different reader–modality combinations (Ishwaran 2000). A somewhat simpler model that also permits incorporation of reader-specific thresholds is described by Johnson and Johnson (2005). Due to its Bayesian formulation, the approach proposed by Ishwaran and Gatsonis (2000) can be applied to both ordinal and commonly encountered 100-point data (Ishwaran and Gatsonis, 2000; Obuchowski et al., 2005).

The distribution-based (indirect ROC inferences) approaches for Bayesian analysis of continuous multireader data can be performed by extending the approaches for single reader inferences (see Chapter 5 for details). These approaches usually impose the assumption of normality of the observed ratings and corresponding conjugate priors, but may be extended to a larger class of distributions using, for example, a Box–Cox transformation (Chapter 3). However, the properties of these approaches in multireader ROC data have not yet been investigated.

In addition to the approaches based on direct and indirect modeling of ROC curves, Bayesian approaches are available for analyzing summary indices as well. Wang and Gatsonis (2007) proposed a hierarchical model for analysis of cross-correlated multireader data based on the index of the overall discriminative ability (area under the ROC curve or AUC). They model the relationship between the covariates and the AUC using a standard generalized linear structure:

$$E\begin{pmatrix} A_r^1 \\ A_r^2 \end{pmatrix} = g(\beta^T Z + \alpha_r), \tag{7-27}$$

where g can be any standard link function such as *logit* or *probit*. The (A_r) reader-specific AUCs are assumed to follow the multivariate normal distribution with a reader-specific covariance matrix (Σ_r), i.e., $A_r \sim N(E(A_r), \Sigma_r)$. The covariance matrix depends upon the mean of AUC and may be estimated using the variability estimated from the original data using conventional approaches (Obuchowski and McClish, 1996; DeLong et al., 1988) and a correlation parameter with a specific prior. The correlation due to readers and the additional variability associated with incomplete sampling of the readers is modeled using the normally distributed random factor α_r shared among the AUCs of the same reader.

The approach by Wang and Gatsonis (2007) has a frequentist analog formulated by Song and Zhou (2005). Both approaches have the same generalized linear structures and account for the cross-correlated nature of the multireader data. However, unlike its frequentist analog, the approach of Wang and Gatsonis (2007) also accounts for the additional variability associated with readers.

7.4 Remarks and Further Reading

The covariate adjustment approaches provide powerful tools for multireader analysis, but many such approaches are limited to fixed reader inferences and scenarios in which the assumption of within-reader independence is reasonable. Only a few model-based approaches may be modified to account for within-reader correlation (Song and Zhou, 2005; Toledano and Gatsonis, 1996). Accounting for uncertainties related to the incomplete sampling of readers in a complex model-based setting presents additional difficulties. For comparing diagnostic modalities, this uncertainty affects a reader-by-modality variance component. Quantification of this component of variability in a model-based setting depends greatly on the structure of the adopted model. Indeed, for the same data, different models may show substantial or minimal technical interaction of reader and modality effects (e.g., a multiplicative model needs an interaction for a truly additive structure and vice versa).

Correlated ROC data may result from many different types of diagnostic accuracy studies. Some of the data structures and approaches share certain similarities with the structures and analyses of multireader studies. One example is the ROC analysis of conventional clustered data in which the observations are correlated within but are independently between the clusters (evaluation of multiple locations on the same image, multireader studies in which readers evaluate different subjects, multicenter studies). In contrast to most multireader methods, ROC analysis of clustered data is typically performed in a population-averaged manner. Two well known non-parametric approaches for ROC analysis of clustered data were proposed by Obuchowski (1997) and Lee and Rosner (2001). Both methods effectively pool the data from different clusters, reflecting clustered structures in the correlation between the observations. The primary difference is that the approach by Obuchowski accounts for the random sizes of clusters while Lee and Rosner's approach treats the sizes as fixed.

ROC analysis of clustered data is closely related to another extension of the ROC analysis known as free-response ROC (FROC) analysis. FROC is designed to analyze the performance of diagnostic systems in detecting and localizing multiple abnormalities within a subject. Under certain study designs of detection and localization performance, the results may be viewed as clustered ROC data. For this study design, Obuchowski et al. (2000) adapted their method for analysis of clustered ROC data. The FROC analysis and different approaches to analyzing detection and localization data are discussed in Chapter 8.

Many concepts and approaches to design and analysis for multireader studies are summarized in detail in books by Swets and Pickett (1982) and Zhou et al. (2002). Some of the topics covered in those books (but not in this one) include design issues, details of implementation of DBM, OR and Swets & Pickett approaches, and sample size estimation. Recent developments on DBM methodology and sample size estimations are discussed in recent papers by Hillis et al. (2008) and Hillis and Obuchowski (2011).

Many of the methods discussed in this chapter may be implemented by using the custom-written code (often written for Stata, SAS, R, and S-Plus packages) provided by the authors of the corresponding approach. Codes and/or references for codes for implementation of many methods described in recent books by Zhou et al. (2002), Pepe (2003), and Gönen (2007) are available via the book websites (see references below). Only a few multireader approaches have corresponding stand-alone software; a notable exception is the procedure for implementing DBM-OR analysis which, along with several other software and SAS codes, is available from the Medical Image Perception Laboratory of the University of Iowa (http://perception.radiology.uiowa.edu/Software/ReceiverOperatingCharacteristicROC/tabid/120/Default.aspx).

References

Arvesen, J.N. 1969. Jack-knifing U-statistics. *Annals of Mathematical Statistics* 40: 2076–2100.

Bamber, D. 1975. The area above the ordinal dominance graph and the area below the receiver operating characteristic graph. *Journal of Mathematical Psychology* 12: 387–415.

Bandos, A.I., Rockette, H.E., and Gur, D. 2005. A permutation test sensitive to differences in areas for comparing ROC curves from a paired design. *Statistics in Medicine* 24: 2873–2893.

Bandos, A.I., Rockette, H.E., and Gur, D. 2006. Resampling methods for the area under the ROC curve. *Proceedings of ICML Workshop on ROC Analysis in Machine Learning* pp. 1–8.

Bandos, A.I., Rockette, H.E., and Gur, D. 2006. A permutation test for comparing ROC curves in multireader studies. *Academic Radiology* 13: 414–420.

Bandos, A.I., Rockette, H.E., and Gur, D. 2007. Exact bootstrap variances of the area under the ROC curve. *Communications in Statistics: Theory & Methods* 36: 2443–2461.

Beam, C.A. 1998. Analysis of clustered data in receiver operating characteristic studies. *Statistical Methods in Medical Research* 7: 324–336.

Beiden, S.V., Wagner, R.F., and Campbell, G. 2000. Components-of-variance models and multiple-bootstrap experiments: an alternative method for random-effects receiver operating characteristic analysis. *Academic Radiology* 7: 341–349.

Davison, A.C. and Hinkley, D.V. 1997. *Bootstrap Methods and Their Application.* Edinburgh: Cambridge University Press.

DBM MRMC software. http://perception.radiology.uiowa.edu/Software/ReceiverOperatingCharacteristicROC/DBMMRMC/tabid/116/Default.aspx (accessed December 29, 2010).

DeLong, E.R., DeLong, D.M., and Clarke-Pearson, D.L. 1988. Comparing the area under two or more correlated receiver operating characteristic curves: a nonparametric approach. *Biometrics* 44: 837–845.

Dorfman, D.D. and Alf, E., Jr. 1969. Maximum likelihood estimation of parameters of signal detection theory and determination of confidence intervals: rating-method data. *Journal of Mathematical Psychology* 6: 487–496.

Dorfman, D.D., Berbaum, K.S., and Metz, C.E. 1992. Receiver operating characteristic rating analysis: generalization to the population of readers and patients with the jack-knife method. *Investigative Radiology* 27: 723–731.

Gallas, B.D., Penello, G.A., and Myers, K.L. 2007. Multireader multicase variance analysis for binary data. *Journal of the Optical Society of America* 24: B70–B80.

Gönen, M. 2007. *Analyzing Receiver Operating Characteristic Curves with SAS®*. Cary, NC: SAS Institute (http://works.bepress.com/mithat_gonen/).

Gu, J., Ghosal, S., and Roy, A. 2008. Bayesian bootstrap estimation of ROC curve. *Statistics in Medicine* 27: 5407–5420.

Gur, D., Bandos, A.I., Fuhrman, C.R. et al. 2007. The prevalence effect in laboratory environment: changing the confidence ratings. *Academic Radiology* 14: 49–53.

Hanley, J.A. and Hajian-Tilaki, K.O. 1997. Sampling variability of nonparametric estimates of the area under the receiver operating characteristic curves: an update. *Academic Radiology* 4: 49–58.

Hedeker, D. and Gibbons, R.D. 1994. A random-effects ordinal regression model for multilevel analysis. *Biometrics* 50: 993–944.
Hillis, S.L. 2007. A comparison of denominator degrees of freedom methods for multiple observer ROC analysis. *Statistics in Medicine* 26: 596–619.
Hillis, S. L. 2009. Multireader ROC analysis In *Handbook of Medical Image Perception and Techniques*, Samei, E. et al., Eds., Cambridge: Cambridge University Press.
Hillis, S.L. and Obuchowski, N.A. 2011. Power estimation for multireader ROC methods: an updated and unified approach. *Academic Radiology* (in press).
Hillis, S.L., Berbaum, K.S., and Metz, C.E. 2008. Recent developments in the Dorfman–Berbaum–Metz procedure for multireader ROC study analysis. *Academic Radiology* 15: 647–661.
Hillis, S.L., Obuchowski, N.A., Schartz, K.M. et al. 2005. Comparison of the Dorfman–Berbaum–Metz and Obuchowski–Rockette methods for receiver operating characteristic (ROC) data. *Statistics in Medicine* 24: 1579–1607.
Hoffman, E.B., Sen, P.K., and Weinberg, C.R. 2001. Within-cluster resampling. *Biometrika* 88: 1121–1134.
Ishwaran H. 2000. Univariate and multirater ordinal cumulative link regression with covariate specific cut points. *Canadian Journal of Statistics* 28: 715–730.
Ishwaran, H. and Gatsonis, C.A. 2000. A general class of hierarchical ordinal regression models with applications to correlated ROC analysis. *Canadian Journal of Statistics* 28: 731–750.
Janes, H. and Pepe, M.S. 2009. Adjusting for covariate effects on classification accuracy using the covariate-adjusted receiver operating characteristic curve. *Biometrika* 96: 371–382.
Lee, M.L.T. and Rosner, B.A. 2001. The average area under correlated receiver operating characteristic curves: a nonparametric approach based on generalized two-sample Wilcoxon statistics. *Applied Statistics* 50: 337–344.
Liang, K.Y. and Zeger, S.L. 1986. Longitudinal data analysis using generalized linear models. *Biometrika* 73: 13–22.
Obuchowski, N.A. 1995. Multireader receiver operating characteristic studies: a comparison of study designs. *Academic Radiology* 2: 709–716.
Obuchowski, N.A. and Rockette, H.E. 1995. Hypothesis testing of the diagnostic accuracy for multiple diagnostic tests: an ANOVA approach with dependent observations. *Communications in Statistics: Simulation and Computation* 24: 285–308.
Obuchowski, N.A. 1997. Nonparametric analysis of clustered ROC curve data. *Biometrics* 53: 567–578.
Obuchowski, N.A. 2009. Reducing the number of reader interpretations in MRMC studies. *Academic Radiology* 16: 209–217.
Obuchowski, N.A., Lieber, M.L., and Powel, K.A. 2000. Data analysis for detection and localization of multiple abnormalities with application to mammography. *Academic Radiology* 7: 516–525.
Obuchowski, N.A. and McClish, D.K. 1997. Sample size determination for diagnostic accuracy studies involving binormal ROC curve indices. *Statistics in Medicine* 16: 1529–1542.
O'Malley, A.J. and Zou, K.H. 2006. Bayesian multivariate hierarchical transformation models for ROC analysis. *Statistics in Medicine* 25: 459–479.
Pepe, M.S.., Urban, N., Rutter, C. et al. 1997. Design of a study to improve accuracy in reading mammograms. *Journal of Clinical Epidemiology* 50: 1327–1338.

Pepe, M.S. 1998. Three approaches to regression analysis of receiver operating characteristic curves for continuous test results. *Biometrics* 54: 124–135.

Pepe, M.S. 2003. *The Statistical Evaluation of Medical Tests for Classification and Prediction*. Oxford: Oxford University Press (http://labs.fhcrc.org/pepe/book/).

Rao, J.N.K. and Scott, A.J. 1992. A simple method for the analysis of clustered binary data. *Biometrics* 48: 577–585.

Rockette, H.E., Campbell, W.L., Britton, C.A. et al. 1999. Empiric assessment of parameters that affect the design of multireader receiver operating characteristic studies. *Academic Radiology* 6: 723–729.

Song, H.H. 1997. Analysis of correlated ROC areas in diagnostic testing. *Biometrics* 53: 370–382.

Song, X. and Zhou, X.H. 2005. A marginal model approach for analysis of multi-reader multi-test receiver operating characteristic (ROC) data. *Biostatistics* 6: 303–312.

Swets, J.A. and Pickett, R.M. 1982. *Evaluation of Diagnostic Systems: Methods from Signal Detection Theory*. New York: Academic Press.

Thompson, M.L. and Zucchini, W. 1989. On the statistical analysis of ROC curves. *Statistics in Medicine* 8: 1277–1290.

Tosteson, A.N.A. and Begg, C.B. 1988. A general regression methodology for ROC curve estimation. *Medical Decision Making* 8: 204–215.

Toledano, A.Y. and Gatsonis, G. 1996. Ordinal regression methodology for ROC curves derived from correlated data. *Statistics in Medicine* 15: 1807–1826.

Toledano, A.Y. 2003. Three methods for analyzing correlated ROC curves: a comparison in real data sets from multi-reader, multi-case studies with a factorial design. *Statistics in Medicine* 22: 2919–2933.

Venkatraman, E.S. and Begg, C.B. 1996. A distribution-free procedure for comparing receiver operating characteristic curves from a paired experiment. *Biometrika* 83: 835–848.

Wagner, R.F., Beiden, S.V., Campbell, G. et al. 2002. Assessment of medical imaging and computer-assist systems: lessons from recent experience. *Academic Radiology* 9: 1264–1277.

Wang, F. and Gatsonis, C.A. 2008. Hierarchical models for ROC curve summary measures: design and analysis of multi-reader, multi-modality studies of medical tests. *Statistics in Medicine* 27: 243–256.

Wieand, H.S., Gail, M.M., and Hanley, J.A. 1983. A nonparametric procedure for comparing diagnostic tests with paired or unpaired data. *IMS. Bulletin* 12: 213–214.

Zeger, S.L., Liang, K.Y., and Albert, P.S. 1988. Models for longitudinal data: a generalized estimating equation approach. *Biometrics* 44: 1049–1060.

Zhou, X.H., Obuchowski, N.A., and McClish, D.K. 2002. Statistical methods in diagnostic medicine. New York: Wiley (ftp://ftp.wiley.com/public/sci_tech_med/statistical_methods).

Appendix 7.A: Closed Form Formulation of DBM Approach for Comparing Two Modalities Using Empirical AUC

We start with deriving a closed-form for the standard (one-sample) jack-knife estimates of the area under the empirical ROC curve (empirical AUC), then consider simplifications for various mean squares used in the DBM approach. Under the completely paired design for comparison of two modalities, the individual empirical AUCs and their difference can be expressed as:

$$A_r^m = \frac{\sum_{i=1}^{n^0}\sum_{j=1}^{n^1} \psi\left(x_{ir}^m, y_{jr}^m\right)}{n^1 n^0} \qquad \psi(x,y) = \begin{cases} 0 & x > y \\ 0.5 & x = y \\ 1 & x < y \end{cases}$$

$$D_r = A_r^1 - A_r^2 = \frac{\sum_{i=1}^{n^0}\sum_{j=1}^{n^1} \psi_{ijr}^1}{n^0 n^1} - \frac{\sum_{i=1}^{n^0}\sum_{j=1}^{N_Y} \psi_{ijr}^2}{n^0 n^1} = \frac{\sum_{i=1}^{n^0}\sum_{j=1}^{n^1} w_{ijr}}{n^0 n^1} = \bar{w}_{\bullet\bullet r} \qquad w_{ijr} = \psi_{ijr}^1 - \psi_{ijr}^2 \tag{7.A-1}$$

To compute the pseudovalues, we first consider the expression for the estimates based on a (jack-knife) sample constructed by removing observations corresponding to a single case c:

$$D_{(-c)r}^* = \begin{cases} \dfrac{\sum_{k=1}^{n^0}\sum_{l=1}^{n^1} w_{klr}}{\left(n^0-1\right)n^1} - \dfrac{\sum_{j=1}^{n^1} w_{ijr}}{\left(n^0-1\right)n^1} = \dfrac{n^0}{n^0-1}\bar{w}_{\bullet\bullet r} - \dfrac{1}{n^0-1}\bar{w}_{i\bullet r} & \text{if } x \text{ is removed } (c = i) \\[2ex] \dfrac{\sum_{k=1}^{n^0}\sum_{l=1}^{n^1} w_{klr}}{n^0\left(n^1-1\right)} - \dfrac{\sum_{k=1}^{n^0} w_{kjr}}{n^0\left(n^1-1\right)} = \dfrac{n^1}{n^1-1}\bar{w}_{\bullet\bullet r} - \dfrac{\bar{w}_{\bullet jr}}{n^1-1} & \text{if } y \text{ is removed } (c = j) \end{cases}.$$

The pseudovalues [distinguished from the original estimates by an asterisk (*) in the superscript] for the difference can be written:

$$\text{if } x \text{ is removed } (c=i) \quad D_{cr}^* = \left(n^0+n^1\right)D_r - \left(n^0+n^1-1\right)D_{(-c)r}^* = \frac{n^0+n^1-1}{n^0-1}\bar{w}_{i\bullet r} - \frac{n^1}{n^0-1}\bar{w}_{\bullet\bullet r},$$

$$\text{if } y \text{ is removed } (c=j) \quad D_{cr}^* = \left(n^0+n^1\right)D_r - \left(n^0+n^1-1\right)D_{(-c)r}^* = \frac{n^0+n^1-1}{n^1-1}\bar{w}_{\bullet jr} - \frac{n^0}{n^1-1}\bar{w}_{\bullet\bullet r}. \tag{7.A-2}$$

Similarly for the individual empirical AUCs:

$$A_{cr}^{*}=\begin{cases}\dfrac{n^0+n^1-1}{n^0-1}\bar{\psi}_{i\bullet r}-\dfrac{n^1}{n^0-1}\bar{\psi}_{\bullet\bullet r} & \text{if } x \text{ is removed } (c=i)\\[2ex] \dfrac{n^0+n^1-1}{n^1-1}\bar{\psi}_{\bullet jr}-\dfrac{n^1}{n^1-1}\bar{\psi}_{\bullet\bullet r} & \text{if } y \text{ is removed } (c=j)\end{cases}. \tag{7.A-3}$$

These formulations illustrate the following relationship, which is natural because of the unbiased nature of the empirical estimates of the AUC for observable ROC curves:

$$\bar{D}^{*}_{\bullet r}=\frac{\sum_{c=1}^{n^0+n^1}D^{*}_{cr}}{n^0+n^1}=\frac{\sum_{i=1}^{n^0}\left(\frac{n^0+n^1-1}{n^0-1}\bar{w}_{i\bullet r}-\frac{n^1}{n^0-1}\bar{w}_{\bullet\bullet r}\right)+\sum_{j=1}^{n^1}\left(\frac{n^0+n^1-1}{n^1-1}\bar{w}_{\bullet jr}-\frac{n^0}{n^1-1}\bar{w}_{\bullet\bullet r}\right)}{n^0+n^1}=\bar{w}_{\bullet\bullet r}=D_r.$$

As a result we obtain the following useful properties:

$$\bar{D}^{*}_{\bullet\bullet}=\bar{w}_{\bullet\bullet\bullet}=\hat{\bar{D}}_{\bullet}$$
$$\text{and} \tag{7.A-4}$$
$$\bar{A}^{*}_{\bullet r}=\bar{\psi}_{\bullet\bullet r}=A_r \quad \bar{A}^{*}_{\bullet\bullet}=\bar{\psi}_{\bullet\bullet\bullet}=\bar{A}_{\bullet}\ .$$

Now, using the above-derived formulations and properties, we can simplify the DBM-ANOVA mean squares for empirical AUCs. In agreement with the literature on the DBM approach (Dorfman et al., 1992; Hillis et al., 2005), we use capital letters T, C, and R and their combinations to identify sources of variability due to modalities, cases, and readers, and their interactions correspondingly. The superscript asterisk (*) reflects that the corresponding mean square is computed on pseudovalues rather than raw observations.

$$MS^{*}(T)=(n^0+n^1)n^R\sum_{m=1}^{2}\left(\bar{A}^{*m}_{\bullet\bullet}-\bar{A}^{*\bullet}_{\bullet\bullet}\right)^2=(n^0+n^1)n^R\sum_{m=1}^{2}\left(A^{m}_{\bullet}-\bar{A}^{\bullet}_{\bullet}\right)^2=\frac{(n^0+n^1)n^R}{2}\left(\bar{D}_{\bullet}\right)^2, \tag{7.A-5}$$

$$MS^{*}(TC)=\frac{n^R}{n^0+n^1-1}\sum_{c=1}^{n^0+n^1}\sum_{m=1}^{2}\left(\bar{A}^{*m}_{c\bullet}-\bar{A}^{*m}_{\bullet\bullet}-\bar{A}^{*\bullet}_{c\bullet}+\bar{A}^{*\bullet}_{\bullet\bullet}\right)^2=\frac{n^R}{2(n^0+n^1-1)}\sum_{c=1}^{n^0+n^1}\left(\bar{D}^{*}_{c\bullet}-\bar{D}^{*}_{\bullet\bullet}\right)^2=\frac{n^R(n^0+n^1)}{2}V_{J1}(\bar{D}_{\bullet}), \tag{7.A-6}$$

where $V_{J1}(\bar{D}_{\bullet})$ is the one-sample jack-knife estimator of the variance of the reader-averaged differences in AUCs ($\bar{D}_{\bullet}$) which can be written as:

$$V_{J1}(\bar{D}_{\bullet}) = \frac{\sum_{c=1}^{n^0+n^1}\left(\bar{D}^{*}_{c\bullet} - \bar{D}^{*}_{\bullet\bullet}\right)^2}{(n^0+n^1-1)(n^0+n^1)} =$$

$$= \frac{1}{(n^0+n^1-1)(n^0+n^1)}\left\{\sum_{i=1}^{n^0}\left(\frac{n^0+n^1-1}{n^0-1}\bar{w}_{i\bullet\bullet} - \frac{n^1}{n^0-1}\bar{w}_{\bullet\bullet\bullet} - \bar{w}_{\bullet\bullet\bullet}\right)^2 + \sum_{j=1}^{n^1}\left(\frac{n^0+n^1-1}{n^1-1}\bar{w}_{\bullet j\bullet} - \frac{n^0}{n^1-1}\bar{w}_{\bullet\bullet\bullet} - \bar{w}_{\bullet\bullet\bullet}\right)^2\right\}$$

$$= \frac{1}{(n^0+n^1-1)(n^0+n^1)}\left\{\left(\frac{n^0+n^1-1}{n^0-1}\right)^2\sum_{i=1}^{n^0}\left(\bar{w}_{i\bullet\bullet} - \bar{w}_{\bullet\bullet\bullet}\right)^2 + \left(\frac{n^0+n^1-1}{n^1-1}\right)^2\sum_{j=1}^{n^1}\left(\bar{w}_{\bullet j\bullet} - \bar{w}_{\bullet\bullet\bullet}\right)^2\right\}$$

$$= \frac{n^0+n^1-1}{n^0+n^1}\left\{\frac{\sum_{i=1}^{n^0}\left(\bar{w}_{i\bullet\bullet} - \bar{w}_{\bullet\bullet\bullet}\right)^2}{(n^0-1)^2} + \frac{\sum_{j=1}^{n^1}\left(\bar{w}_{\bullet j\bullet} - \bar{w}_{\bullet\bullet\bullet}\right)^2}{(n^1-1)^2}\right\}.$$

Furthermore,

$$MS^{*}(TR) = \frac{n^0+n^1}{n^R-1}\sum_{r=1}^{n^R}\sum_{m=1}^{2}\left(\bar{A}^{*m}_{\bullet r} - \bar{A}^{*m}_{\bullet\bullet} - \bar{A}^{*\bullet}_{\bullet r} + \bar{A}^{*\bullet}_{\bullet\bullet}\right)^2 = \frac{n^0+n^1}{2(n^R-1)}\sum_{r=1}^{n^R}\left(\bar{D}^{*}_{\bullet r} - \bar{D}^{*}_{\bullet\bullet}\right)^2 = \frac{n^R(n^0+n^1)}{2(n^R-1)}\frac{\sum_{r=1}^{n^R}\left(D_r - \bar{D}_{\bullet}\right)^2}{n^R},$$

(7.A-7)

$$MS^{*}(TRC) = \frac{1}{(n^R-1)(n^0+n^1-1)}\sum_{c=1}^{n^0+n^1}\sum_{r=1}^{n^R}\sum_{m=1}^{2}\left(A^{*m}_{cr} - \bar{A}^{*m}_{\bullet r} - \bar{A}^{*m}_{c\bullet} - \bar{A}^{*\bullet}_{cr} + \bar{A}^{*m}_{\bullet\bullet} + \bar{A}^{*\bullet}_{c\bullet} + \bar{A}^{*\bullet}_{\bullet r} - \bar{A}^{*\bullet}_{\bullet\bullet}\right)^2$$

$$= \frac{1}{2(n^R-1)(n^0+n^1-1)}\sum_{c=1}^{n^0+n^1}\sum_{r=1}^{n^R}\left(D_{cr} - \bar{D}^{*}_{\bullet r} - \bar{D}^{*}_{c\bullet} + \bar{D}^{*}_{\bullet\bullet}\right)^2$$

$$= \frac{1}{2(n^R-1)(n^0+n^1-1)}\sum_{r=1}^{n^R}\left\{\begin{array}{l}\sum_{i=1}^{n^0}\left(\frac{n^0+n^1-1}{n^0-1}\bar{w}_{i\bullet r} - \frac{n^1}{n^0-1}\bar{w}_{\bullet\bullet r} - \bar{w}_{\bullet\bullet r} - \frac{n^0+n^1-1}{n^0-1}\bar{w}_{i\bullet\bullet} + \frac{n^1}{n^0-1}\bar{w}_{\bullet\bullet\bullet} + \bar{w}_{\bullet\bullet\bullet}\right)^2 \\ +\sum_{j=1}^{n^1}\left(\frac{n^0+n^1-1}{n^1-1}\bar{w}_{\bullet jr} - \frac{n^0}{n^1-1}\bar{w}_{\bullet\bullet r} - \bar{w}_{\bullet\bullet r} - \frac{n^0+n^1-1}{n^1-1}\bar{w}_{\bullet j\bullet} + \frac{n^0}{n^1-1}\bar{w}_{\bullet\bullet\bullet} + \bar{w}_{\bullet\bullet\bullet}\right)^2\end{array}\right\}$$

$$= \frac{(n^0+n^1-1)}{2(n^R-1)}\sum_{r=1}^{n^R}\left\{\frac{\sum_{i=1}^{n^0}\left(\bar{w}_{i\bullet r} - \bar{w}_{\bullet\bullet r} - \bar{w}_{i\bullet\bullet} + \bar{w}_{\bullet\bullet\bullet}\right)^2}{(n^0-1)^2} + \frac{\sum_{j=1}^{n^1}\left(\bar{w}_{\bullet jr} - \bar{w}_{\bullet\bullet r} - \bar{w}_{\bullet j\bullet} + \bar{w}_{\bullet\bullet\bullet}\right)^2}{(n^1-1)^2}\right\}$$

$$= \frac{(n^0+n^1-1)}{2(n^R-1)} \times \frac{n^0+n^1}{n^0+n^1-1}\sum_{r=1}^{n^R}V_{J1}(D_r) - \frac{n^0+n^1-1}{2(n^R-1)} \times \frac{n^0+n^1}{n^0+n^1-1} \times n^R \times V_{J1}(\bar{D}_{\bullet}) = \frac{(n^0+n^1)n^R}{2(n^R-1)}\left\{\overline{V_{J1}(D_r)} - V_{J1}(\bar{D}_{\bullet})\right\}.$$

(7.A-8)

Using the expression for the mean squares in Equations (7.A-5) through (7.A-8), we can formulate the closed-form expressions for the test statistics. The fixed reader test statistic is equivalent to the square of the t-test with the jack-knife estimate of variance, i.e.,

$$F_{fixed} = \frac{MS^*(T)}{MS^*(TC)} = \frac{\frac{(n^0 + n^1)n^R}{2}(\bar{D}_\bullet)^2}{\frac{n^R(n^0 + n^1)}{2}V_{J1}(\bar{D}_\bullet)} = \left(\frac{\bar{D}_\bullet}{\sqrt{V_{J1}(\bar{D}_\bullet)}}\right)^2. \tag{7.A-9}$$

The DBM test statistic for the random readers can also be expressed as a square of the t-statistic where the standard deviation in the denominator accounts for the additional variability due to incomplete sampling of readers, i.e.,

$$F_{random} = \frac{MS^*(T)}{MS^*(TR) + MS^*(TC) - MS^*(TRC)}$$

$$= \frac{\frac{n^R(n^0+n^1)}{2}(D_r)^2}{\frac{n^R(n^0+n^1)}{2(n^R-1)}\frac{\sum_{r=1}^{n^R}(D_r - \bar{D}_\bullet)^2}{n^R} + \frac{n^R(n^0+n^1)}{2}V_{J1}(\bar{D}_\bullet) - \frac{(n^0+n^1)n^R}{2(n^R-1)}\left\{\overline{V_{J1}(D_r)} - V_{J1}(\bar{D}_\bullet)\right\}}$$

$$= \frac{(D_r)^2}{\frac{\sum_{r=1}^{n^R}\left(\hat{D}_r - \bar{\hat{D}}_r\right)^2}{n^R(n^R-1)} + V_{J1}(\bar{D}_\bullet) - \frac{1}{(n^R-1)}\left\{\overline{V_{J1}(D_r)} - V_{J1}(\bar{D}_\bullet)\right\}}$$

$$= \left(\frac{D_r}{\sqrt{\frac{\sum_{r=1}^{n^R}(D_r - \bar{D}_\bullet)^2}{n^R(n^R-1)} + \frac{n^R}{n^R-1}V_{J1}(\bar{D}_\bullet) - \frac{1}{(n^R-1)}\overline{V_{J1}(D_r)}}}\right)^2. \tag{7.A-10}$$

Appendix 7.B: Variance Estimators of Empirical AUCs

As discussed in Appendix 7.A, the empirical AUCs in the completely paired design have closed-form expressions for point estimate and variance under the one-sample jack-knife approach. The variances of individual empirical AUCs may be obtained in a closed form under other case resampling approaches including bootstrap and two-sample jack-knife. Here we discuss the relationships between the commonly encountered variance estimators. For simplicity, we present several formulas for the single-reader difference (7-2). The estimates of fixed reader variance for individual estimates, averages, and pooled estimates can be obtained by replacing w with an appropriate quantity; see Equation (7-3). Note that the presented variance estimators reflect variability due to cases only. Although some resampling approaches use closed-form formulations for random reader variance estimators (Bandos et al., 2005) they have a more complex expression. We now consider the following five variance estimators of AUC differences:

Variance estimator (Wieand et al., 1988) —

$$V_W = \frac{n^1-1}{n^1}\frac{\sum_{i=1}^{n^0}\left(\overline{w}_{i\bullet}-\overline{w}_{\bullet\bullet}\right)^2}{\left(n^0\right)^2}+\frac{n^0-1}{n^0}\frac{\sum_{j=1}^{n^1}\left(\overline{w}_{\bullet j}-\overline{w}_{\bullet\bullet}\right)^2}{\left(n^1\right)^2}-\frac{\sum_{i=1}^{n^0}\sum_{j=1}^{n^1}\left(w_{ij}-\overline{w}_{i\bullet}-\overline{w}_{\bullet j}+\overline{w}_{\bullet\bullet}\right)^2}{\left(n^0\right)^2\left(n^1\right)^2}. \tag{7.B-1}$$

Bootstrap variance —

$$V_B(D)=\frac{\sum_{i=1}^{n^0}\left(\overline{w}_{i\bullet}-\overline{w}_{\bullet\bullet}\right)^2}{\left(n^0\right)^2}+\frac{\sum_{j=1}^{n^1}\left(\overline{w}_{\bullet j}-\overline{w}_{\bullet\bullet}\right)^2}{\left(n^1\right)^2}+\frac{\sum_{i=1}^{n^0}\sum_{j=1}^{n^1}\left(w_{ij}-\overline{w}_{i\bullet}-\overline{w}_{\bullet j}+\overline{w}_{\bullet\bullet}\right)^2}{\left(n^0\right)^2\left(n^1\right)^2}. \tag{7.B-2}$$

Unbiased variance estimator (Bamber, 1975; Wieand et al., 1988) —

$$V_U(D)=\frac{\sum_{i=1}^{n^0}\left(\overline{w}_{i\bullet}-\overline{w}_{\bullet\bullet}\right)^2}{n^0(n^0-1)}+\frac{\sum_{j=1}^{n^1}\left(\overline{w}_{\bullet j}-\overline{w}_{\bullet\bullet}\right)^2}{n^1(n^1-1)}-\frac{\sum_{i=1}^{n^0}\sum_{j=1}^{n^1}\left(w_{ij}-\overline{w}_{i\bullet}-\overline{w}_{\bullet j}+\overline{w}_{\bullet\bullet}\right)^2}{n^0n^1(n^0-1)(n^1-1)}. \tag{7.B-3}$$

Two-sample jack-knife (DeLong et al., 1988) —

$$V_{J2}(D)=\frac{\sum_{i=1}^{n^0}\left(\overline{w}_{i\bullet}-\overline{w}_{\bullet\bullet}\right)^2}{n^0(n^0-1)}+\frac{\sum_{j=1}^{n^1}\left(\overline{w}_{\bullet j}-\overline{w}_{\bullet\bullet}\right)^2}{n^1(n^1-1)}. \tag{7.B-4}$$

One-sample jack-knife (Dorfman et al., 1992; Hanley et al., 1997) —

$$V_{J1}(D) = \frac{n^0+n^1-1}{n^0+n^1}\left\{\frac{\sum_{i=1}^{n^0}\left(\overline{w}_{i\bullet}-\overline{w}_{\bullet\bullet}\right)^2}{\left(n^0-1\right)^2}+\frac{\sum_{j=1}^{n^1}\left(\overline{w}_{\bullet j}-\overline{w}_{\bullet\bullet}\right)^2}{\left(n^1-1\right)^2}\right\}. \quad (7.B\text{-}5)$$

Certain deterministic relationships exist among the considered variance estimators:

$$V_W \le V_U \le V_{J2} \le V_{J1} \text{ and}$$
$$V_W \le V_B. \quad (7.B\text{-}6)$$

The bootstrap variance may be smaller or larger than any of the V_U, V_{J1}, and V_{J2} estimators, depending on the data. The inequalities shown in Equation (7.B-6) may be proved by the following observations:

1. It follows from Equations (7.B-3) and (7.B-4) that the two-sample jack-knife variance estimator is always larger than the unbiased variance estimator (hence upward biased), i.e.,

$$V_U + \frac{\sum_{i=1}^{n^0}\sum_{j=1}^{n^1}\left(w_{ij}-\overline{w}_{i\bullet}-\overline{w}_{\bullet j}+\overline{w}_{\bullet\bullet}\right)^2}{n^0 n^1(n^0-1)(n^1-1)} = V_{J2}.$$

2. To establish relationship $V_{J2} \le V_{J1}$, note that Equation (7.B-4) can be rewritten as:

$$V_{J1} = \frac{\left(n^0+n^1-1\right)n^0}{\left(n^0+n^1\right)\left(n^0-1\right)}\left[\frac{\sum_{k=1}^{n^0}\left(\overline{w}_{k\bullet}-\overline{w}_{\bullet\bullet}\right)^2}{n^0\left(n^0-1\right)}\right]+\frac{\left(n^0+n^1-1\right)n^1}{\left(n^0+n^1\right)\left(n^1-1\right)}\left[\frac{\sum_{l=1}^{n^1}\left(\overline{w}_{\bullet l}-\overline{w}_{\bullet\bullet}\right)^2}{n^1\left(n^1-1\right)}\right].$$

The fact that the two-sample jack-knife variance estimator is never smaller than one-sample follows the next observation:

$$\frac{(n^0+n^1-1)n^0}{(n^0+n^1)(n^0-1)}=\frac{\left(n^0\right)^2+n^0n^1-n^0}{\left(n^0\right)^2+n^0n^1-n^0-n^1}>1$$

and

$$\frac{(n^0+n^1-1)n^1}{(n^0+n^1)(n^1-1)}=\frac{\left(n^1\right)^2+n^0n^1-n^1}{\left(n^1\right)^2+n^0n^1-n^1-n^0}>1.$$

3. If, when multiplied by a smaller-than-unity coefficient, the estimator in Equation (7.B-1) is less than bootstrap variance, we prove the remaining inequality $V_W \le V_B$, indeed:

$$V_W\frac{(n^0-1)(n^1-1)}{n^0n^1}=\frac{n^1-1}{n^1}\frac{\sum_{i=1}^{n^0}\left(\bar{w}_{i\bullet}-\bar{w}_{\bullet\bullet}\right)^2}{\left(n^0\right)^2}+\frac{n^0-1}{n^0}\frac{\sum_{j=1}^{n^1}\left(\bar{w}_{\bullet j}-\bar{w}_{\bullet\bullet}\right)^2}{\left(n^1\right)^2}-\frac{\sum_{i=1}^{n^0}\sum_{j=1}^{n^1}\left(w_{ij}-\bar{w}_{i\bullet}-\bar{w}_{\bullet j}+\bar{w}_{\bullet\bullet}\right)^2}{\left(n^0\right)^2\left(n^1\right)^2}$$

$$\le\frac{\sum_{i=1}^{n^0}\left(\bar{w}_{i\bullet}-\bar{w}_{\bullet\bullet}\right)^2}{\left(n^0\right)^2}+\frac{\sum_{j=1}^{n^1}\left(\bar{w}_{\bullet j}-\bar{w}_{\bullet\bullet}\right)^2}{\left(n^1\right)^2}-\frac{\sum_{i=1}^{n^0}\sum_{j=1}^{n^1}\left(w_{ij}-\bar{w}_{i\bullet}-\bar{w}_{\bullet j}+\bar{w}_{\bullet\bullet}\right)^2}{\left(n^0\right)^2\left(n^1\right)^2}\le V_B.$$

8

Free-Response ROC Analysis

8.1 Introduction

A variety of applications often trigger a need for detection and localization of multiple targets within a single subject. Such diagnostic tasks include, for example, detection and localization of chest nodules (Bunch, 1978; Chakraborty, 1989), detection and localization of military targets (Irvine, 2004), and detection of sound signals in temporal intervals (Egan, 1961). Here we adopt medical imaging terminology; *target* or *abnormality* and *subject* or *image* are used interchangeably.

In an attempt to detect and localize potentially multiple targets, a system (with or without a human interpreter) can produce multiple marks (on imagery or audio records) indicating the estimated locations of suspected targets. Depending on a specific task, a system may or may not have *a priori* information on the maximum possible number of targets, and may or may not have restrictions on the allowed proximities between marks. For example, in a primary diagnostic task of identifying one of the three brain regions (left hemisphere, right hemisphere, and brain stem) that has cerebral infarcts, the number of targets is limited by the three regions. Any of the regions can be marked and the locations of the marks are restricted by the defined regions within an image (Obuchowski et al., 2000). Conversely, in detecting and localizing masses and microcalcifications on mammograms using mammography or acoustic signals in a temporal interval, the locations of different targets may be arbitrarily close to each other, thus allowing an observer to place different marks arbitrarily close to each other.

In general, based on the known locations of all targets and the locations of the produced marks, the accuracy of a system can be characterized by the strength of association of the numbers and locations of the marks and the numbers and locations of the targets. Multiple approaches to characterizing this association are possible. However, from a practical view, the primary interest often lies in the properties of a set of marks to adequately detect and localize the targets for purposes of making decisions about further management. From this perspective, the information carried in targets and marks can be crudely classified as (1) beneficial information represented by adequately localized targets, (2) detrimental information represented by missed or inadequately localized targets, and (3) false cues that do not correspond to any targets of interest. Although it may be possible to distinguish between detection but inadequate localization and pure errors, most approaches do not make such distinctions.

Most practical problems exhibit a certain limit below which the localization error can be ignored (e.g., a target "hit" within a certain area around its center is adequately localized for given practical purposes). This limit, also known as *proximity criterion*, *acceptance radius*, or size of acceptance area is used to determine the type of response. For example, a mark placed closer to the corresponding target than determined by the proximity criterion is considered to adequately localize a target (e.g., the mark is within the acceptance radius of the center of the target). Such a mark is called a *true positive* and the localized target is considered detected (hit). Marks that do not have corresponding targets within the regions determined by a proximity criterion represent errors (due to poor localization or erroneous suspicion) and are classified as *false positives*. A target that has no marks closer than determined by the proximity criterion is a *false negative* (missed target).

Clearly, classifications in terms of true and false positives and negatives depend on the adopted proximity criterion. Furthermore, classification may involve multiple complex issues such as establishing correspondence between marks and targets and handling multiple marks that are adequately close to the same target. This chapter focuses on statistical problems assuming that, for considered proximity criteria, a single target corresponds to a single mark at most.

The analytical methods we discuss in this chapter may involve different approaches to establishing correspondence and determining proximity criteria, but they all use true positive (*TP*), false positive (*FP*), and false negative (*FN*) categories. Note that unlike traditional ROC analysis, this classification does not necessarily include true negative outcomes. The absence of this category is one of the salient features of the conventional free-response ROC (FROC) type of performance assessment. This feature also makes the data obtained from a simple FROC protocol unsuitable for analysis by conventional ROC methods.

It is intuitively appealing that a good diagnostic system tends to produce many *TP* and few *FP* responses. All approaches considered in this chapter assess performance from this perspective, but may use different experimental paradigms and primary summary measures. We consider in detail the frequently used FROC approach and briefly discuss alternative FROC (AFROC), region-of-interest (ROI), and localization ROC (LROC) approaches for assessing performance in detection and localization tasks. The chapter concludes with highlights of important differences and similarities among the approaches.

8.2 FROC Approach

8.2.1 Rating-Free FROC Analysis

The simplest type of data collected via FROC assessment for a single subject describes the numbers and locations of the marks and targets. Based on the locations of t known targets, we can employ the proximity criterion (acceptance radius) to determine which known targets are detected and adequately localized (hit targets, or *TP* marks) and which marks do not correspond to any targets (*FP* marks). We denote the numbers of *TP* and *FP* responses as a realization of the random variables N and M correspondingly:

$$\begin{aligned} &\#TP = M \quad (M \le t), \\ &\#FP = N, \\ &\#FN = t - M. \end{aligned} \tag{8-1}$$

True negative responses correspond to target-free locations not marked. In the FROC paradigm, the number of these responses is undefined. Figure 8.1 provides an example of data contributed by a single subject that has t = 3 targets; the diagnostic system produced a total of three marks (hits). The target at top left is adequately localized with one of the marks. The target at top right was missed (*FN*) for the given proximity criterion; although it can be hypothesized that the target was detected but inadequately localized, as one mark is relatively close. The third target was also missed (*FN*) and likely to be undetected because no marks are in reasonable proximity. Thus, we classify two marks as false positives (n = 2) and one as a true positive (m = 1).

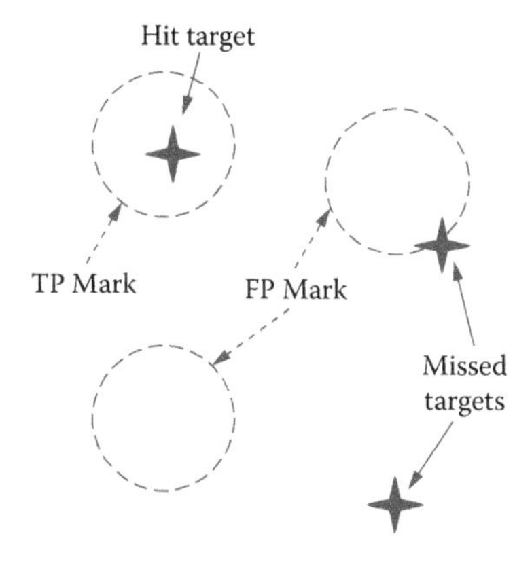

FIGURE 8.1
Classification of marks and targets under FROC paradigm.

Naturally, one would want a system to localize as many targets as possible while producing as few false positives as possible. In traditional FROC analysis, the frequencies of true and false positive responses are characterized by the proportion of detected targets (true positive fraction or *TPF*) and the rate of erroneous responses per subject (false positive rate or *FPR*):

$$FPR = E(N) \quad TPF = \frac{E(M)}{t}. \tag{8-2}$$

Note that due to the generally unknown bounds for the number of *FP* responses, their frequency is quantified with a *rate* rather than a *fraction* (*FPR* instead of *FPF*). Under the assumption that a hit target corresponds to a single mark, *TPF* is often represented in terms of a random variable $\tilde{H}$, indicating detection and adequate localization of a target randomly selected from a population of targets, i.e.:

$$TPF = \frac{E(M)}{t} = \frac{E\left\{\sum_{j=1}^{t} I(H_j = 1)\right\}}{t} = \frac{t \times P(\tilde{H} = 1)}{t} = P(\tilde{H} = 1). \tag{8-3}$$

This formulation implies an interpretation of the *TPF* as a probability of detection and adequate localization of a target. However, it is important to highlight that in a general case this probability represents a marginal probability for a hypothetical population with a given distribution of targets among subjects [conditional on sample composition, i.e., in general $TPF = E(\Sigma M)/\Sigma t$]. It is not necessarily equivalent to the probability of identification of a target randomly selected from an ensemble of targets in a general population of subjects (unconditional space) or to the event of identification of a target randomly selected from a single subject (subject-specific inference).

Because of the interpretation of *TPF* as a probability and the interpretation of *FPR* as a rate, in computer simulations and frequently in estimation models as well, the number of localized targets (*M*) is modeled using a binomial distribution, and the number of false positive responses (*N*) is modeled using a Poisson distribution. Simpler models assume the same parameters for these distributions for all subjects regardless of their characteristics (e.g., number of depicted targets or difficulty of evaluating subjects). More complicated models may consider heterogeneity of the parameters according to readily available characteristics and/or consideration of subject-specific parameters.

The assessment of performance should consider both *TPF* and *FPR* quantities simultaneously, since one can be increased at the expense of the other (see Section 8.2.2). In other words, the frequency of correct decisions should always be assessed relative to the number of errors. Perfect FROC systems identify all targets without making errors, i.e., $M \equiv t$ and $N \equiv 0$ (hence $TPF = 1$ and $FPR = 0$).

The poorest performing systems would yield only erroneous responses regardless of their number, i.e., $M \equiv 0$ (hence $TPF = 0$).

Although the poorest extreme is useful conceptually, a more useful benchmark is the accuracy of a completely random response, i.e., the performance of a guessing process. In an ROC setting, a guessing process is easy to define due to an *a priori* known number of possible responses. Under a random ROC guessing protocol, on average, the number of *TP* responses among all positive responses is proportional to the number of actually positive cases among all subjects in the population. The performance of such a diagnostic test corresponds to a point on a diagonal line in ROC space where specific coordinates of a point depend on the frequency of positive responses (aggressiveness of guessing process). Defining chance performance in an FROC setting is not as straightforward due to the lack of knowledge of the upper bound for the number of responses. One approach for defining an FROC guessing process is to consider a random placement of marks. This approach explicitly requires the relative size of the acceptance radius to the spatial density of targets in the "markable" area that includes all subjects. We discuss one of the approaches for defining a guessing FROC process and its characteristics in Section 8.2.2.

Data collected under a rating-free evaluation of subjects can be represented as:

$$\{t_s, n_s, m_s\}_{s=1}^{S}, \tag{8-4}$$

where s indicates one of S subjects (with and without targets), n_s and m_s are the numbers of *FP* and *TP* marks, respectively, and t_s is the number of targets associated with the sth subject. FROC studies are often conducted using a sample of subjects with *a priori* known numbers of targets and conventional FROC analyses treat the proportion of subjects with a specific number of targets as fixed. Thus, most analyses discussed in this chapter are conditioned on the distribution of targets among the subjects in a specific sample, although some techniques are generalizable to a variable number of targets.

Conventional FROC inferences are conditional on sample composition, effectively considering a sampling scheme in which a new sample consists of the same proportion of subjects with a specific number of targets. In the corresponding target population, the following estimates of the operating characteristics become unbiased by definition:

$$\widehat{FPR} = \frac{\sum_{s=1}^{S} n_s}{S} \quad \widehat{TPF} = \frac{\sum_{s=1}^{S} m_s}{\sum_{s=1}^{S} t_s} \tag{8-5}$$

Statistical inferences about *TPF* and *FPR* can be made via different approaches. The nonparametric estimates of these quantities can be obtained using Equation (8-5) and the variability of these estimates can be assessed using variance estimators for clustered proportions (Rao and Scott, 1992; Obuchowski, 1998).

8.2.2 FROC Space and Use of Guessing Process for Interpretation and Comparison

Performance of a system that marks suspected targets can be characterized with a pair of scalar characteristics: *TPF* and *FPR*. Similar to ROC, FROC coordinates reflect the frequency of false positives on the horizontal axis and the frequency of true positive responses on the vertical axis. However, unlike the *FPF* in ROC analysis, the *FPR* in FROC analysis is *a priori* unbounded. Consequently, the performance level of a mark-only-producing system corresponds to a single point in an infinite band $[0,\infty) \times [0,1]$.

In the ROC space, the performance characteristics may be benchmarked against a diagonal line connecting [0,0] and [1,1] which serves as a reference level for "guessing" performance. Furthermore, comparison of two systems is facilitated by the ability to evaluate minimum reasonable performance at a higher *FPF* using straight lines representing the performance of a simple random process (Norman, 1964; Schisterman et al., 2006; Bandos et al., 2010). In the FROC space, no known finite trivial point is analogous to the trivial ROC point of [1,1] at which everything is classified as positive, and there is no conventional benchmark for negligible performance (except for a system with an *FPR* at 0 which can be compared with [0,0]). These features complicate the assessment of a single diagnostic system and comparisons of several systems. Here we discuss one example of an FROC guessing process that helps interpretations and comparisons in FROC analysis.

A simple approach to characterize the random placement of marks is to consider a homogeneous Poisson process that describes the distribution of a random number η of point marks at random locations within an area of an image of size Σ. The primary parameter of this process is the average number of marks λ (per Σ) which reflects the level of aggressiveness of the random process. For simplicity, we assume that a circle of radius r around a single target is located entirely within the area (of size Σ) in which marks are permitted. A mark "hits" the target ($\delta = 1$) when it falls within an acceptance radius r from its center. Hence the probability of hitting the target by chance is the ratio between the area of a circle of size r and the size of the image, i.e.:

$$p = \frac{\pi r^2}{\Sigma}. \tag{8-6}$$

Under this protocol, multiple marks can hit the same target, and we will consider a target "hit" if at least one mark hits it. Multiple marks hitting the same target are counted as one. Then, for a given rate λ, the frequency of targets hit (*TPF*) and the frequency of false positives (*FPRs*) can be written as:

$$TPF = 1 - P\left(\sum_{i=1}^{\eta} \delta_i = 0\right) = 1 - E\left[(1-p)^{\eta}\right] = 1 - \sum_{k=0}^{\infty} (1-p)^k \times \frac{\lambda^k}{k!} e^{-\lambda} = 1 - e^{-\lambda p}$$

$$FPR = E\left[\eta - \sum_{i=1}^{\eta} \delta_i\right] = \lambda(1-p). \tag{8-7}$$

The benchmark curve of this process has the following parametric form (see Figure 8.2):

$$TPF = 1 - \exp(-FPR \times \varphi) \quad \text{where} \quad \varphi = \frac{p}{1-p}. \tag{8-8}$$

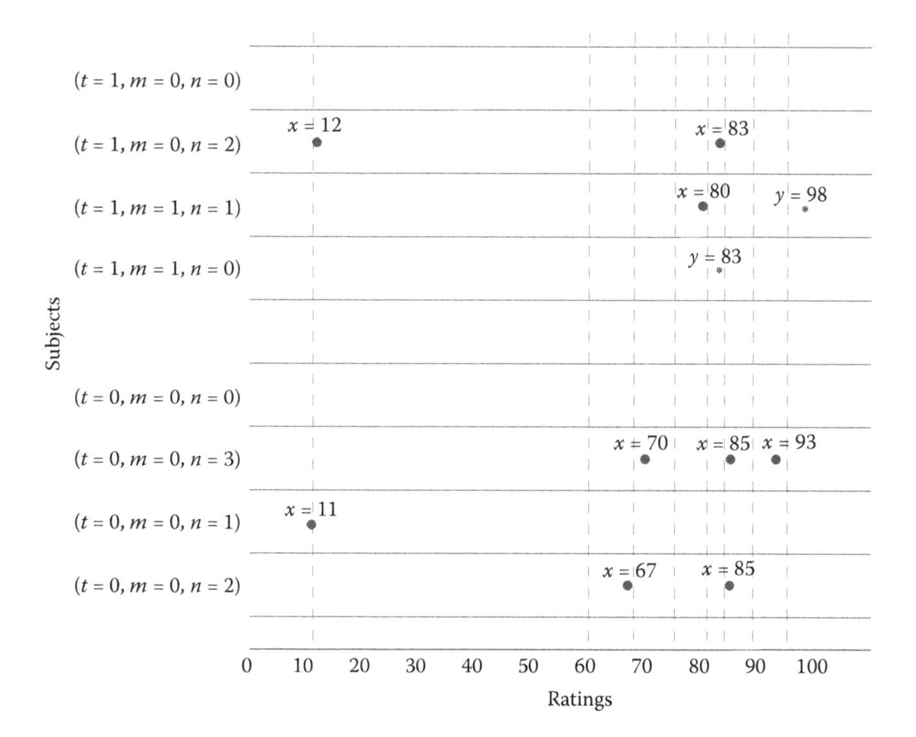

FIGURE 8.2
Example of FROC rating data (Bandos et al., 2009).

The general case that includes multiple targets would lead to a more complicated expression for the guessing curves, but the general principles remain. With a guessing curve, one can interpret the level of performance achieved by a given diagnostic system (fpr_0, tpf_0) by comparing tpf_0 to a *TPF* coordinate of a point on the guessing curve corresponding to fpr_0. For example, assuming that the density of targets corresponds to a φ of 0.11, a point with coordinates $FPR = 1.6$, $TPF = 0.7$ corresponds to a system with reasonable performance since the guessing process with the parameter $\varphi = 0.11$ at $FPR = 1.6$ would produce a *TPF* of only 0.163. Thus, the evaluated system performs about four times better than a guessing process that produces on average the same number of false positive marks.

Another useful application of a guessing process lies in enabling an objective comparison of diagnostic systems, one of which has a higher *TPF* (0.72 versus 0.7) and sufficiently higher *FPR* (3 versus 1.6). Systems with such characteristics are difficult to compare without introducing explicit (e.g., with utility function) or implicit (e.g., linear combination of *FPR–TPF*) tradeoff between *TP* and *FP* marks. In ROC analysis, an objective comparison of systems with similar characteristics may be performed at times with the help of a guessing process (Norman, 1964; Egan 1975; Bandos et al., 2010). The same general approach can be applied to FROC analysis in which a system with smaller *FPR* and *TPF* values can be considered better in terms of expected performance characteristics, if the characteristic of the guessing augmentation achieves higher *TPF* at the *FPR* of the second system. The rationale is that in such a case the second system can be outperformed on average by adding a random number of marks at the subjects previously evaluated by the first system. For example, in the case of the guessing process in Equation (8-8), the guessing augmentation of the system with characteristics ($fpr_0 = 1.6$; $tpf_0 = 0.7$) under an acceptance radius resulting in $\varphi = 0.11$ is described with the following curve (dotted extension on Figure 8.3):

$$\forall FPR > fpr_0 \quad TPF = 1 - \left\{(1 - tpf_0) \times e^{\varphi \times fpr_0}\right\} \times e^{-\varphi \times FPR}. \tag{8-9}$$

Thus, when augmented with a guessing process, this system achieves on average $TPF = 0.74$ at cost of $FPR = 3$. Hence any diagnostic system with true $FPR = 3$ and $TPF < 0.74$ is inferior in terms of the expected performance characteristics.

One advantage of using the above guessing process is that it reflects the magnitude of the proximity criterion (acceptance radius). In cases where substantially different acceptance radii may be adopted, interpretation of the FROC performance level without considering the magnitude of the proximity criterion would be questionable. Indeed, an increasing acceptance radius can result in reclassification of previous *FP* marks (outside the original acceptance area) as *TP* (within the new acceptance area), thus increasing the estimated performance level. The same system evaluated under a larger

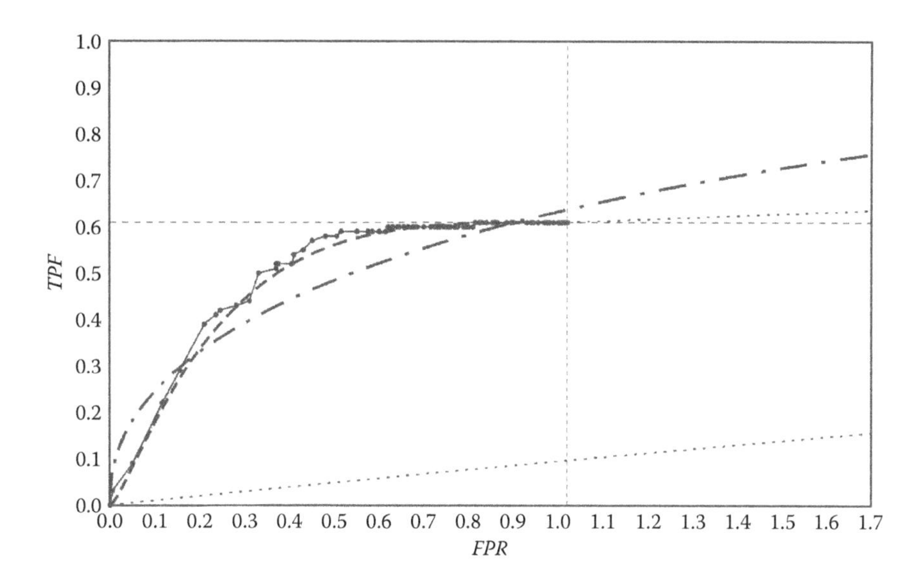

FIGURE 8.3
Parametric, empirical, and guessing FROC curves. Dots represent empirical points. The empirical FROC curve connects consecutive empirical points with a solid line. The largest dot indicates the pruning point. The dotted line corresponds to guessing processes: pure guessing FROC curves start at 0; guessing augmentation of the empirical FROC curve starts at the pruning point. The smooth dashed curve ending at the pruning point is the finite parametric Poisson–binomial–normal FROC curve. The smooth FROC curve extending to infinity is the parametric Poisson–normal FROC curve.

acceptance radius may appear better. The proximity criteria-dependent guessing process described above offers an adjustment for differing magnitudes of proximity criteria. However, in many practical scenarios the adjustments are only approximate.

Two limitations of guessing processes in FROC analysis are (1) the multiplicity of possible functional forms and (2) alternative approaches for computing guessing parameters. Thus, it is a good practice to verify the consistency of the results for a range of values of the parameters of a specific guessing process.

8.2.3 FROC Curve

Often a simple mark-producing diagnostic test represents a specific tune-up of a more general system that is capable of performing at different levels of aggressiveness. However, a change in aggressiveness level typically results in improvement of one parameter (*TPF* or *FPR*) at the expense of the other. Thus, if a diagnostic system is "forced" to produce a larger number of marks, the likely results will be both an increase in *FPR* (larger number of false positive errors) and an increase in *TPF* (improvement of number of detected targets). As with a conventional ROC analysis, it is important in FROC to recognize that a system with larger *TPF* and *FPR* values may have the same, or even worse intrinsic accuracy (underlying performance curve) as a system with smaller *TPF* and *FPR*, while merely operating at a more aggressive mode.

Similar to the traditional ROC approach, we can characterize the overall performances of a system by considering multiple FROC points (*FPR*, *TPF*) obtained at different levels of aggressiveness. The set of FROC points obtained by considering all aggressiveness settings is a traditional FROC curve that summarizes performance at all aggressiveness modes simultaneously (Bunch, 1978). Similar to the ROC curve, the FROC curve is nondecreasing because adoption of a more aggressive mode leads to expanding the set of reported marks. Figure 8.3 illustrates several FROC curves, a detailed discussion of which will be provided later.

One of the unique features of the FROC approach is the absence of *a priori* known finite *FPR-TPF* characteristics of the trivial mode at which everything is classified as positive (analogous to the ROC point [1,1]). The absence of this finite trivial point increases the importance of the "limiting" (pruning) point of the FROC curve that corresponds to the characteristics that the system is currently able to achieve. The concept and ramifications of a pruning point bear a close relationship to limits of detection (Perkins et al., 2007) and mass at zero (Schisterman et al., 2006) in ROC analysis.

8.2.4 Rating-Based FROC Analysis

In some cases, one can assess the FROC curve by forcing a system to operate multiple times at different aggressiveness levels. Under certain assumptions, it is possible to employ a more cost effective rating-based approach. Namely, a system is requested to evaluate every subject only once, but in addition to indicating suspicious locations, it is required to supplement each mark with a multicategory score (rating) reflecting a degree of confidence regarding the presence of a target in the marked location. The data contributed by a single random subject represent a realization of the following random variables:

$$\{X_i\}_{i=1}^{N}, \{Y_j\}_{j=1}^{M}, \tag{8-10}$$

where X and Y represent the ratings of *FP* and *TP* marks, respectively. Without loss of generality we will assume that ratings are always positive (>0). Under the rating-based approach, the response of a system at any aggressiveness setting is assumed to be modeled by the marks that rated above a corresponding rating threshold. The *TPF* and *FPR* characteristics can then be expressed as functions of a varying rating threshold ξ, i.e.:

$$FPR_{\rho\circ\pi}(\xi) = E\left\{ N(\xi) \right\} = E\left\{ \sum_{i=1}^{N} I(X_i > \xi) \right\}$$

$$\text{and} \quad TPF_{\rho\circ\pi}(\xi) = \frac{E\left\{ \sum_{j=1}^{M} I(Y_j > \xi) \right\}}{t}. \tag{8-11}$$

We use subscript $\rho\circ\pi$ to indicate rating-based FROC characteristics of a diagnostic system. The meaning of this subscript will be made clear later in this section.

Many ramifications and properties of the rating-based FROC curve are similar to those of a rating-based ROC curve. Similar to ROC curves, a rating-based FROC curve is always nondecreasing and invariant with respect to order-preserving transformations of the ratings. However, as discussed previously and as apparent from the formulation above, different FROC curves can "end" at different points ($\xi = -\infty$ may relate to different results for different systems), while conventional ROC curves always end at [1,1]. This may appear to generate a conceptual difference from conventional ROC analysis, but in reality, the underlying structure is very similar.

Our choice of the convention that the ratings are positive (strictly greater than 0) was made specifically to highlight this similarity. If, in an abstract rating-based ROC analysis, we consider rating thresholds only in [0,100], omitting a threshold below the lowest rating of 0, the resulting curve would end at a point different from [1,1], (corresponding to $\xi = 0$). In other words, the FROC rating protocol is analogous to an ROC rating protocol where the least suspicious response (e.g., 0 on a scale of 0 to 100) is indicated by the absence of a corresponding mark (Chakraborty and Winter, 1990).

The characteristics of the last nontrivial point under an FROC or ROC paradigm are determined by the accuracy achieved with responses rated greater than 0, or alternatively by the accuracy associated with the lowest- or default-rated responses. Multiple responses at the default rating (corresponding to missed targets in FROC) may be manifestations of certain latent phenomena. For example, as related to the FROC paradigm, eye tracking experiments clearly suggest that some of the areas unmarked by human observers actually drew attention but were not considered suspicious enough to warrant reporting (Chakraborty, 2006). The analog ROC problem is a hidden distinction between two types of 0-rated subjects: completely nonsuspicious subjects (missed) and subjects with some suspicious level but ultimately perceived as completely non-target-related. A more common phenomenon under the ROC paradigm relates to lower limits of detection (Perkins et al., 2007). Regardless of the presence of latent phenomena, the characteristics of the point corresponding to $\xi = 0$ are as important in FROC analysis as they are in conventional ROC analysis (Gur et al., 2008; Schisterman et al., 2006).

The importance of the point in FROC analysis is reflected in the representation of the FROC rating process as a composition of two distinct processes: the first describing the detection and localization of suspicious locations and the second describing the ratings of the reported locations according to the degree of suspicion. The terminology for these processes varies, depending on the specific type of application. The process describing rating-free detection and localization of suspicious areas can be called candidate selection (Edwards et al., 2002), pre-attentive analysis (Chakraborty, 2006), or (as in this book) a pruning process or π (Bandos et al., 2009). The second process may be termed candidate analysis (Edwards et al., 2002), cognitive evaluation (Chakraborty, 2006), or (as in this book) a rating process or ρ (Bandos et al., 2009). The representation of FROC performance as a combination of the two processes does not limit its applicability to a specific area, but rather offers a convenient way to represent the FROC characteristics of a system. However, for some types of diagnostic systems (e.g., automated systems), the pruning and rating processes correspond to explicit methods employed in producing actually rated marks. The pruning characteristics (subscript π) are reflected by a point (FPR_π, TPF_π). According to our conventions, these can be written as:

$$FPR_\pi = FPR_{\rho\circ\pi}(0) = E\left\{\sum_{i=1}^{N} I(X_i > 0)\right\} = E\{N\},$$
$$TPF_\pi = TPF_{\rho\circ\pi}(0) = \frac{E\left\{\sum_{j=1}^{M} I(Y_j > 0)\right\}}{t} = \frac{E\{M\}}{t}. \tag{8-12}$$

The rating characteristics are obtained by standardizing the FROC characteristics in Equation (8-11) with pruning characteristics, Equation (8-12), i.e.:

$$FPF_{\rho|\pi}(\xi) = \frac{FPR_{\rho\circ\pi}(\xi)}{FPR_\pi} = \frac{E\left\{\sum_{i=1}^{N} I(X_i > \xi)\right\}}{E(N)},$$
$$TPF_{\rho|\pi}(\xi) = \frac{TPF_{\rho\circ\pi}(\xi)}{TPF_\pi} = \frac{E\left\{\sum_{j=1}^{M} I(Y_j > \xi)\right\}}{E(M)}. \tag{8-13}$$

The subscript $\rho|\pi$ highlights the fact that the distribution of X, Y generally depends on the characteristics of the pruning process π. The subscript $\rho\circ\pi$ reflects the representation of FROC characteristics in Equation (8-11) as a composition of pruning characteristics (subscript π) and rating characteristics (subscript $\rho|\pi$). Using appropriately redefined random variables $\tilde{X},\tilde{Y}$, the characteristics in Equation (8-13) can be rewritten in a form more traditional for ROC analysis, i.e., $FPF_{\rho|\pi}(\xi) = P(\tilde{X} > \xi)$, $TPF_{\rho|\pi}(\xi) = P(\tilde{Y} > \xi)$. Due to a possible correlation between the observations obtained from the same subject, these characteristics fall into the realm of clustered ROC analysis. However, in the rest of the chapter we will use more explicit definitions in terms of *X* and *Y*, Knowledge of the joint distribution of *X*, *N*, *M*, and *Y* variables yields complete information for the assessment of an FROC-type performance, thereby providing the basis for various types of inferences (Popescu, 2009).

8.2.5 Estimation of FROC Curve

A performance assessment study conducted under the conventional FROC paradigm typically results in data that can be represented as follows:

$$\left\{\left\{x_{si}\right\}_{i=1}^{n_s}, \left\{y_{sj}\right\}_{j=1}^{m_s}, t_s\right\}_{s=1}^{S}, \tag{8-14}$$

where *s* indicates one of *S* subjects used in the study associated with the number of targets t_s; the number of detected and correctly localized targets (equivalently the number of *TP* marks) m_s ($m_s \leq t_s$); the number of *FP* marks n_s;, and ensembles of ratings for *TP* and *FP* marks, respectively, $\left\{y_{sj}\right\}_{j=1}^{m_s}$ and $\left\{x_{si}\right\}_{i=1}^{n_s}$.

The FROC data summarized in Figure 8.2 consist of eight observations demonstrating various combinations of *TP* and *FP* marks per subject (Bandos et al., 2009). These data are based on four subjects depicting a single target and four subjects not depicting targets that result in examinations (1) without marks, (2) with only false positive marks, (3) with only true positive marks, and (4) with both true positive and false positive marks.

Similar to the ROC methodology, techniques to estimate FROC curves may incorporate a varying number of assumptions and involve different levels of complexity. Here we distinguish only parametric and nonparametric approach classifications, although more detailed classification is possible (Pepe, 2003). Parametric approaches rely on complete specification of the distribution of observable (and in some instances latent) data. This includes structural assumptions about the relationships of the random variables (e.g., independent or identical distribution) and the complete specification of the distribution of relevant random variables (e.g., normal distribution for the ratings). Nonparametric approaches rely on empirically observed data and may include some structural assumptions.

Parametric assumptions were introduced early in the development of FROC analysis (Bunch,1976). Some of these assumptions, such as the use of a Poisson distribution for the number of *FP* marks, remain central to many current parametric approaches. One of the first estimation methods for the FROC curve was a parametric approach based on Poisson and normal distributions (Chakraborty, 1989). This method relies on the structural assumption of mutual independence between the latent ratings X^* and Y^* for FP and TP marks and the observable number of false positive marks N:

$$\max_{i=1,..,N}\left(X_i^*\right) \sim N(\tilde{\mu}_x,\tilde{\sigma}_x^2), \qquad Y^* \sim N(\mu_y,\sigma_y^2), \qquad N(\xi) \sim Poisson(\lambda_\xi),$$

$$where \qquad \lambda_\xi = -\log\{\Phi((\tilde{\mu}_x - \xi)/\tilde{\sigma}_x)\} \quad or \quad \xi = \tilde{\mu}_x + \tilde{\sigma}_x \Phi^{-1}\left(1 - e^{-\lambda_\xi}\right). \tag{8-15}$$

Observable ratings X,Y are binned versions of the latent ratings X^*,Y^*, i.e.:

$$X = \sum_{c=1}^{C} cI\left(\xi_{c-1} < X^* \le \xi_c\right), \quad Y = \sum_{c=1}^{C} cI\left(\xi_{c-1} < Y^* \le \xi_c\right),$$
$$where \quad \xi_0 = -\infty, \quad \xi_C = +\infty. \tag{8-16}$$

Parameter λ_ξ reflects the FPR corresponding to the threshold ξ. The corresponding FROC curve is smooth, extends to infinity, and has the following form:

$$TPF(\xi) = \Phi\left\{\tilde{a} + \tilde{b} \times \Phi^{-1}\left(1 - e^{-FPR(\xi)}\right)\right\},$$
$$\text{where} \quad \tilde{a} = \frac{\mu_y - \tilde{\mu}_x}{\sigma_y} \quad \tilde{b} = \frac{\tilde{\sigma}_x}{\sigma_y} \quad and \quad FPR(\xi) = \lambda_\xi\,. \tag{8-17}$$

Despite the similarity of parameters $\tilde{a}$ and $\tilde{b}$ to the traditional parameters of a binormal ROC model (Zhou et al., 2002), they have different ranges of values. For example, the parameter a of a reasonable binormal ROC curve should be greater than 0; but for a reasonable FROC model, $\tilde{a}$ may have a value below 0. This reflects the fact that even if FP ratings are stochastically smaller than a TP rating, the maximum of several false positive ratings may be stochastically larger.

A simple approach for fitting an FROC curve to a model Equation (8-15), can be based on conventional methods for a binormal ROC curve under the assumption of independence among all ratings. To implement this approach, the ROC-type data is generated from the complete FROC data by selecting all TP ratings and the maximum of FP ratings for each subject and augmenting the data with the default ratings for missed targets or unmarked subjects.

Augmentation with the default ratings is a convenient way to represent the total number of subjects and targets. The corresponding FROC curve is the binormal ROC curve stretched to an infinite band $[0,\infty] \times [0,1]$ by transforming the horizontal axis of the ROC with $-\log(1 - fpf)$. This approach is closely related to the alternative FROC (AFROC; Section

8.3.1). An approach for fitting the model [Equation (8-15)] based on complete FROC data, albeit still under the assumption of independence, is described by Chakraborty (1989).

The FROC curve in Equation (8-17) and the originally described conceptual FROC curve (Bunch, 1978) extend to infinity, implying that a system potentially may detect any given fraction of targets at the cost of a defined number of *FP* responses. However, many practical problems focus on the immediately achievable characteristics described by an FROC curve ending at the pruning point (FPR_π, TPF_π).

Edwards et al. (2002) considered a model for a finite FROC curve (under a two-stage pruning rating representation) in which the individual (as opposed to maximum) ratings for the marks follow a traditional binormal model whose total number of marks (candidates) follows a Poisson distribution. All random variables are considered mutually independent and multiple *FP* or *TP* ratings are assumed to be i.i.d. In terms of latent ratings X^*, Y^* for *FP* and *TP* marks, respectively [see Equation (9-16)], the model can be formally written as:

$$N \sim Poisson(fpr_\pi) \quad M \sim Bin(t, tpf_\pi) \quad X^* \sim N(\mu_x, \sigma_x^2) \quad Y^* \sim N(\mu_y, \sigma_y^2). \tag{8-18}$$

The approach is based on constructing an ROC curve corresponding to marks treated as diagnostic units. For known parameters, the FROC curve can be obtained as follows:

$$\begin{gathered} for \quad FPR \leq fpr_\pi \quad TPF = \Phi\left\{a + b\Phi^{-1}\left(\frac{FPR}{fpr_\pi}\right)\right\} \times tpf_\pi \\ where \quad a = \frac{\mu_y - \mu_x}{\sigma_y} \quad b = \frac{\sigma_x}{\sigma_y}. \end{gathered} \tag{8-19}$$

In other words, the ROC curve for marks considered diagnostic units is scaled to the rectangle determined by the pruning characteristics (fpr_π, tpf_π). Because of the assumed mutual independence of variables *X*, *Y*, *N*, and *M*, the parameters of the corresponding FROC curve may be estimated in two steps. First, without any additional modification, binormal parameters *a* and *b* can be estimated using standard ROC techniques for corresponding types of ratings (Dorfman and Alf, 1969; Tosteson and Begg, 1988 Zou and Hall, 2000; Zou et al., 1997; Pepe, 2003). Second, binomial and Poisson assumptions used for the numbers of marks lead to the usual empirical estimates of pruning characteristics $\left(\widehat{fpr}_\pi, \widehat{tpf}_\pi\right)$ that may be obtained as in Equation (8-5). The estimated FROC curve is then obtained by stretching the fitted binormal ROC curve using the estimates of the pruning characteristics.

Clearly, using different parametric and structural assumptions, it is possible to build a number of models for FROC curves (Swensson, 1996; Irvin, 2004; Hutchinson, 2007). Depending on the specific method used, it could be of interest to model more complex latent structures such as the number of detected but not rated lesions (Chakraborty, 2006). Parametric approaches provide the ability to extrapolate and increase efficiency of the inferences if the assumed model is in fact correct. However, justification of the appropriateness of parametric assumptions is frequently a difficult task. In addition, parametric approaches for fitting FROC curves often rely on the difficult-to-justify assumptions of independence of different observations corresponding to the same subject. Although less restrictive parametric approaches to the estimation of FROC curves are possible (e.g., adjusting for correlation within a generalized linear model framework), none of these seem to have been comprehensively investigated as of this date.

One straightforward FROC curve estimate that does not require the assumption of independence is the empirical FROC curve, which can be formulated as follows:

$$\widehat{FPR}_{\rho\circ\pi}(\xi) = \frac{\sum_{s=1}^{S}\sum_{i=1}^{n_s} I(x_{si} > \xi)}{S} \qquad \widehat{TPF}_{\rho\circ\pi}(\xi) = \frac{\sum_{s=1}^{S}\sum_{j=1}^{m_s} I(y_{sj} > \xi)}{\sum_{s=1}^{S} t_s}. \tag{8-20}$$

Without any additional assumptions, nonparametric characteristics can be represented as products of empirical pruning and rating characteristics (as in Section 8.2.4), i.e.:

$$\begin{aligned} \widehat{FPR}_{\rho\circ\pi}(\xi) &= \widehat{FPF}_{\rho|\pi}(\xi) \times \widehat{FPR}_{\pi} \\ \widehat{TPF}_{\rho\circ\pi}(\xi) &= \widehat{TPF}_{\rho|\pi}(\xi) \times \widehat{TPF}_{\pi}, \end{aligned} \tag{8-21}$$

where the empirical pruning characteristics FPR_{π}, TPF_{π} are estimated as in Equation (8-5), and the empirical rating characteristics $FPF_{\rho|\pi}$, $TPF_{\rho|\pi}$ can be expressed as follows:

$$\widehat{FPF}_{\rho|\pi}(\xi) = \frac{\sum_{s=1}^{S}\sum_{i=1}^{n_s} I(x_{si} > \xi)}{\sum_{s=1}^{S} n_s} \qquad \widehat{TPF}_{\rho|\pi}(\xi) = \frac{\sum_{s=1}^{S}\sum_{j=1}^{m_s} I(y_{sj} > \xi)}{\sum_{s=1}^{S} m_s}. \tag{8-22}$$

An empirical FROC curve connects the empirical FROC points [Equation (8-20)] with straight lines (Figure 8.3). Similar to the interpretation of an empirical ROC curve, a point on a straight line connecting two empirical FROC points may be interpreted as an average performance of the guessing process that randomly relabels discordant marks at the two thresholds. The straight lines also provide a lower bound for a concave FROC curve, thereby conveying the interpretation that it is "locally better than chance." Similarly, the extension of the FROC curve beyond the pruning point with the help of a guessing process (e.g., Section 8.2.2) may be interpreted as a lower bound for hypothetical performance levels under more aggressive diagnostic settings.

8.2.6 Summary Indices

FROC curves are often summarized using scalar summary indices. These indices are frequently easier to comprehend than an entire FROC curve but are inevitably associated with some loss of information that may mask differences between certain types of nonidentical curves. However, in some instances, based on the specific question of interest, a summary index may provide relevant information in a more usable and understandable form.

One of the most practically relevant summary indices is a specific point on the FROC curve. Since diagnostic systems are usually developed for eventual implementation in practice, the primary interest often lies in how accurately the marks produced in a specific setting (e.g., at a given rating threshold) detect and localize the targets. Depending on the specific application, a point of interest on an FROC curve may be determined as a function of different parameters of interest (e.g., specified levels of *TPF* or *FPR*, number of marks, or maximum expected utility). For example, for applications in diagnostic radiology, it may be of interest to consider a point corresponding to an *FPR* of 0.1 (Chakraborty and Winter, 1990). Statistical inferences for this parameter can be easily made with one of the parametric models for the infinite FROC curve; nonparametric inferences are more complicated.

Under the assumption of independence between the numbers and ratings of the marks, the representation of the FROC curve as a scaled ROC curve can be used to make inferences about any FROC point at a given *FPR* by adopting traditional procedures for estimating sensitivity at a given specificity in ROC analysis (Pepe, 2003, Zhou et al., 2000; Platt et al., 2000). The nonparametric estimates can be obtained by scaling corresponding ROC estimates. For inferences that consider correlation as well as a variable number of marks, one can use subject resampling techniques (e.g., subject-based bootstrap) for nonparametric statistical inferences that are free from the assumptions of within-subject independence.

One of the primary limitations of a single-point index is the subjectivity in selecting the *FPR* level. Indeed, by adopting different *FPR* levels of interest, one can sometimes obtain different conclusions for the same system. The subjectivity in selecting a particular *FPR* level may be alleviated with indices summarizing performance over multiple thresholds simultaneously.

Similar to ROC analysis, it is possible to define a partial area under the FROC curve that summarizes FROC performance levels corresponding to multiple thresholds. Although summarizing over more than one threshold, this index still requires selection of a range of interest (e.g., in terms of *FPR*).

One approach that uses a partial area index (for comparison of FROC curves) while circumventing the necessity to specify a range was considered by Samuelson and Petrick (2006). They suggested using the area under the empirical FROC curves over the entire "common range" of the empirically observed *FPR*. Hence, the range for integrating the FROC curve is driven by the observed data rather than investigator's choice. The statistical analysis proposed by Samuelson and Petrick is based on bootstrap or permutation methodology. The estimate of partial area is typically not available in a closed form even for parametric approaches, and its computation often requires numerical integration.

It is important to note that without the restriction to the common range, the area under the (entire) empirical FROC curve may be misleading. Indeed, a large estimated area under the empirical FROC curve may correspond to a very "good" or very "poor" FROC curve, depending on the last observed empirical point (fpr_π, tpf_π).

A useful property of the indices summarizing FROC curves is the ability to reflect salient features of the curve, hence minimizing the possibility for inconsistencies such as obtaining a smaller index for a higher curve. One approach to elicit essential features of the entire FROC curve stems from the two-stage representation. Since the FROC curve is an ROC curve scaled by the pruning characteristics in this representation, the obvious essential components are the pruning characteristics tpf_π, fpr_π and separability between the ratings of *TP* and *FP* marks—$AUC_{\rho|\pi}$ (area under the $\rho|\pi$ ROC curve).

Similar parameters are also emphasized in studies focused on more complicated characteristics of human behavior in performance assessments (Chakraborty, 2006). Ideally, a better diagnostic system would have a higher tpf_π and $AUC_{\rho|\pi}$ and lower fpr_π. Hence, a reasonable index summarizing the FROC curve should increase with increasing tpf_π and $AUC_{\rho|\pi}$, and decrease with increasing fpr_π. However, when using these properties, the three conditions may be combined in a number of ways without any particular combination performing "better" for all purposes. For example, more efficient inferences about $AUC_{\rho|\pi}$ may be made with an estimate of AUC alone (e.g., using 0s for coefficients of other quantities in the linear combination). Thus, an important objective of constructing a specific combination may be related to obtaining an index that has an interpretation related to the observed FROC curves, hence increasing chances that the results of comparisons are consistent with visual representation of the FROC curves. An approach proposed by Bandos et al. (2009) explicitly combines the three salient FROC components described above in an index that has a convenient geometric interpretation in terms of the observable FROC curve. It can be written as follows:

$$\Lambda = AUC_{\rho|\pi} \times fpr_{\pi} \times tpf_{\pi} - fpr_{\pi} + \frac{tpf_{\pi}}{\varphi}, \tag{8-23}$$

where φ is a parameter reflecting the "liberalness" of the proximity criteria adopted for a given sample. The nonparametric estimator of Λ can be obtained by using the estimators for FPR_{π} and TPF_{π} (e.g., 9-5) and the nonparametric estimator of the $AUC_{\rho|\pi}$:

$$\widehat{AUC_{\rho|\pi}} = \frac{\sum_{\bar{s}=1}^{S}\sum_{s=1}^{S}\sum_{i=1}^{n_{\bar{s}}}\sum_{j=1}^{m_s}\psi\left(x_{\bar{s}i}, y_{sj}\right)}{\left(\sum_{\bar{s}=1}^{S} n_{\bar{s}}\right)\times\left(\sum_{s=1}^{S} m_s\right)} \quad \textit{where} \quad \psi\left(x_{\bar{s}i}, y_{sj}\right) = \begin{cases} 1 & x_{\bar{s}i} < y_{sj} \\ \frac{1}{2} & x_{\bar{s}i} = y_{sj} \\ 0 & x_{\bar{s}i} > y_{sj} \end{cases}. \tag{8-24}$$

Λ can be interpreted as the area between the augmented FROC curve and a guessing process. The augmented FROC curve coincides with the empirical curve until the estimated pruning point $\left(\widehat{fpr}_{\pi}, \widehat{tpf}_{\pi}\right)$. Beyond the estimated pruning point, it coincides with the exponential guessing curve (Figure 8.3), thereby providing a benchmark for the *lowest* expected performance level. One can prove this interpretation by noting that the estimator of the first term in Equation (8-23) is exactly the area under the empirical FROC curve, while the areas above the guessing curve [Equation (8-8)] and guessing extension [Equation (8-9)] are $1/\varphi$ and $1 - tpf_{\pi}/\varphi$, respectively.

Statistical inferences based on Λ can be performed using subject-based resampling. A conventional structure of the nonparametric estimator of Λ permits one to compute the ideal bootstrap variance exactly, thereby avoiding resampling errors.

In addition to the summary indices derived directly from the FROC curve, several indices were developed to summarize FROC data without directly relating the index to the actual FROC curve. One popular type of index is JAFROC (Chakraborty and Berbaum, 2004). The general structure resembles the U-statistic used for estimating the area under the ROC curve. Two of the better known indices of this type are $JAFROC^{I}$ and $JAFROC^{II}$ that can be written as follows, in the case of homogeneous weighting ($1/t_s$):

$$JAFROC^{I} = \frac{\sum_{\tilde{s}=1}^{S_0+S_1} \sum_{s=1}^{S_1} \frac{\sum_{j=1}^{t_s} \psi(\chi_{\tilde{s}}, h_{sj})}{t_s}}{(S_0+S_1)S_1}$$

$$JAFROC^{II} = \frac{\sum_{\tilde{s}=1}^{S_0} \sum_{s=1}^{S_1} \frac{\sum_{j=1}^{t_s} \psi(\chi_{\tilde{s}}, h_{sj})}{t_s}}{S_0 S_1} = \frac{\sum_{\tilde{s}=1}^{S_0} \sum_{s=1}^{S_1} \phi_{\tilde{s}s}}{S_0 S_1}, \tag{8-25}$$

where

$$\phi_{\tilde{s}s} = \frac{\sum_{j=1}^{t_s} \psi(\chi_{\tilde{s}}, h^{*}_{sj})}{t_s} \qquad \chi_{\tilde{s}} = \begin{cases} \max\limits_{i=1,\ldots n}(x_{\tilde{s}i}), & n_s > 0 \\ 0, & n_s = 0 \end{cases} \qquad h_{sj} = \begin{cases} y_{sj}, & j \le m_s \\ 0, & m_s < j \end{cases}$$

where S_0 and S_1 denote the numbers of target-free and target-depicting subjects, correspondingly (total number of subjects $S=S_0+S_1$). The similarity of the above structure to the area under the empirical ROC curve is not surprising, given that for a sample where subjects have either 0 or t targets, $JAFROC^{I}$ is equivalent to the area under the ROC curve based on the maximum *FP* ratings per subject and all *TP* ratings (see Section 8.3.1). Due to data reduction, this type of ROC curve can be substantially different from the transformation of the empirical FROC curve. $JAFROC^{I}$ is only indirectly related to the observed FROC curve. For a reasonable FROC curve, $JAFROC^{I}$ increases with increasing $\widehat{tpf_\pi}$ and $\widehat{AUC_{\rho|\pi}}$. A decrease of $JAFROC^{I}$ with increasing $\widehat{fpr_\pi}$ is not automatic and must be assured by additional assumptions (e.g., i.i.d. for *FP* ratings). In general, $JAFROC^{II}$ is considered inferior to $JAFROC^{I}$ since it ignores the *FP* responses on the target-depicting subjects.

Another approach for summarizing FROC data is based on traditional ROC tools. One can generate pseudoROC ratings by taking the maximum of the ratings for *all* marks produced for a subject (i.e., most suspicious finding) and use this maximum as an overall subject rating in a conventional ROC analysis. The area under such an ROC curve reflects the probability of correct discrimination between subjects with and without targets in a forced choice experiment. With some parametric FROC models, one can estimate such an AUC directly as one of the parameters (Chakraborty, 2006). Nonparametric estimation and inferences about the probability of correct discrimination can be performed according to the general pattern described below.

Some of the indices, including AUCs based on maximum ratings and $JAFROC^{II}$, may be represented in the form of a *U*-statistic with a specific type of two-sample kernel function defined for a pair of subjects with and without targets, namely:

$$\hat{A} = \frac{\sum_{\bar{s}=1}^{S_0}\sum_{s=1}^{S_1} w_{\bar{s}s}}{S_0 S_1}, \tag{8-26}$$

where $w_{\bar{s}s}$ depends on a specific index represented, for example, $w_{\bar{s}s} = \psi[\max(\{x_{\bar{s}i}\}) \times I(n_{\bar{s}} > 0), \max(\{x_{si}\}_{i=1}^{n_s}, \{y_{sj}\}_{j=1}^{t_s} \times I(t_s n_s > 0)]$ for the AUC based on maximum ratings and $w_{\bar{s}s} = \phi_{\bar{s}s}$ for $JAFROC^{II}$. Regardless of the specific form of $w_{\bar{s}s}$ the two-sample jack-knife variance estimator (Arvesen, 1969) can be written as:

$$V(\hat{A}) = \frac{\sum_{\bar{s}=1}^{S_0}(\bar{w}_{\bar{s}\bullet} - \bar{w}_{\bullet\bullet})^2}{S_0(S_0-1)} + \frac{\sum_{s=1}^{S_1}(\bar{w}_{\bullet s} - \bar{w}_{\bullet\bullet})^2}{S_1(S_1-1)}$$

$$\textit{where} \quad \bar{w}_{\bar{s}\bullet} = \frac{\sum_{s=1}^{S_1} w_{\bar{s}s}}{S_1} \quad \bar{w}_{\bullet s} = \frac{\sum_{\bar{s}=1}^{S_0} w_{\bar{s}s}}{S_0} \quad \textit{and} \quad \bar{w}_{\bullet\bullet} = \frac{\sum_{s=1}^{S_1}\sum_{\bar{s}=1}^{S_0} w_{\bar{s}s}}{S_0 S_1} = \hat{A}. \tag{8-27}$$

Properties of this type of variance estimator for conventional ROC data are well understood (Delong et al., 1989). For FROC data, the properties of these types of variance estimators were verified for pseudoROC summary indices (Song et al., 2008). For *A*-like indices, it is also possible to derive a closed-form expression for various estimators of the variance, some of which are in exact algebraic relationship to one another. For example, one can derive a conventional one-sample jack-knife variance, which is always smaller than the two-sample jack-knife variance (Bandos et al., 2006) in Equation (8-27) but larger than the unbiased variance estimator (Wieand et al., 1983) then biased upward. The ideal bootstrap variance estimator that also has a closed-form for *A*-like indices does not have a constant order relationship with others and tends to be slightly positively biased (Bandos et al., 2006).

The indices that are similar to *A* but apply the kernel function to the overlapping samples ($JAFROC^{I}$ or the area under the empirical FROC curve) typically require more elaborate procedures for adequate assessment of variability. However, some also permit closed-form expression for simple resampling procedures (Bandos et al., 2009). In general, even when analyzed in a similar manner, different indices may yield different and sometimes contradictory answers. Therefore, it is important to carefully select appropriate indices for the problem at hand.

8.2.7 Comparison of FROC Performance Levels

Comparisons of diagnostic systems using FROC data are often based on summary indices discussed above. In an unpaired design, the assessment of the uncertainty of the difference in the two indices can often be performed using the sum of the variance estimators. In many instances, comparisons are conducted under a paired design in which systems compared assess the same subjects. Under the paired design, the variance of the difference also includes a covariance term or terms. However, comparison of many indices under a paired design can be conveniently formulated similar to a paired t-test, avoiding the need for estimating covariance terms.

For example, the difference in empirical estimates of Λ^k indices (superscript indicates the system) can be written as a two-sample index with a structure similar to an estimate of a single Λ, i.e.,

$$\hat{\Lambda}^1 - \hat{\Lambda}^2 = \frac{\sum_{\tilde{s}=1}^{S_0}\sum_{s=1}^{S_1}\left\{w_{\tilde{s}s}^1 - w_{\tilde{s}s}^2\right\}}{S_0 S_1} - \frac{\sum_{\tilde{s}=1}^{S_0+S_1}\left(n_{\tilde{s}}^1 - n_{\tilde{s}}^2\right)}{S_0 + S_1} + \frac{1}{\varphi} \times \frac{\sum_{s=1}^{S_1}\left(m_s^1 - m_s^2\right)}{\sum_{s=1}^{S_1} t_s} \tag{8-28}$$

$$\text{where } w_{\tilde{s}s}^k = \frac{S_0 S_1}{\left(S_0 + S_1\right)\left(\sum_{s=1}^{S_1} t_s\right)} \sum_{j=1}^{m_s}\left(\sum_{\tilde{i}=1}^{n_{\tilde{s}}} \psi\left(x_{\tilde{s}\tilde{i}}^k, y_{sj}^k\right) + \sum_{i=1}^{n_s} \psi\left(x_{si}^k, y_{sj}^k\right)\right).$$

The closed-form variance estimators can be obtained by replacing the averaged quantities (w, n, m) with their corresponding differences. A similar approach can be employed for A-like indices like $JAFROC^{II}$ [Equation (8-26)] or similar indices like $JAFROC^{I}$. Thus, the technical comparison of indices, whether correlated or not, can often be performed using techniques for statistical assessment of individual indices.

Aside from estimating the statistical uncertainty, other important issues relate to the implications of comparisons. One feature of an FROC analysis that complicates the comparison of diagnostic systems is the presence of an important design parameter known as the proximity criterion. As we described in previous sections, a proximity criterion (e.g., acceptance radius) is a necessary parameter that enables classifying each mark as a true positive or a false positive.

The strictness of the proximity criterion affects a number of performance indices and can bias the result of comparison. Since most conventional summary measures do not include explicit mechanisms for adjusting for differences in proximity criteria, investigators typically must ensure that the proximity criteria used for the systems compared are similar (would result in a relevant comparison) before proceeding to a formal assessment. Calibrating proximity criteria is rarely a simple task. The problem of comparing diagnostic technologies while accounting for the proximity criterion has been a driving force for developing techniques independent from the acceptance radius (Chakraborty et al., 2007). However, since the classification imposed by the proximity criterion is inherently linked to the practically relevant characteristics, standard approaches based on proximity criteria remain desirable, even if analytically problematic. Thus, an essential problem for many comparisons of diagnostic systems continues to be an adjustment for possible differences in proximity criteria adopted by the diagnostic systems compared.

One approach that helps adjust the comparison of two diagnostic systems with respect to the proximity criterion is to explicitly incorporate the criterion in the summary measure. For example, index Λ, discussed previously in this chapter, reflects the proximity criterion in terms of weights for the pruning detection characteristic TPF_{π} in a manner that attempts to compensate for changes in the number of correct localizations due to changes in acceptance radii. The specific manner in which the proximity criterion is incorporated in this index permits a useful interpretation of Λ as an average relative improvement over a certain guessing process. Thus, comparison of systems using this index can be interpreted as comparing which system is better over the guessing process under the condition of the specific adopted proximity criterion.

Aside from the comparison of diagnostic systems based on the summary index, one may want to compare the FROC curves. A salient problem of comparing FROC curves is their frequently different lengths. Indeed, even when the shorter of the two curves is higher in the empirically observed range, the relative performance levels beyond the pruning point of the shorter curve are not always easy to assess (Figure 8.4). This may become a problem when greater detection and localization accuracies are achieved by the longer curve. Guessing processes may in some cases help resolve this problem by extending the FROC curve in a manner that provides a lower bound for its possible performance at a more aggressive setting (associated with a higher rate of false positives). If the longer curve is lower than the shorter curve in the common range and lower than the guessing extension of the shorter curve beyond the common range (straight lines on Figure 8.7), one can conclude that the performance of the system described by the longer curve is worse. Indeed, a diagnostic system corresponding to a longer curve at any given *FPR* has a lower *TPF* than could be obtained when the other diagnostic system (corresponding to a shorter curve) is augmented with a guessing process. The guessing process is of less use when augmented curves cross.

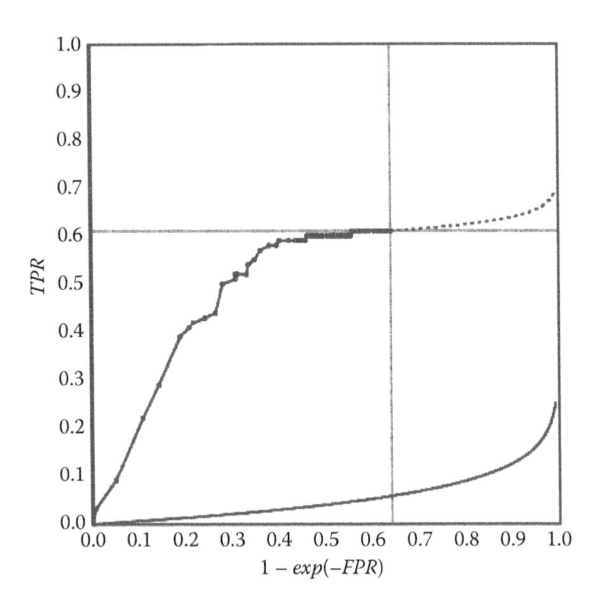

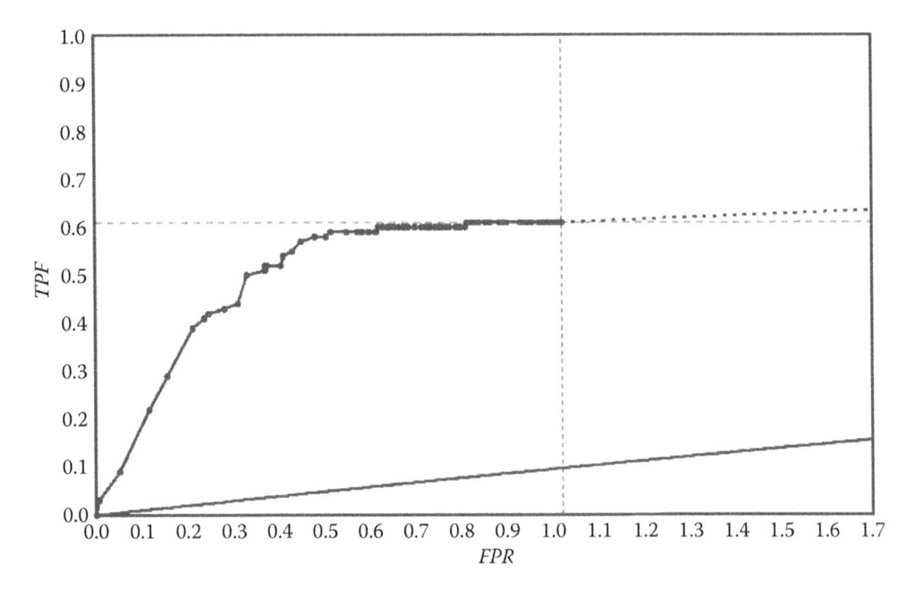

FIGURE 8.4
Top: AFROC representation of empirical and guessing FROC curves. Bottom: FROC representation. Dots indicate empirical points. Solid lines without dots describe performance of guessing process. Dotted lines correspond to guessing augmentation of empirical FROC curve.

In that case, a comparison of the systems may be more appropriate to base on the analysis of a relevant part of the curve.

8.3 Other Approaches of Detection–Localization Performance Assessment

8.3.1 Alternative FROC (AFROC)

One of the alternative methods for analyzing the FROC-type problem is the alternative free-response ROC approach (AFROC; Bunch, 1978; Chakraborty and Winter, 1990). The primary tool of this approach is the AFROC curve which, like the ROC curve, resides in a unit square. The ordinate in the AFROC space is the same as in FROC space ($TPF_{\rho\pi}$). Its abscissa (denoted *AFP*) represents an alternative way to quantify false positive responses and varies between 0 and 1.

One possible use of the AFROC curve is to summarize FROC data [see Equation (8-14)]. In this case, the AFROC curve is a monotonically transformed FROC curve (Figure 8.4) in which the transformation maps an infinite band $[0,\infty) \times [0,1]$ to $[0,1] \times [0,1]$ (Chakraborty, 1989). Specifically, the abscissa of the FROC curve $FPR_{\rho\pi}$, is transformed as follows:

$$AFP = 1 - e^{-FPR}. \quad (8\text{-}29)$$

Another type of implementation of AFROC analysis is based on an AFROC curve constructed as an ROC curve from the data consisting of ratings of the targets (using a default rating for missed targets) and the highest rated *FP* marks on each subject.

When using the similarities with an ROC curve, it is tempting to construct the empirical AFROC curve by extending it with a straight line or use a diagonal line as a benchmark. This, however, may often be inappropriate as these straight lines correspond to performance of overly optimistic guessing processes, thereby generating a potential for practically useful systems to appear worse than "guess" results indicate. For example, in terms of the guessing process discussed in Section 8.2, the straight lines in AFROC space correspond to a process that has a 50% probability ($\varphi = 1$) of hitting a target by chance.

Under some parametric FROC models, the transformation-defined *AFP*, Equation (8-29), can be interpreted as the probability of observing an image with at least one false positive mark [$N \sim Poisson(\lambda)$]. This interpretation led to an alternative analysis of FROC-type data (Chakraborty and Winter, 1990). Under this system, the FROC data are reduced to ROC-type data in which the ratings for targets are treated as ratings for actually positive diagnostic units, and the highest ratings for false positive responses are treated as actually negative diagnostic units (default rating 0 represents subjects with no responses and missed targets). The corresponding ROC curve is also known as the AFROC curve, although the horizontal coordinate $P\{\max_{i=1...N}(X_i) > \xi\}$ is generally different from the original *AFP* (8-29).

Under the assumption of independence between ratings, AFROC-reduced FROC data may be analyzed via conventional ROC methods. When such methods are based on fitting a binormal ROC curve, the resulting AFROC curve is equivalent to a transformation of the Poisson–max–normal FROC curve (Section 8.2.5). Alternatively, AFROC-type data can also be analyzed by clustered nonparametric ROC analysis. One such example is the *JAFROC*-type approach. Indeed, for data where all target-depicting subjects contain the same number of targets, the area under the empirical ROC curve obtained from AFROC-type pseudoROC data is equivalent to the $JAFROC^{I}$ index with homogeneous weights [Equation (8-25)]. A nonparametric analysis of the $JAFROC^{I}$ index accounting for within-subject correlations and variability of numbers of marks may be performed with subject-based resampling techniques (Chakraborty, 2008).

In general, the AFROC reduction of FROC data leads to loss of part of the data (multiple false positive ratings from an subject are replaced with their maximum). This can result in conclusions inconsistent with those obtained from the analysis of the FROC curve. For example, a uniformly higher FROC curve does not necessarily result in a uniformly higher AFROC curve. As a result, one can always find scenarios in which a uniformly higher FROC curve results in a smaller area under the AFROC curve.

The use of the AFROC curve merely as a transformation of an FROC curve has its own limitation, since the greater complexity of the AFROC space complicates the development of simple nonparametric methods. On the other hand, AFROC methodology can and should be preferred over FROC if the false positive marks of the lower tier (those rated lower than one of the *FP* marks on the same subject) are of no practical interest. In this case, AFROC analysis could lead to more practically relevant and/or efficient assessment.

8.3.2 Localization ROC (LROC)

One of the earlier approaches for performance analysis that included detection and localization tasks focused on the detection and localization of a single abnormality on radiographic images (Starr et al., 1975). To address both detection and localization characteristics, this approach requires a system to mark the location of a suspected target in addition to rating the entire subject. The event of correct identification of an subject as containing a target $\{+|D\}$ is split into two mutually exclusive events: (1) correct identification with true positive localization $\{+, TP|D\}$, and (2) correct identification with false positive localization *{+, FP|D}*. Consequently, the probability of correct identification of a target-depicting subject can be represented as:

$$P(+\mid D)=P(TP\mid D)+P(FP\mid D). \tag{8-30}$$

The generalized ROC curve for detection and localization tasks may be represented by a curve in a three-dimensional space determined by a conventional ROC coordinate $P(+_{\xi}\mid \bar{D})$—the fraction of target-free subjects rated higher than a predetermined threshold ξ—and two probabilities of correct identification: one with correct *P[TP|D]* or simply *P[TP]*, and the other with incorrect *P[FP|D]* localization (Starr et al., 1975). The projection of the generalized ROC curve on the plane $[P(+\mid \bar{D}),P(TP\mid D)]$ is called the localization ROC or LROC curve (Figure 8.5, top). The LROC curve can be viewed as a hybrid combining the abscissa of an subject-based ROC curve $FPF_{ROC}(\xi)=P(+_{\xi}\mid \bar{D})$ and the ordinate of a conventional FROC curve $TPF_{\rho\pi}(\xi)$. Indeed, since *TP* findings are possible only on target-depicting subjects, $P[TP|D]= P[TP]= TPF_{\rho\pi}$. The analog to the pruning characteristic TPF_{π} in LROC analysis is sometimes called localization accuracy (Swensson, 2000).

Under the LROC paradigm each subject has a single mark so we can treat interchangeably the rating for the mark and the corresponding subject (as a whole). The data from the LROC experiment can be represented in a manner traditional for FROC:

$$\{x_{s1}\}_{s=1}^{S_0} \quad \{y_{s`1}\}_{s`=1}^{L} \; L<S_1 \quad and \quad \{x_{s`1}\}_{s`=L+1}^{S_1}, \tag{8-31}$$

where x is an *FP* rating for a mark, y is a rating corresponding to a correctly localized target (*TP* rating), and L is the number of subjects with correctly localized targets (equivalent to the sum of all *m*s in FROC data). As in FROC, the decision about adequate localization is made using a predetermined proximity criterion. The coordinates of the LROC curve can be estimated in a nonparametric manner as:

$$\hat{P}(FP_{\xi}\mid \bar{D})=F\hat{P}F_{ROC}(\xi)=\frac{\sum_{s=1}^{S_0} I(x_{s1}>\xi)}{S_0} \quad \hat{P}(TP_{\xi}\mid D)=T\hat{P}F_{\rho\pi}(\xi)=\frac{\sum_{s`=1}^{L} I(y_{s`}>\xi)}{S_1}. \tag{8-32}$$

This formulation of the LROC curve highlights the fact that ratings of S_1-L *FP* marks on subjects with targets $\{x_{s`}\}_{s`=L+1}^{S_1}$ are completely ignored in this analysis. The maximum value of *P[TP]* is the estimate of the TPF_{π} under the FROC representation. The area under the empirical LROC curve may be estimated similarly to the area under the ROC curve, but unlike a conventional

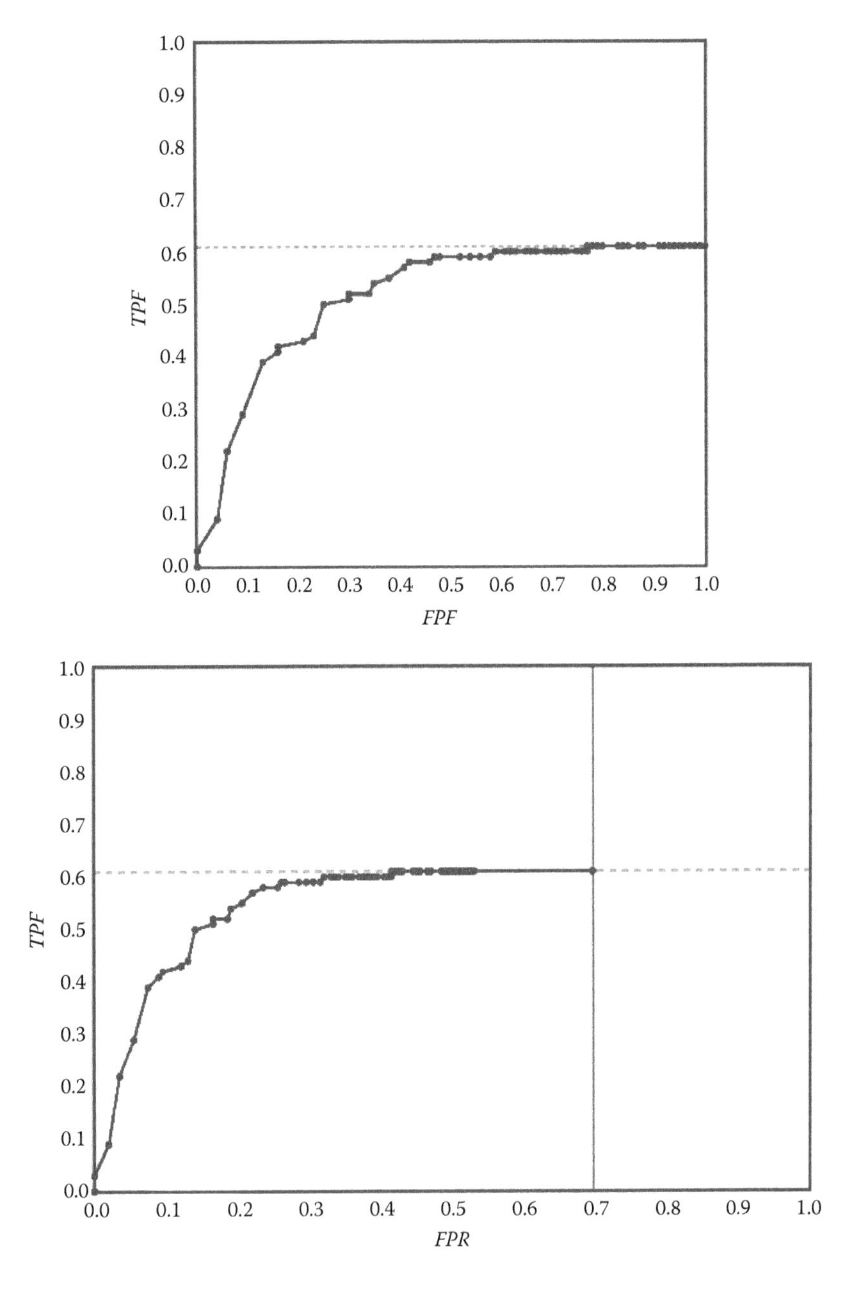

FIGURE 8.5
LROC curve (top) and corresponding FROC curve for LROC data (bottom).

ROC, a reasonable LROC curve may have areas less than 0.5. An extension of standard ROC technique for variance estimation of the area under the LROC curve can be obtained (Popescu, 2006; Tang et al., 2011).

Similar to an FROC curve, an LROC curve can be considered a scaled ROC curve. One can estimate the ROC curve from the subset of data composed of ratings from target-free subjects ($\{x_s\}_{s=1}^{S_0}$) and ratings for correctly localized targets ($\{y_{s`}\}_{s`=1}^{L}$) and then scale it vertically to a rectangle with height L/S_1 (localization accuracy). This representation of the LROC curve opens multiple possibilities to extend conventional approaches typically used in ROC analyses.

The LROC approach can be applied to FROC data by using a default rating for the unmarked subjects and making certain data reduction assumptions such as reducing multiple findings to a single most suspicious one (Swensson, 1996; Chakraborty and Yoon, 2008). As a result of data reduction, it is possible to construct examples in which the conclusions based on LROC and FROC curves differ. Where FROC analysis is applied to data acquired under the LROC paradigm (exactly one mark per subject), the ordinates of both performance curves are exactly the same, but the abscissae differ ($FPR_{\text{po}\pi}$ versus FPF_{ROC}; see Figure 8.5). Under the LROC paradigm, every subject contributes only one FROC mark (*FP* or *TP*) and the *TPF* and *FPR* of FROC representation of the LROC curve are constrained, for example:

$$FPR_{\pi} = \frac{S_0}{S_0 + S_1} + \frac{S_1}{S_0 + S_1}\left(1 - TPF_{\pi}\right). \tag{8-33}$$

However, it is possible for specific summary indices to construct scenarios under which conclusions of LROC and FROC analysis of the same data disagree.

For many applications, the LROC approach offers limited flexibility because of the restriction to a single target and single response per subject. Furthermore, even when the LROC assessment protocol is natural, the applicability of the approach is limited to tasks in which ratings for *FP* marks on target-depicting subjects represent nuisances because the corresponding $S_1 - L$ ratings are ignored in LROC analysis. An extension of the LROC concept was later developed for analyzing multiple targets per image, albeit under strong structural and parametric assumptions (Metz et al., 1976). This approach formed the basis for the more flexible nonparametric method discussed in the next section.

8.3.3 Regions of Interest (ROI) Approach

An alternative to the FROC approach is the region of interest (ROI) analysis (Obuchowski et al., 2000) that may be viewed as a natural extension of the parametric approach proposed by Metz et al. (1976). Its original version required a diagnostic system to assess separately every region of interest

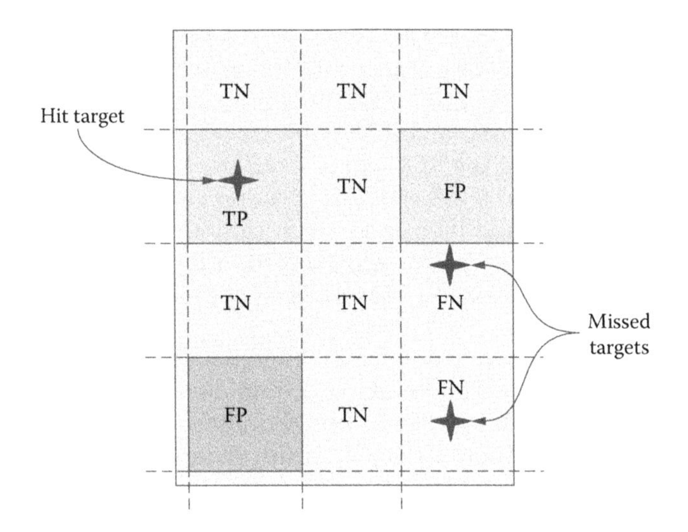

FIGURE 8.6
Classification of marks and targets under ROI paradigm.

(ROI) within an subject. Primarily because of the required assessment of all predefined ROIs, the original version was criticized as an artificial protocol that could alter estimated performance summary measures.

A natural modification of the ROI approach (Obuchowski et al., 2000) offers the freedom to assess performance under a more natural FROC-like protocol by superimposing an ROI grid on an subject (partitioning an entire area) evaluated by the system. Based on the task of interest, the superimposed grid may be defined to minimize the possibility that any region will contain more than one target or any target will span more than one region. The resolutions of these problems depend on the specific applications and this chapter does not address them. In scenarios in which ROIs are driven by clinical relevance and are large enough to host multiple targets and/or responses, some straightforward modifications can be developed (Obuchowski et al., 2010). Here we focus on a scenario of one target and response per ROI.

As with a conventional FROC paradigm, assessment with a modified ROI paradigm (Obuchowski et al., 2000) consists of marking an unconstrained number of locations for an subject and supplementing each with a confidence rating. A target located somewhere within a marked ROI is considered hit and the corresponding region considered a true positive (Figure 8.6). The ROIs that were not marked are assigned a default rating lower than any of the ratings used to indicate the degree of suspiciousness of actually marked locations (0 according to our convention). Depending on the presence or absence of a target, each unmarked ROI corresponds to an *FP* or *TN* response. Data from a simple ROI experiment may be expressed in a form very similar to FROC data representation:

$$\left\{\underbrace{\{x_{si}\}_{i=1}^{n_s}}_{FP},\underbrace{\{y_{sj}\}_{j=1}^{m_s}}_{TP}\right\}_{s=1}^{S} \cup \left\{\underbrace{\{x_{si}=0\}_{i=n_s+1}^{R-t_s}}_{TN},\underbrace{\{y_{sj}=0\}_{j=m_s+1}^{t_s}}_{FN}\right\}_{s=1}^{S} \quad n_s \le R-t_s$$

$$and \quad m_s \le t_s \quad or \tag{8-34}$$

$$\left\{\{x_{si}\}_{i=1}^{R-t_s},\{h_{sj}\}_{j=1}^{t_s}\right\} \quad where \quad h_{sj}=\begin{cases} y_{sj}, & j \le m_s \\ 0, & m_s < j \end{cases},$$

where R is the number of ROIs on each subject, and the remaining quantities have the same meaning as the corresponding quantities in FROC representation. Note that unlike FROC analysis, ROI has a known upper bound for the possible number of *FP* responses: $R - t_s$. This enables an assessment of performance using conventional ROC tools for clustered data (clustering of subject-specific responses) by using a default rating for unmarked target-free locations. Then the empirical *TP* and *FP* fractions can be estimated as follows:

$$FPF_{ROI}(\xi)=\frac{\sum_{s=1}^{S}\sum_{i=1}^{R-t_s} I(x_{si}>\xi)}{SR-\sum_{s=1}^{S} t_s} \qquad TPF_{ROI}(\xi)=\frac{\sum_{s=1}^{S}\sum_{j=1}^{m_s} I(y_{sj}>\xi)}{\sum_{s=1}^{S} t_s}$$

$$=\frac{\sum_{s=1}^{S}\sum_{j=1}^{t_s} I(h_{sj}>\xi)}{\sum_{s=1}^{S} t_s}. \tag{8-35}$$

The traditional summary index of the ROI-ROC curve is the AUC which has the same expression as if all x and y values are independent:

$$AUC_{ROI}=\frac{\sum_{\tilde{s}=1}^{S}\sum_{s=1}^{S_1}\sum_{i=1}^{R-t_s}\sum_{j=1}^{t_s}\left\{I\left(x_{\tilde{s}i}<h_{sj}\right)+0.5\times I\left(x_{\tilde{s}i}=h_{sj}\right)\right\}}{\left(SR-\sum_{s=1}^{S_1} t_s\right)\left(\sum_{s=1}^{S_1} t_s\right)}$$

$$=\frac{\sum_{\tilde{s}=1}^{S}\sum_{s=1}^{S_1}\sum_{i=1}^{R-t_s}\sum_{j=1}^{t_s}\psi_{\tilde{s}isj}}{\left(SR-\sum_{s=1}^{S_1} t_s\right)\left(\sum_{s=1}^{S_1} t_s\right)}. \tag{8-36}$$

The variability of ROI-based AUC is affected by the variable numbers of target-free and target-depicting ROIs within each subject. The variance estimator may be based on the extension and combination of the techniques for *FPF* and *TPF* variance estimation and estimation of the variance of a two-sample U-statistic (Obuchowski, 1997; Zhou et al., 2002). Alternative approaches for estimating the uncertainty of the estimator from clustered ROC data include jack-knife (Hajian-Tilaki et al., 1997; Beam, 1998) and bootstrap (Rutter, 2000). These resampling techniques account for correlations among the random numbers of observations within the same subject by resampling the entire ensemble of observations associated with a given subject.

As a specific type of general clustered ROC data, ROI data may be analyzed by various techniques developed for clustered ROC analysis. A powerful method for analyzing correlated ROC data is based on the GEE technique (Toledano and Gatsonis, 1996). However, the validity of the standard GEE approach is questionable when cluster sizes are informative (Hoffman et al., 2001), and this limits the applicability of this approach for ROI studies. Mixed model techniques suitable for informative cluster sizes have not yet gained widespread popularity for performance assessment.

Interestingly, for a scenario in which each region of interest contains at most a single target and response, ROI and FROC analysis can be closely related under very general conditions. As noted above, under the ROI paradigm the *TP* and *FP* classifications are determined via a predefined grid of regions of interest. Technically, this may produce a classification different from that imposed by the proximity criterion used in FROC classification for the same responses. However, by adopting regions of interest of similar sizes for ROI and FROC (calibrating proximity criteria), the data processed with ROI and FROC may be made equivalent for most practical purposes. The ROI rating data [Equation (8-34)] differs from FROC rating data [Equation (8-14)] only by the presence of a finite set of 0-rated marks or, equivalently, knowledge of the upper limit for the false positive marks. Thus, ROI data can be analyzed using FROC methodology. Conversely, data acquired and processed under the FROC paradigm can be analyzed with ROI methods if we establish the upper limit for the *FP* marks. For the same data, there exists a one-to-one correspondence between the empirical points of ROI-ROC and FROC curves:

$$FPF_{ROI}(\xi)=\frac{\sum_{s=1}^{S}\sum_{i=1}^{n_s} I(x_{si}>\xi)}{S}\times\frac{S}{SR-\sum_{s=1}^{S_1} t_s}=FPR_{\rho\circ\pi}(\xi)\times\frac{S}{SR-\sum_{s=1}^{S_1} t_s}. \qquad (8\text{-}37)$$

$$TPF_{ROI}(\xi)=\sum_{s=1}^{S_1}\sum_{j=1}^{m_s} I(y_{sj}>\xi)\Big/\sum_{s=1}^{S_1} t_s = TPF_{\rho\circ\pi}(\xi)$$

In other words, the empirical FROC curve can be obtained from the ROI-based ROC curve (up to the last observed operating point) by a fixed horizontal scaling. This correspondence assures agreement of inferences based on the empirical points of the FROC and ROI-based ROC curves. We term the representation of the ROI curve in the FROC coordinates is known as the ROI-FROC curve.

As a specific application of clustered ROC analysis, ROI is often based on the entire empirical ROC curve that includes a straight-line extrapolation from the empirical point corresponding to $\xi = 0$ to the trivial point [1,1] where everything is considered positive. The ROI-FROC curve maintains this representation and connects the rightmost empirical point to the trivial point $(R - \Sigma t_s/S, 1)$ with a straight line. For a pure FROC curve, a default trivial point where everything is positive is infinite $[\infty,1]$, and the extrapolation beyond the point with $\xi = 0$ has an exponential shape (Section 8.2.3). This difference in the extensions beyond *[FPR(0) and TPF(0)]* (i.e., the difference in random augmentations of ROI and FROC processes) generates the possibility of a difference between results even when all empirical points are exactly the same (e.g., Figure 8.7). However, if the parameters of ROI and FROC are appropriately calibrated, the differences in conclusions are not likely to be prevalent in practice.

Thus, when regions of interest are sufficiently small, the ROI is closely related to FROC analysis and likely to lead to similar results when the data processing procedures and parameters are appropriately calibrated. ROI offers a wide range of tools and techniques of clustered ROC analysis, making ROI more readily adoptable. At the same time, compared with FROC, the ROI approach requires a somewhat more rigid protocol for processing the observed responses. The summary tools for the two techniques exhibit many structural, conceptual, and numerical similarities. However, unlike FROC, the ROI approach may be used to focus performance assessment on the practically (clinically) relevant regions of interest that may include multiple targets. In this case, the detection and localization performance within an ROI is superseded by the importance of the correct classification of the ROIs.

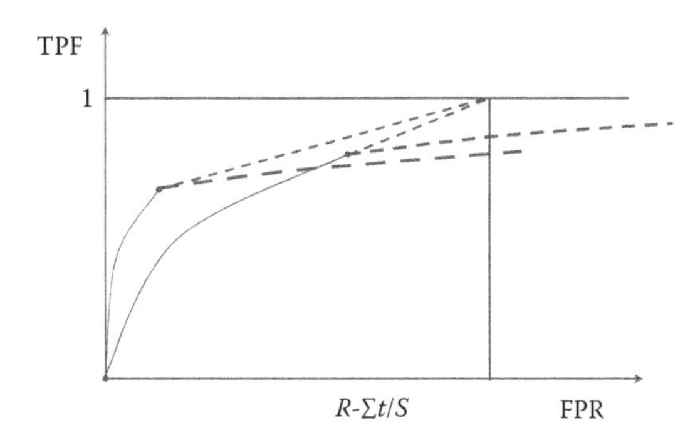

FIGURE 8.7
ROI-FROC and augmented conventional FROC curves. The ROI-FROC curve has a straight-line extension to the fixed point. The FROC curve has a curved augmentation extended to infinity.

8.4 Remarks and Further Reading

The performance assessment field utilizes a large number of approaches that were developed at different times and motivated by different applications and purposes. Although all the techniques are related, and more than one can be applied to assess performance characteristics of a single diagnostic system, they frequently emphasize different aspects of performance and may yield different conclusions.

Most techniques belong to one of two broad categories: those addressing only detection (conventional ROC approach) and those addressing both detection and localization (conventional FROC approach). A detection-only task corresponds to the assessment of an subject as a whole based on the presence of targets. Detection and localization tasks are based on the assessment of individual targets within an subject. Although these tasks are interrelated, the exact relationship is often unknown and the results of assessing the same diagnostic systems may lead to contradicting conclusions.

Clearly when a diagnostic system exhibits neither detection nor localization errors, it is perfect with respect to the assessment of subjects for the presence of targets. Conversely, an imperfect system can be better for assessing detection and localization than performing detection only. For example, a system that is perfect in localization of only a few presented targets it can detect may appear superior to another system under the FROC paradigm, but may perform poorly under the ROC paradigm. Without additional information, one should not assume that better detection and localization performance (higher FROC curve) automatically implies better performance in terms of detection alone (higher ROC curve). However, this does not exclude the possibility that the two methods agree, as they frequently do. Several types of relationships were considered by various investigators in attempts to link ROC to FROC data such as (1) reduction of FROC findings to a single rating using the maximum of ratings, and (2) using the minimum of the ratings or the averaged ratings (Swensson, 1996; Obuchowski et al., 2000; Song et al., 2008). None of these guarantees concordance between ROC and FROC-type performance characteristics for all circumstances and scenarios. However, these data reduction approaches may form stand alone methods of analyzing FROC data in that manner, and may be appropriate for assessing performance in specific diagnostic tasks.

For example, it is intuitively appealing in some applications to presume that the assessment of an subject is driven by the most suspicious finding within an subject (Swensson 1996; Chakraborty, 1989). Under this assumption, FROC data may be reduced to a single observation per subject without loss of information relevant to the overall assessment of the subject as a whole. Data can then be analyzed via standard ROC methods without additional assumptions because the information related to each subject is reduced to a single observation. However, this type of reduced FROC data loses all information about target localization, and the method thus tends to be less sensitive to differences in localization performance than analysis using more complete data (Chakraborty, 2002). Of course it is possible to construct examples in which pseudoROC indices are better for detecting specific types of differences. In addition, one should be cautious in extrapolating the results and properties of pseudoROC structures to actual ROC experiments. In a real ROC experiment, the mechanism by which the system (with or without human observer) generates decisions for each subject may be more complex than simply translating a decision based solely on the most suspicious finding within an subject. Similar considerations are applicable to other methods of performance assessment based on data reduction.

Important differences may also arise among methods used in a detection and localization performance assessment. We previously discussed four approaches for such performance assessments, namely FROC, AFROC, LROC, and ROI. Although some approaches require more rigid assessment protocols, they may be applied to data acquired under a natural free-response protocol, sometimes after data reduction. Conversely, FROC analysis may be applied to data collected under other paradigms for detection and localization performance assessment, but even when applied to the same data, different conclusions may result.

The performance assessment approaches discussed in this chapter address different but interrelated problems. Although specific cases may exhibit a natural relationship between different approaches, this principle is not generally true. There is no methodology that is "optimal" under all circumstances. Thus, care should be taken in selecting a method appropriate for the specific problem to be investigated; generalization of the results to those that may be obtained by other approaches should be avoided.

Specific approaches for detection–localization and FROC methodology are scattered in a number of papers. The earlier concepts and approaches are described in Egan (1961), Bunch et al. (1978), and Starr et al. (1975). Parametric methods of fitting smooth FROC curves are described in Chakraborty (1989), Edwards et al. (2002), Swensson (1996), Irvine (2004), Chakraborty (2006), Hutchinson (2007), and Chakraborty et al. (2007). Nonparametric approaches are cited by Obuchowski et al. (2000), Chakraborty and Berbaum (2004), Popescu (2007), Tang and Balakrishnan (2011), Samuelson and Petrick (2006), and Bandos et al. (2009).

References

Arvesen, J.N. 1969. Jackknifing U-statistics. *Annals of Mathematical Statistics* 40: 2076–2100.

Bandos, A.I., Rockette H.E., and Gur D. 2010. Use of likelihood ratios for comparisons of binary diagnostic tests: underlying ROC curves. *Medical Physics* 37: 5821–5830.

Bandos, A.I., Rockette, H.E., and Gur, D. 2006. Resampling methods for the area under the ROC curve. *Proceedings of ICML Workshop on ROC Analysis in Machine Learning*, pp. 1–8.

Bandos, A.I., Rockette, H.E., Song, T. et al. 2009. Area under the free-response ROC curve (FROC) and a related summary index. *Biometrics* 65: 247–256.

Beam, C.A. 1998. Analysis of clustered data in receiver operating characteristic studies. *Statistical Methods in Medical Research* 7: 324–336.

Bunch, P.C., Hamilton, J.F., Sanderson, G.K. et al. 1978. A free-response approach to the measurement and characterization of radiographic-observer performance. *Journal of Applied Photographic Engineering* 4: 165–171.

Chakraborty, D.P. 1989. Maximum likelihood analysis of free-response receiver operating characteristic (FROC) data. *Medical Physics* 16: 561–568.

Chakraborty, D.P. 2000. Data analysis for detection and localization of multiple abnormalities with application to mammography. *Academic Radiology* 7: 553–556.

Chakraborty, D.P. 2006. A search model and figure of merit for observer data acquired to the free-response paradigm. *Physics in Medicine and Biology* 51: 3449–3462.

Chakraborty, D.P. 2008. Validation and statistical power comparison of methods for analyzing free-response observer performance studies. *Academic Radiology* 15: 1554–1566.

Chakraborty, D.P. and Berbaum, K.S. 2004. Observer studies involving detection and localization: modeling, analysis and validation. *Medical Physics* 31: 2313–2330.

Chakraborty, D.P. and Winter, L.H.L. 1990. Free-response methodology: alternate analysis and a new observer-performance experiment. *Medical Physics* 174: 873–881.

Chakraborty, D.P. and Yoon, H.J. 2008. Operating characteristics predicted by models for diagnostic tasks involving lesion localization. *Medical Physics* 35: 435–445.

Chakraborty, D.P. and Yoon, H.J. 2009. JAFROC analysis revisited: figure-of-merit considerations for human observer studies. In *Proceedings of SPIE Conference on Medical Imaging: Perception, Observer Performance, and Technology Assessment*.

Chakraborty, D.P., Yoon, H.J., and Mello-Thoms, C. 2007. Spatial localization accuracy of radiologists in free-response studies: inferring perceptual FROC curves from mark-rating data. *Academic Radiology* 14: 4–18.

Dorfman, D.D. and Alf, E., Jr. 1969. Maximum likelihood estimation of parameters of signal detection theory and determination of confidence intervals: rating-method data. *Journal of Mathematical Psychology* 6: 487–496.

Edwards, D.C., Kupinski, M.A., Metz, C.E. et al. 2002. Maximum likelihood fitting of FROC curves under an initial-detection-and-candidate-analysis model. *Medical Physics* 29: 2861–2870.

Egan, J.P., Greenberg, G.Z., and Schulman, A.I. 1961. Operating characteristics, signal delectability, and the methods of free response. *Journal of the Acoustical Society of America* 33: 993–1007.

Gallas, B.D., Penello, G.A., and Myers, K.L. 2007. Multireader multicase variance analysis for binary data. *Journal of the Optical Society of America* 24: B70–B80.

Gur, D., Bandos, A.I., and Rockette, H.E. 2008. Comparing areas under the receiver operating characteristic curves: the potential impact of the "last" experimentally measured operating point. *Radiology* 247: 12–15.

Gur, D. and Rockette, H.E. 2008. Performance assessments of diagnostic systems under the FROC paradigm: experimental, analytical and results interpretation issues. *Academic Radiology* 15: 1312–1315.

Hajian-Tilaki, K.O., Hanley, J.A., Lawrance, J. et al. 1997. Extension of receiver operating characteristics analysis to data concerning multiple signal detection tasks. *Academic Radiology* 4: 222–229.

Hoffman, E.B., Sen, P.K., and Weinberg, C.R. 2001. Within-cluster resampling. *Biometrika* 88: 1121–1134.

Hutchinson, T.P. 2007. Free-response operator characteristic models for visual search. *Physics in Medicine and Biology* 52: L1–L3.

Irvine, J.M. 2004. Assessing target search performance: the free-response operator characteristic model. *Optical Engineering* 43: 2926–2934.

Metz, C.E., Herman, B.A., and Shen, J. 1998. Maximum likelihood estimation of receiver operating characteristic (ROC) curves from continuously distributed data. *Statistics in Medicine* 17: 1033–1053.

Metz, C.E., Starr, S.J., and Lusted, L.B. 1976. Observer performance in detecting multiple radiographic signals. *Radiology* 121: 337–347.

Norman, D.A. 1964. A comparison of data obtained with different false-alarm rates. *Psychological Review* 71: 243–246.

Obuchowski, N.A. 1997. Nonparametric analysis of clustered ROC curve data. *Biometrics* 53: 567–578.

Obuchowski, N.A. 1998. On the comparison of correlated proportions for clustered data. *Statistics in Medicine* 17: 1495-1507.

Obuchowski, N.A., Mazzone, P.J., and Dachman, A.H. 2010. Bias, underestimation of risk, and loss of statistical power in patient-level analyses of lesion detection. *European Radiology* 20: 584–594.

Obuchowski, N.A., Lieber, M.L., and Powel, K.A. 2000. Data analysis for detection and localization of multiple abnormalities with application to mammography. *Academic Radiology* 7: 516–525.

Perkins, N.J., Schisterman, E.F., and Vexler, A. 2007. Receiver operating characteristic curve inference from a sample with a limit of detection. *American Journal of Epidemiology* 165: 325–333.

Popescu, L.M. 2007. Nonparametric ROC and LROC analysis. *Medical Physics* 34: 1556–1564.

Popescu, L.M. 2008. Model for the detection of signals in images with multiple suspicious locations. *Medical Physics* 35: 5565–5574.

Rao, J.N.K. and Scott, A.J. 1992. A simple method for the analysis of clustered binary data. *Biometrics* 48: 577–585.

Samuelson, F.W. and Petrick, N. 2006. Comparing image detection algorithms using resampling. In *Proceedings of Third IEEE International Symposium, Biomedical Imaging: Macro to Nano*, Arlington, VA, pp. 1312–1315.

Schisterman, E.F., Reiser, B., and Faraggi, D. 2006. ROC analysis for markers with mass at zero. *Statistics in Medicine* 25: 623–638.

Song, T., Bandos, A.I., Rockette, H.E. et al. 2008. On comparing methods for discriminating between actually negative and actually positive subjects with FROC type data. *Medical Physics* 35: 1547–1558.

Starr, S.J., Metz, C.E., Lusted, L.B. et al. 1975. Visual detection and localization of radiographic images. *Radiology* 116: 533–538.

Swensson, R.G. 1996. Unified measurement of observe performance in detecting and localizing target objects on images. *Medical Physics* 23: 1709–1725.

Swensson, R.G. 2000. Using localization data from image interpretations to improve estimates of performance accuracy. *Medical Decision Making* 20: 170–185.

Swensson, R.G., King, J.L., and Gur, D. 2001. A constrained formulation for the receiver operating characteristic (ROC) curve based on probability summation. *Medical Physics* 28: 1597–1609.

Tang, L. and Balakrishnan N. 2011. A random-sum Wilcoxon statistic with applications to various types of diagnostic data. *Journal of Statistical Planning and Inference* 141: 335–344.

Toledano, A.Y. and Gatsonis, G. 1996. Ordinal regression methodology for ROC curves derived from correlated data. *Statistics in Medicine* 15: 1807–1826.

Tosteson, A.N.A. and Begg, C.B. 1988. A general regression methodology for ROC curve estimation. *Medical Decision Making* 8: 204–215.

Wieand, H.S., Gail, M.M., and Hanley, J.A. 1983. A nonparametric procedure for comparing diagnostic tests with paired or unpaired data. *IMS Bulletin* 12: 213–214.

Yoon, H.J., Zheng, B., Sahiner, B. et al. 2007. Evaluating computer-aided detection algorithms. *Medical Physics* 34: 2024–2038.

Zheng, B., Chakraborty, D.P., Rockette, H.E. et al. 2005. Comparison of two data analyses from two observer performance studies using jackknife ROC and JAFROC. *Medical Physics* 32: 1031–1034.

Zhou, X.H., Obuchowski, N.A., and McClish, D.K. 2002. *Statistical Methods in Diagnostic Medicine*. New York: Wiley.

Zou, K.H. and Hall, W.J. 2000. Two transformation models for estimating an ROC curve derived from continuous data. *Journal of Applied Statistics* 27: 621–631.

Zou, K.H., Hall, W.J., and Shapiro, D.E. 1997. Smooth non-parametric receiver operating characteristic (ROC) curves for continuous diagnostic tests. *Statistics in Medicine* 16: 2143–2156.

9

Machine Learning and Predictive Modeling

9.1 Introduction

As described in Chapter 4, ROC analysis has many applications in biomarker evaluation. The predictive ability of biomarkers for diagnostic and prognostic purposes relies heavily on their ability to produce an accurate estimate of the probability of disease or disease progression.

We have so far refrained from commenting on the types of classifiers that generate the estimates evaluated by ROC analysis. For example, in multivariate analysis, some of these models may help explain how particular covariates affect the dependent variable in a particular data set. However, the models may not necessarily be useful for predictive analyses if their constructions are not based on certain principles that help ensure generalization to previously unseen observations. Binary classifiers have been widely used in biomedical applications to explain and predict outcomes. Throughout this chapter, *machine learning* will encompass predictive models developed by the computer science and medical informatics communities and researchers of statistical learning models. Later in this chapter, resampling techniques such as the bootstrap will be presented to aid assessments of the appropriateness of classifiers for predicting outcomes of new cases.

ROC analysis is often used to compare predictive models, both in model selection and model evaluation. Matheny et al. (2005) compared different models for predicting complications following percutaneous coronary interventions using ROC analysis. Tsai et al. (2004) proposed ROC analysis to determine the optimal cutoff to demonstrate which genes are differentially expressed across various samples. Before we discuss ROC analysis to compare machine learning models for biomedicine, it is important to note that outputs from different types of classifiers perform differently. Some models are designed to output estimates of the probability of a given class; others produce estimates that are simply transformed into a probabilistic scale between 0 and 1 but were not originally intended to estimate class probabilities.

For example, while logistic regression classifiers are usually constructed using MLEs to output predicted class probabilities [also true for certain types of artificial neural networks (ANNs)], support vector machines (SVMs) often utilize the logistic function to transform the distances from each point to the optimal separating plane determined by the support vectors (Smola, 2000). While these SVM outputs are constrained within 0 and 1 and may be used in ROC analysis to evaluate the discrimination of a particular classifier, they were not designed to represent class probabilities although they are often inadvertently used this way. This has implications on how SVMs should be used in practice. ROC analysis does not evaluate the quality of class probability predictions; it only evaluates the ranks of these estimates. It focuses on the performance evaluation of the discrimination abilities of machine learning models, not on their calibration (assessment of the adequacy of the estimates of class probabilities per se). Adequate discrimination is a necessary but not sufficient condition to build a good predictive model.

9.2 Predictive Modeling

The methodologies used to estimate parameters for different types of classifiers depend on their intended uses—typically classified as explanatory or predictive. Explanatory models are intended to determine the relative importance of particular set of covariates for a given outcome using a data set of existing cases. Predictive models estimate outcomes for new cases. The differences can be subtle, and multivariate models such as logistic regression and classification trees are often used for both explanation and prediction.

Machine learning methods such as ANNs and SVMs proved successful for predicting outcomes in various biomedical fields (Ohno-Machado, 1997; Rowland et al., 1998; Ohno-Machado and Rowland, 1999; Nimgaonkar et al. 2004; Matheny et al., 2007). However, these models do not allow interpretation of the importance of covariates and are not very useful for explaining processes. In other words, they may be able to predict well but do not offer additional insights into the biological processes that determine particular outcomes. For example, they may allow the discovery of multivariate molecular "signatures" for particular disease states but do not help researchers understand which genes are the most important markers for these states.

For this reason, the best known predictive models in clinical medicine are based on logistic regression analysis. Applications include cardiovascular risk calculators derived from the Framingham study (Fox et al., 2010), models for prediction of breast cancer (Asiago et al., 2010; Claus, 2001), the MELD model for ranking liver transplant recipients (Martin et al., 2007), the APACHE system for ICU mortality prediction (Knaus et al., 1985), models predicting resectability of neurological tumors (Talos et al., 2006), prediction of complications after percutaneous coronary interventions (Resnic et al., 2001; Zou et al., 2005; Matheny et al., 2007), predicting pregnancy based on characteristics of embryos derived from assisted reproductive technology

(Racowsky et al., 2009), diagnosing true bacteremia from blood cultures (Wang et al., 2000), and a variety of other uses.

A review by Lasko et al. (2005) discusses main uses of ROC analysis in medical matters. Conversely, researchers interested in predictive modeling for bioinformatics rarely use logistic regression for building predictive models to determine molecular signatures from high-throughput gene expressions (Liao and Chin, 2007) or single nucleotide polymorphism measurements (Ayers and Cordell, 2010). As a practical issue, these data sets invariable, contain many more variables than there are observations, so it is not possible to use logistic regression unless a strategy such as stepwise forward selection is used to reduce the number of variables.

Regardless of the type of model used for prediction, an important aspect of predictive modeling is the ability of a model to generalize to new cases. To assess this ability in situations in which the number of observations is not very large, cross-validation and bootstrap strategies are useful.

9.3 Cross-Validation

A simple but not ideal strategy for assessing performance on previously unseen cases is to divide the sample into nonoverlapping training (or validation) and test sets, for example, the commonly used random 2:1 split (2/3 training and validation samples versus 1/3 testing samples) found in Gönen (2007). The training and validation sets are used to estimate parameters of the models and perform model selection. The test set evaluates the performance of the final model. Using all cases available at a certain point in time and evaluating performance on prospective cases is a variant of this procedure frequently utilized for biomedical applications. However, a simple split into one training and one test set if often insufficient to evaluate predictive performance.

Cross-validation is one of the most common resampling techniques for evaluating predictive models. It consists of splitting a sample into several pairs of training and test sets. Usually only one random split into k groups is utilized, although some authors prefer to repeat the procedure several times. Cross-validation can be used to estimate *TPF*s and *FPF*s, respectively, from which ROC curves can be derived and corresponding AUCs calculated. Cross-validation requires that a sample be partitioned into k parts for each randomization. Then k models are generated, each of them built without the cases in the kth partition, which is used for evaluation. The *TPF* and *FPF* are calculated for each k model and averaged for each possible threshold. The resulting ROC is used to calculate the AUC. That is, each observation x_i is part of one of the k partitions, with (κ) returning the partition to which x_i belongs. A special case when $k = n$ is called leave-one-out cross-validation or the jack-knife procedure. The cross-validation estimate for the *TPF*, *FPF*, and

ROC are given below, following notation similar to that of Hastie et al. (2009) and Adler and Lausen (2009):

$$TPF_{CV}(\xi) = \frac{1}{n^1} \sum_{x_i \in Z_1} I(\kappa \hat{f}^{-\kappa(i)}(x_i) > \xi),$$

$$FPF_{CV}(\xi) = \frac{1}{n^0} \sum_{x_i \in Z_0} I(\kappa \hat{f}^{-\kappa(i)}(x_i) > \xi), \tag{9-1}$$

$$ROC_{CV} = \{FPF_{CV}(\xi), TPF_{CV}(\xi)\}, \ \forall \xi \in R,$$

where Z_1 is the set of positive observations, ξ is the threshold, *I(.)* is the indicator function, and $\hat{f}^{-\kappa(i)}(x_i)$ is the model built without using observations from the partition ξ containing x_i. The same procedure may be used several times to generate different data splits, and the results are then aggregated as above.

As discussed in Hastie et al. (2009), the leave-one-out cross-validation procedure in which $k = N$ produces estimates with low bias and high variance, whereas a small k produces the reverse. Many applications use k = 5 or 10 (Hastie et al., 2009), and perform only one random data split. Although the rationale to construct ROC_{CV} as above is clear, the machine learning community often uses other strategies to calculate the cross-validation AUC. For example, Bradley pointed out that some averaged AUCs from ROC curves correspond to each partition and others aggregated the outputs of all folds first, producing one ROC and calculating its AUC (Bishop, 2006).

$$AUC_{CV} = \frac{1}{k} \sum_{i=1}^{k} AUC_i. \tag{9-2}$$

All the above approaches are problematic for very small or very large numbers of partitions.

9.4 Bootstrap Resampling Methods

Unlike cross-validation, the bootstrap allows re-utilization of samples in training sets. Samples with replacements are drawn from the observations into a large number k of groups. The size of this bootstrap group is predetermined, usually consisting of the same number of observations (n) as in the original sample. The bootstrap samples are drawn with replacements into a particular training set. Some observations are not included in the sample and are used as a test set for evaluation (Efron, 1993). As in cross-validation, the *TPF* and *FPF* values generated for each sample in the test set at each threshold are averaged, resulting in a ROC from which the AUC is calculated. The ROC is calculated as follows

$$TPF_B(\xi) = \frac{1}{N^1}\sum_{i=1}^{N}\frac{I(y_i = 1)}{|C_1^{-i}|}\sum_{b \in C_1^{-i}} I(\kappa\hat{f}^{-b}(x_i) > \xi),$$

$$FPF_B(\xi) = \frac{1}{N^0}\sum_{i=1}^{N}\frac{I(y_i = 0)}{|C_0^{-i}|}\sum_{b \in C_0^{-i}} I(\kappa\hat{f}^{-b}(x_i) > \xi), \qquad (9\text{-}3)$$

$$ROC_B = \{FPF_B(\xi), TPF_B(\xi)\},\ \forall \xi \in R,$$

where b is the set of cases not included in the training set, C_1^{-i} is the set of positive observations used for testing, and $\hat{f}^{-b}(x_i)$ is the model built without using observations from the set containing x_i.

Similar to the cross-validation method shown in Equation (9-3), alternative approaches such as averaging the AUCs resulting from each group or aggregating all overlapping test set estimates into a large collection and calculating the ROC from the collection were also used by Dorfman et al. (1995).

9.4.1 Bootstrap Method 1

The apparent true positive fraction $\overline{TPF}$ results from the use of the model in the training cases. The *TPF* is optimistic (because the MLE was optimized for the cases in the training set), while the bootstrap estimate TPF_B is pessimistic so a weighted average of these indices was proposed by Efron (1997).

$$TPF_{0.632}(\xi) = 0.368\overline{TPF} + 0.632TPF_B,$$

$$FPF_{0.632}(\xi) = 0.368\overline{FPF} + 0.632FPF_B,$$

$$ROC_{0.632} = \{FPF_{0.632}(\xi), TPF_{0.632}(\xi)\},\ \forall \xi \in R.$$

However, this measure is also not ideal, as it was shown to depend on the degree of overfitting from the model by Dorfman et al. (1995).

9.4.2 Bootstrap Method 2

If a high degree of overfitting is present, Efron and Tibshirani (1997) proposed the .632+ version of this estimator that takes into account the relative rate of overfitting. The rate is calculated using the proportion $q(\xi)$ of predictions considered positive depending on the threshold ξ in situations that exhibit no dependence between class membership and predictions (e.g., by randomly permuting class labels; Gerds and Cai, 2008). This proportion $q(\xi)$ is known as the no-information value. Relative overfitting rates are defined as:

$$R_{TPF}(\xi) = \frac{\overline{TPF(\xi)} - TPF_B(\xi)}{\overline{TPF(\xi)} - q(\xi)},$$

$$R_{FPF}(\xi) = -\frac{\overline{FPF(\xi)} - FPF_B(\xi)}{\overline{FPF(\xi)} - q(\xi)}.$$

Adler and Lausen (2009) proposed the calculation of *TPF, FPF,* and *ROC* for .632+ estimation as follows:

$$TPF_{.632+}(\xi) = TPF_{0.632}(\xi) + \left[TPF_B(\xi) - \overline{TPF}\right]\left[\frac{0.368 \times 0.632 R_{TPF}(\xi)}{1 - 0.368 R_{TPF}(\xi)}\right],$$

$$FPF_{.632+}(\xi) = FPF_{0.632}(\xi) + \left[FPF_B(\xi) - \overline{FPF}\right]\left[\frac{0.368 \times 0.632 R_{FPF}(\xi)}{1 - 0.368 R_{FPF}(\xi)}\right],$$

$$ROC_{.632+}(\xi) = \{FPF_{0.632+}(\xi), TPF_{0.632+}(\xi)\}, \ \forall \xi \in R.$$

Since it is possible for $R_{.}(\xi)$ to be outside the [0,1] interval, Adler and Lausen (2007) proposed modifications such that:

$$TPF' = \max(TPF(\xi), q(\xi)),$$

$$FPF' = \min(FPF(\xi), q(\xi)),$$

$$R'_{TPF}(\xi) = \frac{\overline{TPF(\xi)} - TPF'(\xi)}{\overline{TPF(\xi)} - q(\xi)},$$

$$R'_{FPF}(\xi) = -\frac{\overline{FPF(\xi)} - FPF'(\xi)}{\overline{FPF(\xi)} - q(\xi)},$$

except when $TPF' > \overline{TPF}$, in which case $R'_{TPF} = 0$, or when $FPF' < \overline{FPF}$, in which case $R'_{FPF} = 0$.

9.5 Overfitting and False Discovery Rate

The cross-validation and bootstrap procedures gained popularity in biomedical data analyses because of the concern that present high-dimensional data methods may easily produce overfitted models that fail to be generalized to new data. In fact, considerable research on controlling false discovery rates (FDRs) in high-dimensional data analyses was published (Storey, 2003; Benjamini et al., 1995).

Resampling methods will continue to be important as more data are generated and predictions for several conditions are produced by "personalized medicine" initiatives in which the absolute risk produced by predictive models has more importance than the relative rank of the predictions. Hence, ROC analysis is not the main factor determining whether models are considered successful. Nevertheless, it plays an important role in model selection and preliminary model evaluation.

Models that overfit existing data are unlikely to be useful for prediction tasks. It is thus particularly important to control overfitting and obtain a realistic estimate of model performance. Particularly for bioinformatics, overfitting is a real threat because many experiments use high-throughput technologies—thousands of measurements are performed for a single sample. The number of such samples is often one or two orders of magnitude smaller than the number of covariates due to the relatively high cost of processing a single sample.

9.6 Remarks and Further Reading

We concentrated our discussion on ROC and AUC as predictive performance indicators and on resampling techniques for minimizing the overfitting problem. Other ways to control overfitting rely on shrinkage of coefficients when building regression models (Steyerberg et al., 2004) or selecting models based on indices that penalize the use of a high number of covariates (Hosmer and Lemeshow, 2000).

The use of high-throughput technologies and the desire to determine a small set of genes (among thousands of candidates) associated with particular diseases or conditions generated a lot of attention for indices that control for rates of false positives. As a result, controlling for false discovery rates (Pawitan et al, 2005) became an important aspect of defining the necessary sample size for microarrays and other types of high-throughput technologies. However, since sensitivity in such studies must not be neglected, ROC analysis has been proposed as an additional strategy to determine which genes should be considered differentially expressed (Chen et al., 2007).

Several techniques have been used to mitigate the overfitting problem, including regularization (establishing penalties for including a large number of predictors) and resampling techniques that sequester cases from the model building phase, utilize them to evaluate model performance in the testing phase, and rebuild a model if necessary, as discussed in this chapter.

The basic concept is that if all available data are used to build, select, and evaluate a model, the results will be too optimistic.

Conversely, if few samples are available, reserving them exclusively for evaluation impairs the construction of a model. The choices of model building, selection, and evaluation methods are important to achieve predictive models that generalize to new cases. However, an important consideration is that ROC analysis evaluates only the discrimination ability of models, not their calibration. Discrimination is important but not sufficient for predictive models. To cover the evaluation of personalized medicine models effectively, ROC analysis must be combined with techniques that evaluate model calibration.

References

Adler, W. and Lausen, B. 2009. Bootstrap estimated true and false positive rates and ROC curve. *Computational Statistics and Data Analysis* 53: 718–729.

Asiago, V.M., Alvarado, L.Z., Shanaiah, N. et al. 2010. Early detection of recurrent breast cancer using metabolite profiling. *Cancer Research* 70: 8309–8318.

Ayers, K.L. and Cordell, H.J. 2010. SNP Selection in genome-wide and candidate gene studies via penalized logistic regression. *Genetic Epidemiology* 34: 879–891.

Benjamini, Y. and Hochberg, Y. 1995. Controlling the false discovery rate: a practical and powerful approach to multiple testing. *Journal of the Royal Statistical Society Series B* 57: 289–300.

Bishop, C.M. 2006. *Pattern Recognition and Machine Learning*. New York: Springer.

Bradley, A.P. 1997. The use of the area under the ROC curve in the evaluation of machine learning algorithms. *Pattern Recognition* 30: 1145–1159.

Chen, J.J., Wang, S.J., Tsai, C.A. et al. 2007. Selection of differentially expressed genes in microarray data analysis. *Pharmacogenomics Journal*. 7: 212–220.

Claus, E.B. 2001. Risk models used to counsel women for breast and ovarian cancer: a guide for clinicians. *Familial Cancer* 1: 197–206.

Dorfman, D.D., Berbaum. K.S., and Lenth, RV. 1995. Multireader, multicase receiver operating characteristic methodology: a bootstrap analysis. *Academic Radiology* 2: 626–633.

Efron, B. and Tibshirani, R. 1993. *Introduction to the Bootstrap*. New York: Chapman & Hall.

Efron, B. and Tibshirani, R. 1997. Improvements on cross-validation: the .632+ bootstrap method. *Journal of the American Statistical Association* 92: 548–560.

Fox, C.S., Massaro, J.M, Schlett, C.L. et al. 2010. Periaortic fat deposition is associated with peripheral arterial disease: the Framingham Heart Study. *Circulation: Cardiovascular Imaging* 3: 515–519.

Gerds, T.A. and Cai, T.X. 2008. The performance of risk prediction models. *Biometrical Journal* 50: 457–479.

Gönen, M. 2007. Analyzing Receiver Operating Characteristic Curves with SAS®. Cary, NC: SAS Institute.

Hastie, T., Tibshirani, R., and Friedman, J.H.2009. *The Elements of Statistical Learning: Data Mining, Inference, and Prediction*, 2nd ed. New York: Springer.

Hosmer, D.W, and Lemeshow, S. 2000. *Applied Logistic Regression*. 2nd ed. New York: Wiley.

Knaus ,W.A., Draper, E.A., Wagner, D.P. et al. 1985. APACHE II: a severity of disease classification system. *Critical Care Medicine* 13: 818–829.

Lasko, T.A., Bhagwat, J.G., Zou, K.H. et al. 2005. The use of receiver operating characteristic curves in biomedical informatics. *Journal of Biomedical Informatics* 38: 404–415.

Liao, J.G. and Chin, K.V. 2007. Logistic regression for disease classification using microarray data: model selection in a large p and small n case. *Bioinformatics* 23: 1945–1951.

Martin, A.P., Bartels, M., Hauss, J. et al. 2007. Overview of MELD score and UNOS adult liver allocation system. *Transplantation Proceedings* 39: 3169–3174.

Matheny, M.E., Arora, N., Ohno-Machado, L. et al. 2007. Rare adverse event monitoring of medical devices with the use of an automated surveillance tool. *AMIA Annual Symposium Proceedings*, pp. 518–522.

Matheny, M.E., Ohno-Machado, L., and Resnic, F.S. 2005. Discrimination and calibration of mortality risk prediction models in interventional cardiology. *Journal of Biomedical Informatics* 38: 367–375.

Matheny, M.E., Resnic, F.S., Arora, N. et al. 2007. Effects of SVM parameter optimization on discrimination and calibration for post-procedural PCI mortality. *Journal of Biomedical Informatics* 40: 688–697.

Nimgaonkar, A., Karnad, D.R., Sudarshan, S. et al. 2004. Prediction of mortality in an Indian intensive care unit: comparison between APACHE II and artificial neural networks. *Intensive Care Medicine* 30: 248–253.

Ohno-Machado, L. and Rowland, T. 1999. Neural network applications in physical medicine and rehabilitation. *American Journal of Physical Medicine and Rehabilitation* 78: 392–398.

Ohno-Machado, L. 1997. A comparison of Cox proportional hazards and artificial neural network models for medical prognosis. *Computers in Biology and Medicine* 27: 55–65.

Pawitan, Y., Michiels, S., Koscielny, S. et al. 2005. False discovery rate, sensitivity and sample size for microarray studies. *Bioinformatics* 21: 3017–3024.

Racowsky, C., Ohno-Machado, L., Kim, J. et al. 2009. Is there an advantage in scoring early embryos on more than one day? *Human Reproduction* 24: 2104–2113.

Resnic, F.S., Ohno-Machado, L., Selwyn, A. et al. 2001. Simplified risk score models accurately predict the risk of major in-hospital complications following percutaneous coronary intervention. *American Journal of Cardiology* 88: 5–9.

Rowland, T., Ohno-Machado, L., and Ohrn, A. 1998. Comparison of multiple prediction models for ambulation following spinal cord injury. *Proceedings of AMIA Symposium*, pp. 528–532.

Smola, A.J. 2000. *Advances in Large Margin Classifiers*. Cambridge: MIT Press.

Steyerberg, E.W., Borsboom, G.J.J.M., van Houwelingen, H.C. et al. 2004. Validation and updating of predictive logistic regression models: a study on sample size and shrinkage. *Statistics in Medicine* 23: 2567–2586.

Storey, J.D. 2003. The positive false discovery rate: a Bayesian interpretation and the q-value. *Annals of Statistics* 31: 2013–2035.

Talos, I.F., Zou, K.H., Ohno-Machado, L. et al. 2006. Supratentorial low-grade glioma resectability: statistical predictive analysis based on anatomic MR features and tumor characteristics. *Radiology* 239: 506–513.

Tsai, C.A. and Chen, J.J. 2004. Significance analysis of ROC indices for comparing diagnostic markers: applications to gene microarray data. *Journal of Biopharmaceutical Statistics* 14: 985–1003.

Wang, S.J., Kuperman, G.J., Ohno-Machado, L. et al. 2000. Using electronic data to predict the probability of true bacteremia from positive blood cultures. *Proceedings of AMIA Symposium*, pp. 893–897.

Zou, K.H., Resnic, F.S, Talos, I.F. et al. 2005. A global goodness-of-fit test for receiver operating characteristic curve analysis via the bootstrap method. *Journal of Biomedical Informatics* 38: 395–403.

Section IV

Discussions and Extensions

10

Summary and Challenges

10.1 Summary and Discussion

The problems of classification and prediction arise frequently. In recent decades, one of the most common approaches has been ROC analysis for assessing the performance of diagnostic systems, technologies, and practices (collectively called diagnostic systems in this chapter). Many topics related to the evaluation of diagnostic tests have been thoroughly discussed in recent textbooks and have been examined in this book. However, the field of classification is still developing and evolving. The area of ROC analysis, in particular, has increasingly been enriched with approaches that address new and challenging problems with innovative techniques that better address old but challenging questions. The complex nature of those problems encountered in medical and other diagnostic disciplines has led to the development of extensions of the conventional ROC analysis.

10.2 Future Directions in ROC Analysis

Diagnostic systems are designed to classify a unit of assessment into one of a predefined set of classes (normal and abnormal) or express confidence in the presence of certain predefined abnormalities within a unit. The unit of assessment is sometimes called a diagnostic unit. In medical imaging, a diagnostic unit may be, for example, an individual (patient), body organ (breast, lung, etc.), or a suspicious location within an organ (a suspected nodule in the left upper lobe of a lung). A specific diagnostic unit considered in a study may include multiple units of interest. The assessments of an overall unit and nested diagnostic units (e.g., assessment of nodules within each lung and an overall classification of the patient) are related. Several types of relationships have been hypothesized, but in the context of observer performance studies, these relationships in the best defined problems may not have been thoroughly explored and may not be fully understood. To date, many such studies consider only one diagnostic unit at a time.

The simplest assessment of diagnostic systems is through a binary classifier. For example, suspected presence and absence of a disease would indicate the true status of a given diagnostic unit. The results of a binary diagnostic test are expressed as positive or a negative. A positive result indicates the suspected presence of the condition of interest. To distinguish the true status, units showing that a condition of interest is truly present or absent are usually designated actually positive or negative. The evaluation of binary diagnostic tests is primarily based on estimating sensitivity and specificity. The performance of diagnostic tests can be assessed and compared using a direct comparison of sensitivity and specificity, a combined index such as the Youden index, or an expected utility. Other relevant measures of performance of binary diagnostic tests include positive and negative predictive values. However, such measures depend on the prevalence of the condition of interest in a sample and thus often require very careful sampling.

Several diagnostic tests yield more than two possible results. Any diagnostic system involving multicategory test results may be converted into a binary diagnostic system by dichotomizing the test results. In the most common case in which test results are ordinal (may be ordered), dichotomization is achieved by labeling the results as positive or negative, depending on whether they are greater or smaller than a prespecified threshold.

The standard approach for assessing the accuracy of a diagnostic system with ordinal test results is based on estimating its ROC curve—a depiction of the tradeoff between sensitivity and specificity when the corresponding threshold is varied. The ROC curve comprehensively reflects intrinsic performance characteristics and is independent to the prevalence of the condition of interest. This provides a foundation for assessments and comparisons of various performance measures such as sensitivity at given specificity, AUC, and pAUC. Although the ROC curve is completely determined by the distribution of test results, the reverse is not true. A well-known example is the binormal ROC curve that may be obtained from both normally distributed test results and from any order-preserving transformation thereof. This invariance property of an ROC curve is an important feature of ROC analysis.

The ROC curve and all performance indices derived from it may be estimated using assumptions of variable strength. Nonparametric and distribution-free methods use the least number of assumptions, that is, they do not assume any functional form of the ROC curve or distribution of the test results. Completely nonparametric approaches enable the construction of both jagged (e.g., empirical) ROC curves and smooth ROC curves (e.g., semiparametric, distribution-free methods that use parametric smoothing components). The next level of assumption is made by fully parametric methods. The most common method is fitting a convenient binormal ROC curve among choices of parametric models. Finally, most parametric and semiparametric distribution-based approaches assume a known distribution of test results and predict the shape of the curve. However, fully parametric approaches without optimal transformation of the measurement scales may lead to a poor fit.

In addition to the invariance property of the ROC curve that requires specific adjustments to some of the fitting methods, there are several other desirable but challenging properties. First, the ROC curve is by definition monotonic. Although all parametric approaches automatically account for this property, some nonparametric and semiparametric approaches need adjustments to ensure monotonicity. Second, a practical assumption for many applications, in particular those depicting the performances of observers, should be concave downward, because the convexity of an ROC curve would imply that at a certain threshold the observer would perform at a level worse than chance. The problem of convexity of the estimated ROC curve is relevant in both parametric and nonparametric systems but newer approaches may provide remedies.

Methods for fitting ROC curves must be flexible enough to permit adjustments for covariates that potentially affect the ability of a system to diagnose a condition of interest (e.g., severity of a disease). An approach for covariate adjustment includes distribution-based methods in which the effects of the covariates are first determined for the distribution of the test results and then transformed to determine the effects on the ROC curve. Additional approaches include parametric and semiparametric distribution-free methods that model the effects of covariates on the ROC curve directly. The effects of covariates may also be modeled on the summary measures of the ROC curve or alternatively on other basic measures such as sensitivity and specificity.

10.3 Future Directions in Reliability Analysis

In the course of ROC analysis, investigators often face the problem of correlated data where observations from the same groups are more alike than observations from different groups. Correlated data typically result from a set of assessments performed on the same subject (patient or medical image) by the same human observer (radiologist) or within the same evaluation environment (medical center). When dealing with repeated pixel or voxel data, additional complexity may be encountered due to both spatial and temporal correlations.

Correlated data are often imposed by a specific study design, for example, a paired design that evaluates the same subjects under different modalities. However, correlated data may be a consequence of evaluations performed in the field, for example, multireader data collected from a clinical environment and observations obtained from the same reader or center may be correlated. The analysis of correlated data is complicated by the need to account for all relevant correlations and variabilities. The simplest correlated structure comes from data obtained from a reader-free or single-reader comparison of two diagnostic systems in a paired design. Several nonparametric, parametric, and regression-based approaches may be developed to analyze such data.

A more complicated correlated data structure may arise from a multi-reader and multimodality study design. Such studies are typically planned to estimate the performance of diagnostic tests in the presence of highly variable reader-specific performance levels. Because of differences in experience, training, and other relevant characteristics of individual observers, the results of observations made by the same observer are likely to be more alike than results from different observers. Similar to the scenario of a paired study design, multireader studies are often designed to have the same set of cases evaluated by different readers to alleviate the effect of between-case variability. The corresponding data are sometimes called cross-correlated, based on use of the same readers and cases, and pose additional analytical challenges. Multiple approaches have been developed to enable analyses of cross-correlated multireader data.

One problem that is closely-related to multireader analysis is the assessment of the predictive ability of statistical classifiers. One may develop a statistical model for predicting a binary outcome and attempt to assess the ability of the specific model to predict binary outcomes such as the presence or absence of a specific condition. A specific feature of statistical models is that they are estimated using a set of subjects with a known binary outcome—sometimes called a training sample. A sample of subjects with known true status that is used to assess the predictive ability of a model is often termed a testing sample. Naturally, the assessed performance of the model depends heavily on both the training and the testing samples. This is analogous to the dependence of assessed performance of a diagnostic system on sampled observers and sampled test cases. Specific methods must be used to ensure that the performance of a statistical model is assessed in an efficient and unbiased manner.

Another level of complexity in correlated data results from evaluating specific parts and organs of the subject in question. In the simplest case, these data are correlated due to clustering within a subject. Furthermore, in complicated multireader studies, the correlation structure is complicated by potential correlation arising from use of the same readers and subjects.

Clustered diagnostic (e.g., imaging) data often result when the main goal is to consider multiple abnormalities within a subject. A major approach for acquiring and analyzing such data within an ROC is the ROI approach that assumes a separate assessment of all predefined regions of an image that was criticized for being artificial and different from the actual practice.

However, the ROI approach may be implemented according to the same free-response data acquisition paradigm used in FROC studies. That is, observers may mark a suspicious location anywhere on a raw image and a fine predefined grid segmenting the image is hidden from the observer at the time of evaluation. While methods for ROI analyses are almost entirely based on the original nonparametric method for clustered ROC data analysis, the methods for FROC analysis develop continually.

Several aspects of experimentally ascertained ROC data present specific challenges. Therefore, appropriate analytical techniques for evaluating reliability and reproducibility must be developed to address the challenges. A number of problems arise in practice: (1) the need for case verification where only specific subsets of test cases have verified true status, (2) an imperfect gold standard that allows only approximations of the true status of test cases, and (3) incomplete data—evaluation results for certain subjects under certain modalities or observers are not completely known.

The extensions of the kappa statistic and intraclass correlation coefficient may include (1) incorporation of the location and multiple correlations where the goal is assessing the performance of a system for classifying more than two true states over time, and (2) time-dependent reproducibility analysis.

10.4 Final Remarks

In closing, toolsets and techniques for analyzing classification data are constantly under development. An important component of the ROC and reliability analyses relates to designing a study that allows the acquisition of relevant information in the most efficient manner. Among primary issues in classification tasks, challenges in medical imaging arise from multiple factors including the selection of cases and readers, relative merits of different sampling strategies, training observers for studies, using a specific rating scale, possible effects of prevalence and how it impacts the performance of human observers, high-dimensional data analysis, hierarchical data structures, and multiple types of spatial and temporal correlations. Consequently, investigators who adopt such complex designs must develop and extend novel and most likely highly computationally intensive methods to improve classification accuracy and reliability. The methodologies reviewed in this book hopefully provide relevant toolsets for dealing with problems arising from complex diagnostic data.

Appendix: Notation List

2.1 General Notations

Θ, θ	Parameter space and parameter
D, d	Disease status for binary truth: $D = 1$ indicates actually positive, diseased, or abnormal; $D = 0$ indicates actually negative, nondiseased, healthy, or normal
BC	Box–Cox transformation
T, t	Result of diagnostic test
T', t'	Result of diagnostic test after a monotone transformation
k	Kernel used for density smoothing
S_k	Survival function of kernel function
W	Bandwidth
h	Monotone transformation
λ	Power coefficient in Box–Cox transformation
log	Unless specified, *log* is a logarithm based in *e*, often written as *ln*.
log_B	Logarithm based in *B*
l	Log likelihood function
X, x	Test result for actually negative diagnostic unit (equivalent to $T\|D = 0$)
X', x'	Monotone-transformed test result, $X' = h(X)$, for actually negative diagnostic unit (equivalent to $T'\|D = 0$) after monotone transformation
Y, y	Test result for actually positive diagnostic unit (equivalent to $T\|D = 1$)
Y', y'	Monotone-transformed test result, $Y' = h(Y)$ for actually positive diagnostic unit (equivalent to $T'\|D = 1$) after monotone transformation
$\bar{x}, \bar{y}$	Sample means of healthy or diseased sample
s_X, s_Y	Sample standard deviation of healthy or diseased sample
Z, z	Secondary covariates
ξ	Threshold (belongs to scale of observed or latent test result)
ξ'	Monotone-transformed threshold (belongs to scale of observed or latent test result)
g	Link function in generalized linear model

$F_X(\xi), f_X(\xi)$	Cumulative distribution and probability density functions of test results for actually negative diagnostic units
$F_Y(\xi), f_Y(\xi)$	Cumulative distribution and probability density functions of test results for actually positive diagnostic units
$S_X(\xi)$	Survival function of test results for actually negative diagnostic units
$S_Y(\xi)$	Survival function of test results for actually positive diagnostic units
$I(\ldots)$	Indicator of event
$P(\ldots)$	Probability of event
$\Phi(\ldots)$	Cumulative distribution function of standard normal distribution
$E(\ldots)$	Expectation; subscript indicates random variable averaged over; conditioning can be indicated in subscript or within parentheses after vertical line
$V(\ldots)$	Variance; subscript indicates random variable; conditioning can be indicated in subscript or within parentheses after vertical line
$COV(\ldots, \ldots)$	Covariance; subscript indicates random variable; conditioning can be indicated in subscript or within parentheses after vertical line
$\Sigma(\ldots, \ldots, \ldots)$	Variance and covariance matrix
$TPF(\xi)$, TPF	True positive fraction (without an argument corresponds to binary test)
$FPF(\xi)$, FPF	False positive fraction
$PV^{+}(\xi)$, PV^{+}	Positive predictive values
$PV^{-}(\xi)$, PV^{-}	Negative predictive values
$DLR^{+}(\xi)$, DLR	Positive disease likelihood ratio (at given threshold)
$DLR^{-}(\xi)$	Negative disease likelihood ratio (at given threshold)
$DLR(t)$	Disease Likelihood Ratio of a given test result t
$ROC(fpf)$	Receiver operating characteristics function
$rank(\ldots)$	Ranks of data
$TPF\|_{fpf^0}$	True positive fraction corresponding to given false positive fraction [equivalent to $ROC(fpf^0)$]
N^0, n^0	Number of actually negative diagnostic units
N^1, n^1	Number of actually positive diagnostic units
i	Subscript index for normal diagnostic units ($I = 1,\ldots, {}^0$)
j	Subscript index for abnormal diagnostic units ($j = 1,\ldots, n^1$)
κ	Kappa statistic
ICC	Intraclass correlation coefficient
p	Probability; without subscript corresponds to prevalence of a disease in a population [$P(D = 1)$]
$\Sigma\ldots$	Summation
$\Pi\ldots$	Product
c	Constant

2.2 Specialized Notations

s	Index for subject (cluster) containing multiple diagnostic units
r	Subscript index for reader such as a radiologist ($r = 1,\ldots,n^r$)
c	Index for case
nr	Number of readers (e.g., radiologists)
n_S^0	Number of subjects without abnormal diagnostic units
n_S^1	Number of subjects with some abnormal diagnostic units
n_i^0	Number of normal diagnostic units within *ith* subject
n_i	Number of abnormal diagnostic units within *ith* subject
$\mathcal{T},\tau$	Number of actual abnormalities within subject ($\tau \geq n_i^1$)

Index

For Product Safety Concerns and Information please contact our EU representative GPSR@taylorandfrancis.com
Taylor & Francis Verlag GmbH, Kaufingerstraße 24, 80331 München, Germany

www.ingramcontent.com/pod-product-compliance
Ingram Content Group UK Ltd.
Pitfield, Milton Keynes, MK11 3LW, UK
UKHW021119180425
457613UK00005B/151
9781439812228